Pharmacology for Anaesthesia and Intensive Care

THIRD EDITION

D1343319

Tom Peck, Sue Hill and Mark Williams

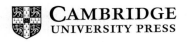

CAMBRIDGE
UNIVERSITY PRESS

CAMBRIDGE UNIVERSITY PRESS

Cambridge, New York, Melbourne, Madrid, Cape Town, Singapore, São Paulo, Delhi

Cambridge University Press
The Edinburgh Building, Cambridge CB2 8RU, UK

Published in the United States of America by Cambridge University Press, New York

www.cambridge.org
Information on this title: www.cambridge.org/9780521704632

© Tom Peck Sue Hill and Mark Williams 2008

First published 2000
Second edition 2003
Third edition 2008

Printed in the United Kingdom at the University Press, Cambridge

A catalogue record for this publication is available from the British Library

Library of Congress Cataloging-in-Publication Data

Peck, T. E.
Pharmacology for anaesthesia and intensive care / Tom Peck, S. Hill, Mark Williams. – 3rd ed.
p. ; cm.
Includes bibliographical references and index.
ISBN 978-0-521-70463-2 (pbk.)
1. Pharmacology.   2. Anesthetics.   3. Anesthesia.   4. Critical care medicine.
   I. Hill, S. A. (Sue A.)   II. Williams, Mark (Mark Andrew) 1965-   III. Title.
[DNLM: 1. Anesthetics–pharmacology.   2. Cardiovascular Agents–pharmacology.
   3. Intensive Care. QV 81 P367p 2007]

RM300.P396   2007
615'.1–dc22

2007029048

ISBN 978-0-521-70463-2 paperback

CONTENTS

CONTRIBUTOR

Dr. A.S. Grice, BSc, DCH, FRCA, Consultant Anaesthetist, Exeter

PREFACE

The third edition has seen further changes. The mathematics section has been overhauled and expanded to give a better base for the kinetics. An additional chapter has been added on intravenous fluids, and the chapters on intravenous and volatile anaesthetics have been combined with an expanded section on the molecular mechanism of anaesthesia.

We have tried to maintain the style of the previous two editions with an emphasis on clarity both in terms of presentation and content. In addition we have tried very hard to eliminate those small errors that are disproportionately irritating. We hope that this book will continue to be a helpful aid to the wide range of readers it appears to have attracted.

Tom Peck
Sue Hill
Mark Williams

FOREWORD

I can remember my first day as an anaesthetic senior house officer, back in August 1985, and the advice that I received on that first day is still relevant for the twenty first century anaesthetist. "Anaesthesia is based on three basic sciences, physiology, physics and pharmacology," said my first college tutor. The following weekend I took a trip to Lewis's book shop in Gower Street to buy the recommended texts of the day. None of those I bought are still in print, but the pharmacology text has certainly been replaced by "Pharmacology for Anaesthesia and Intensive Care."

The first two editions established themselves as the core pharmacology text for aspiring anaesthetists. It has evolved with each edition and the third edition has continued this trend, with some interesting new features. The mathematics and pharmacokinetics chapter is particularly well presented, and explains the concepts concisely and clearly. This is core knowledge that appears in the examinations of the Royal College of Anaesthetists but should be retained for all clinical anaesthetists and intensive care specialists.

Perhaps the title of the book should be changed for future editions as there has been a large change in medical education in the UK since the second edition, namely Modernising Medical Careers. This book is relevant to all foundation trainees who rotate through anaesthesia, intensive care and acute medical specialties. The new chapter on fluids is especially relevant to those at the start of their careers. The core knowledge presented should help to encourage good prescribing practice on all acute medical and surgical wards and avoid fluid management errors.

In summary the new edition is essential reading for those embarking on an anaesthetic career and is a core text for the FRCA. The authors come from district general and teaching hospital backgrounds but this book offers concise common sense pharmacology knowledge to all grades, even those who started anaesthesia before propofol was introduced!!

Richard Griffiths MD FRCA
Consultant in Anaesthesia & Intensive Care Medicine
Peterborough & Stamford Hospitals NHS Trust.
Chairman of Structured Oral Examination I for the FRCA Pt I

SECTION I **Basic principles**

1

Drug passage across the cell membrane

Many drugs need to pass through one or more cell membranes to reach their site of action. A common feature of all cell membranes is a phospholipid bilayer, about 10 nm thick, arranged with the hydrophilic heads on the outside and the lipophilic chains facing inwards. This gives a sandwich effect, with two hydrophilic layers surrounding the central hydrophobic one. Spanning this bilayer or attached to the outer or inner leaflets are glycoproteins, which may act as ion channels, receptors, intermediate messengers (G-proteins) or enzymes. The cell membrane has been described as a 'fluid mosaic' as the positions of individual phosphoglycerides and glycoproteins are by no means fixed (Figure 1.1). An exception to this is a specialized membrane area such as the neuromuscular junction, where the array of post-synaptic receptors is found opposite a motor nerve ending.

The general cell membrane structure is modified in certain tissues to allow more specialized functions. Capillary endothelial cells have fenestrae, which are regions of the endothelial cell where the outer and inner membranes are fused together, with no intervening cytosol. These make the endothelium of the capillary relatively permeable; fluid in particular can pass rapidly through the cell by this route. In the case of the renal glomerular endothelium, gaps or clefts exist between cells to allow the passage of larger molecules as part of filtration. Tight junctions exist between endothelial cells of brain blood vessels, forming the blood–brain barrier (BBB), intestinal mucosa and renal tubules. These limit the passage of polar molecules and also prevent the lateral movement of glycoproteins within the cell membrane, which may help to keep specialized glycoproteins at their site of action (e.g. transport glycoproteins on the luminal surface of intestinal mucosa) (Figure 1.2).

Methods of crossing the cell membrane

Passive diffusion

This is the commonest method for crossing the cell membrane. Drug molecules move down a concentration gradient, from an area of high concentration to one of low concentration, and the process requires no energy to proceed. Many drugs are weak acids or weak bases and can exist in either the unionized or ionized form, depending on the pH. The unionized form of a drug is lipid-soluble and diffuses easily by dissolution in the lipid bilayer. Thus the rate at which transfer occurs depends on

1

Extracellular

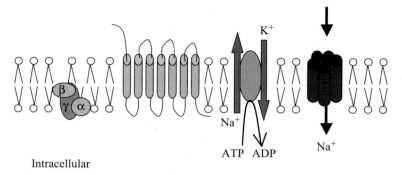

Intracellular

ATP ADP

Figure 1.1. Representation of the cell membrane structure. The integral proteins embedded in this phospholipid bilayer are G-protein, G-protein-coupled receptors, transport proteins and ligand-gated ion channels. Additionally, enzymes or voltage-gated ion channels may also be present.

the pK_a of the drug in question. Factors influencing the rate of diffusion are discussed below.

In addition, there are specialized **ion channels** in the membrane that allow intermittent passive movement of selected ions down a concentration gradient. When opened, ion channels allow rapid ion flux for a short time (a few milliseconds) down relatively large concentration and electrical gradients, which makes them suitable to propagate either ligand- or voltage-gated action potentials in nerve and muscle membranes.

The acetylcholine (ACh) receptor has five subunits (pentameric) arranged to form a central ion channel that spans the membrane (Figure 1.3). Of the five subunits, two (the α subunits) are identical. The receptor requires the binding of two ACh molecules to open the ion channel, allowing ions to pass at about 10^7 s^{-1}. If a threshold flux is achieved, depolarization occurs, which is responsible for impulse transmission. The ACh receptor demonstrates selectivity for small cations, but it is by no means specific for Na$^+$. The GABA$_A$ receptor is also a pentameric, ligand-gated

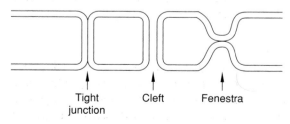

Tight   Cleft   Fenestra
junction

Figure 1.2. Modifications of the general cell membrane structure.

1 Drug passage across the cell membrane

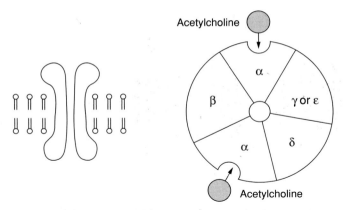

Figure 1.3. The acetylcholine (ACh) receptor has five subunits and spans the cell membrane. ACh binds to the α subunits, causing a conformational change and allowing the passage of small cations through its central ion channel. The ϵ subunit replaces the fetal-type γ subunit after birth once the neuromuscular junction reaches maturity.

channel, but selective for anions, especially the chloride anion. The NMDA (N-methyl D-aspartate) receptor belongs to a different family of ion channels and is a dimer; it favours calcium as the cation mediating membrane depolariztion.

Ion channels may have their permeability altered by endogenous compounds or by drugs. Local anaesthetics bind to the internal surface of the fast Na^+ ion channel and prevent the conformational change required for activation, while non-depolarizing muscle relaxants prevent receptor activation by competitively inhibiting the binding of ACh to its receptor site.

Facilitated diffusion

Facilitated diffusion refers to the process where molecules combine with membrane-bound carrier proteins to cross the membrane. The rate of diffusion of the molecule–protein complex is still down a concentration gradient but is faster than would be expected by diffusion alone. Examples of this process include the absorption of steroids and amino acids from the gut lumen. The absorption of glucose, a very polar molecule, would be relatively slow if it occurred by diffusion alone and requires facilitated diffusion to cross membranes (including the BBB) rapidly.

Active transport

Active transport is an energy-requiring process. The molecule is transported against its concentration gradient by a molecular pump, which requires energy to function. Energy can be supplied either directly to the ion pump, or indirectly by coupling pump-action to an ionic gradient that is actively maintained. Active transport is encountered commonly in gut mucosa, the liver, renal tubules and the BBB.

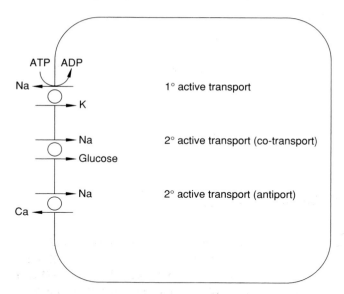

Figure 1.4. Mechanisms of active transport across the cell membrane.

Na^+/K^+ ATPase is an example of a direct energy-dependent pump – the energy in the high-energy phosphate bond is lost as the molecule is hydrolysed, with concurrent ion transport against the respective concentration gradients. It is an example of an antiport, as sodium moves in one direction and potassium in the opposite direction. The Na^+/amino acid symport (substances moved in the same direction) in the mucosal cells of the small bowel or on the luminal side of the proximal renal tubule is an example of secondary active transport. Here, amino acids will only cross the mucosal cell membrane when Na^+ is bound to the carrier protein and moves down its concentration gradient (which is generated using Na^+/K^+ ATPase). So, directly and indirectly, Na^+/K^+ ATPase is central to active transport (Figure 1.4).

Active transport is more specific for a particular molecule than is the process of simple diffusion and is subject to specific antagonism and blockade. In addition, the fixed number of active transport binding sites may be subject to competition or saturation.

Pinocytosis

Pinocytosis is the process by which an area of the cell membrane invaginates around the (usually large) target molecule and moves it into the cell. The molecule may then be released into the cell or may remain in the vacuole so created, until the reverse process occurs on the opposite side of the cell.

The process is usually used for molecules that are too large to traverse the membrane easily via another mechanism (Figure 1.5).

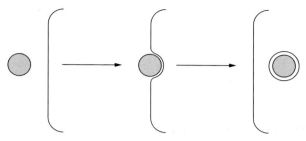

Figure 1.5. Pinocytosis.

Factors influencing the rate of diffusion

Molecular size

The rate of passive diffusion is inversely proportional to the square root of molecular size (Graham's law). In general, small molecules will diffuse much more readily than large ones. The molecular weights of anaesthetic agents are relatively small and anaesthetic agents diffuse rapidly through lipid membranes to exert their effects.

Concentration gradient

Fick's law states that the rate of transfer across a membrane is proportional to the concentration gradient across the membrane. Thus increasing the plasma concentration of the unbound fraction of drug will increase its rate of transfer across the membrane and will accelerate the onset of its pharmacological effect. This is the basis of Bowman's principle, applied to the onset of action of non-depolarizing muscle relaxants. The less potent the drug, the more required to exert an effect – but this increases the concentration gradient between plasma and active site, so the onset of action is faster.

Ionization

The lipophilic nature of the cell membrane only permits the passage of the uncharged fraction of any drug. The degree to which a drug is ionized in a solution depends on the molecular structure of the drug and the pH of the solution in which it is dissolved and is given by the Henderson–Hasselbalch equation.

The pK_a is the pH at which 50% of the drug molecules are ionized – thus the concentrations of ionized and unionized portions are equal. The value for pK_a depends on the molecular structure of the drug and is independent of whether it is acidic or basic.

The Henderson–Hasselbalch equation is most simply expressed as:

$$pH = pK_a + \log \left\{ \frac{[\text{proton acceptor}]}{[\text{proton donor}]} \right\}.$$

Hence, for an acid (XH), the relationship between the ionized and unionized forms is given by:

$$pH = pK_a + \log\left\{\frac{[X^-]}{[XH]}\right\},$$

with X^- being the ionized form of an acid.

For a base (X), the corresponding form of the equation is:

$$pH = pK_a + \log\left\{\frac{[X]}{[XH^+]}\right\},$$

with XH^+ being the ionized form of a base.

Using the terms 'proton donor' and 'proton acceptor' instead of 'acid' or 'base' in the equation avoids confusion and the degree of ionization of a molecule may be readily established if its pK_a and the ambient pH are known. At a pH below their pK_a weak acids will be more unionized; at a pH above their pK_a they will be more ionized. The reverse is true for weak bases, which are more ionized at a pH below their pK_a and more unionized at a pH above their pK_a.

Bupivacaine is a weak base with a tertiary amine group in the piperidine ring. The nitrogen atom of this amine group is a proton acceptor and can become ionized, depending on pH. With a pK_a of 8.1, it is 83% ionized at physiological pH.

Aspirin is an acid with a pK_a of 3.0. It is almost wholly ionized at physiological pH, although in the highly acidic environment of the stomach it is essentially unionized, which therefore increases its rate of absorption. However, because of the limited surface area within the stomach more is absorbed in the small bowel.

Lipid solubility

The lipid solubility of a drug reflects its ability to pass through the cell membrane; this property is independent of the pK_a of the drug. However, high lipid solubility alone does not necessarily result in a rapid onset of action. Alfentanil is nearly seven times less lipid-soluble than fentanyl, yet it has a more rapid onset of action. This is a result of several factors. First, alfentanil is less potent and has a smaller distribution volume and therefore initially a greater concentration gradient exists between effect site and plasma. Second, both fentanyl and alfentanil are weak bases and alfentanil has a lower pK_a than fentanyl (alfentanil = 6.5; fentanyl = 8.4), so that at physiological pH a much greater fraction of alfentanil is unionized and available to cross membranes.

Lipid solubility affects the rate of absorption from the site of administration. Thus, fentanyl is suitable for transdermal application as its high lipid solubility results in effective transfer across the skin. Intrathecal diamorphine readily dissolves into, and fixes to, the local lipid tissues, whereas the less lipid-soluble morphine remains in the cerebrospinal fluid longer, and is therefore liable to spread cranially, with an increased risk of respiratory depression.

1 Drug passage across the cell membrane

Protein binding

Only the unbound fraction of drug in plasma is free to cross the cell membrane; drugs vary greatly in the degree of plasma protein binding. In practice, the extent of this binding is of importance only if the drug is highly protein-bound (more than 90%). In these cases, small changes in the bound fraction produce large changes in the amount of unbound drug. In general, this increases the rate at which drug is metabolized, so a new equilibrium is re-established with little change in free drug concentration. For a very small number of highly protein-bound drugs where metabolic pathways are close to saturation (such as phenytoin) this cannot happen and plasma concentration of unbound drug will increase and possibly reach toxic levels.

Both albumin and globulins bind drugs, each has many binding sites, the number and characteristics of which are determined by the pH of plasma. In general, albumin binds neutral or acidic drugs (e.g. barbiturates), and globulins (in particular, $\alpha-1$ acid glycoprotein) bind basic drugs (e.g. morphine).

Albumin has two important binding sites: the warfarin and diazepam. Binding is usually readily reversible, and competition for binding at any one site between different drugs can alter the active unbound fraction of each. Binding is also possible at other sites on the molecule, which may cause a conformational change and indirectly influence binding at the diazepam and warfarin sites.

Although $\alpha-1$ acid glycoprotein binds basic drugs, other globulins are important in binding individual ions and molecules, particularly the metals. Thus, iron is bound to $\beta-1$ globulin and copper to $\alpha-2$ globulin.

Protein binding is altered in a range of pathological conditions. Inflammation changes the relative proportions of the different proteins and albumin concentration falls in any acute infective or inflammatory process. This effect is independent of any reduction in synthetic capacity resulting from liver impairment and is not due to protein loss. In conditions of severe hypoalbuminaemia (e.g. in end-stage liver cirrhosis or burns), the proportion of unbound drug increases markedly such that the same dose will have a greatly exaggerated pharmacological effect. The magnitude of these effects may be hard to estimate and drug dose should be titrated against clinical effect.

Absorption, distribution, metabolism and excretion

Absorption

Drugs may be given by a variety of routes; the route chosen depends on the desired site of action and the type of drug preparations available. Routes used commonly by the anaesthetist include inhalation, intravenous, oral, intramuscular, rectal, epidural and intrathecal. Other routes, such as transdermal, subcutaneous and sublingual, also can be used. The rate and extent of absorption after a particular route of administration depends on both drug and patient factors.

Drugs may be given orally for local as well as systemic effects, for example, oral vancomycin used to treat pseudomembranous colitis is acting locally; antacids also act locally in the stomach. In such cases, systemic absorption may result in unwanted side effects.

Intravenous administration provides a direct, and therefore more reliable, route of systemic drug delivery. No absorption is required, so plasma levels are independent of such factors as gastrointestinal (GI) absorption and adequate skin or muscle perfusion. However, there are disadvantages in using this route. Pharmacological preparations for intravenous therapy are generally more expensive than the corresponding oral medications, and the initially high plasma level achieved with some drugs may cause undesirable side effects. In addition, if central venous access is used, this carries its own risks. Nevertheless, most drugs used in intensive care are given by intravenous infusion this way.

Oral

After oral administration, absorption must take place through the gut mucosa. For drugs without specific transport mechanisms, only unionized drugs pass readily through the lipid membranes of the gut. Because the pH of the GI tract varies along its length, the physicochemical properties of the drug will determine from which part of the GI tract the drug is absorbed.

Acidic drugs (e.g. aspirin) are unionized in the highly acidic medium of the stomach and therefore are absorbed more rapidly than basic drugs. Although weak bases (e.g. propranolol) are ionized in the stomach, they are relatively unionized in the duodenum, so are absorbed from this site. The salts of permanently charged drugs (e.g. vecuronium, glycopyrrolate) remain ionized at all times and are therefore not absorbed from the GI tract.

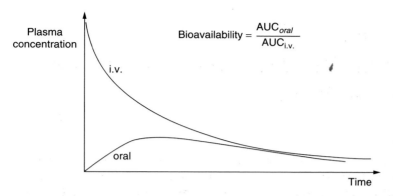

Figure 2.1. Bioavailability may be estimated by comparing the areas under the curves.

In practice, even acidic drugs are predominantly absorbed from the small bowel, as the surface area for absorption is so much greater due to the presence of mucosal villi. However, acidic drugs, such as aspirin, have some advantages over basic drugs in that absorption is initially rapid, giving a shorter time of onset from ingestion, and will continue even in the presence of GI tract stasis.

Bioavailability

Bioavailability is generally defined as the fraction of a drug dose reaching the systemic circulation, compared with the same dose given intravenously (i.v.). In general, the oral route has the lowest bioavailability of any route of administration. Bioavailability can be found from the ratio of the areas under the concentration–time curves for an identical bolus dose given both orally and intravenously (Figure 2.1).

Factors influencing bioavailability

- *Pharmaceutical preparation* – the way in which a drug is formulated affects its rate of absorption. If a drug is presented with a small particle size or as a liquid, dispersion is rapid. If the particle size is large, or binding agents prevent drug dissolution in the stomach (e.g. enteric-coated preparations), absorption may be delayed.
- *Physicochemical interactions* – other drugs or food may interact and inactivate or bind the drug in question (e.g. the absorption of tetracyclines is reduced by the concurrent administration of Ca^{2+} such as in milk).
- *Patient factors* – various patient factors affect absorption of a drug. The presence of congenital or acquired malabsorption syndromes, such as coeliac disease or tropical sprue, will affect absorption, and gastric stasis, whether as a result of trauma or drugs, slows the transit time through the gut.
- *Pharmacokinetic interactions and first-pass metabolism* – drugs absorbed from the gut (with the exception of the buccal and rectal mucosa) pass via the portal

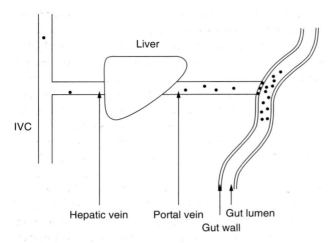

Figure 2.2. First-pass metabolism may occur in the gut wall or in the liver to reduce the amount of drug reaching the circulation.

vein to the liver where they may be subject to first-pass metabolism. Metabolism at either the gut wall (e.g. glyceryl trinitrate (GTN)) or liver will reduce the amount reaching the circulation. Therefore, an adequate plasma level may not be achieved orally using a dose similar to that needed intravenously. So, for an orally administered drug, the bioavailable fraction (F_B) is given by:

$$F_B = F_A \times F_G \times F_H.$$

Here F_A is the fraction absorbed, F_G the fraction remaining after metabolism in the gut mucosa and F_H the fraction remaining after hepatic metabolism. Therefore, drugs with a high oral bioavailability are stable in the gastrointestinal tract, are well absorbed and undergo minimal first-pass metabolism (Figure 2.2). First-pass metabolism may be increased and oral bioavailability reduced through the induction of hepatic enzymes (e.g. phenobarbital induces hepatic enzymes, reducing the bioavailability of warfarin). Conversely, hepatic enzymes may be inhibited and bioavailability increased (e.g. cimetidine may increase the bioavailability of propranolol).

Extraction ratio
The extraction ratio (ER) is that fraction of drug removed from blood by the liver. ER depends on hepatic blood flow, uptake into the hepatocyte and enzyme metabolic capacity within the hepatocyte. The activity of an enzyme is described by its Michaelis constant, which is the concentration of substrate at which it is working at 50% of its maximum rate. Those enzymes with high metabolic capacity have Michaelis constants very much higher than any substrate concentrations likely to be found

clinically; those with low capacity will have Michaelis constants close to clinically relevant concentrations. Drugs fall into three distinct groups:

Drugs for which the hepatocyte has rapid uptake and a high metabolic capacity, for example, propofol and lidocaine. Free drug is rapidly removed from plasma, bound drug is released to maintain equilibrium and a concentration gradient is maintained between plasma and hepatocyte because drug is metabolized very quickly. Because protein binding has rapid equilibration, the total amount of drug metabolized will be independent of protein binding but highly dependent on liver blood flow.

Drugs that have low metabolic capacity and high level of protein binding (>90%). This group includes phenytoin and diazepam. Their ER is limited by the metabolic capacity of the hepatocyte and not by blood flow. If protein binding is altered (e.g. by competition) then the free concentration of drug increases significantly. This initially increases uptake into the hepatocyte and rate of metabolism and plasma levels of free drug do not change significantly. However, if the intracellular concentration exceeds maximum metabolic capacity (saturates the enzyme) drug levels within the cell remain high, so reducing uptake (reduced concentration gradient) and ER. Those drugs with a narrow therapeutic index may then show significant toxic effects; hence the need for regular checks on plasma concentration, particularly when other medication is altered. Therefore for this group of drugs extraction is influenced by changes in protein binding more than by changes in hepatic blood flow.

Drugs that have low metabolic capacity and low level of protein binding. The total amount of drug metabolized for this group of drugs is unaffected by either by hepatic blood flow or by changes in protein binding.

Sublingual

The sublingual, nasal and buccal routes have two advantages – they are rapid in onset and, by avoiding the portal tract, have a higher bioavailability. This is advantageous for drugs where a rapid effect is essential, for example, GTN spray for angina or sublingual nifedipine for the relatively rapid control of high blood pressure.

Rectal

The rectal route can be used to avoid first-pass metabolism, and may be considered if the oral route is not available. Drugs may be given rectally for their local (e.g. steroids for inflammatory bowel disease), as well as their systemic effects (e.g. diclofenac suppositories for analgesia). There is little evidence that the rectal route is more efficacious than the oral route; it provides a relatively small surface area, and absorption may be slow or incomplete.

Intramuscular

The intramuscular (i.m.) route avoids the problems associated with oral administration and the bioavailable fraction approaches 1.0. The speed of onset is generally more rapid compared with the oral route, and for some drugs approaches that for the intravenous route.

The rate of absorption depends on local perfusion at the site of i.m. injection. Injection at a poorly perfused site may result in delayed absorption and for this reason the well-perfused muscles deltoid, quadriceps or gluteus are preferred. If muscle perfusion is poor as a result of systemic hypotension or local vasoconstriction then an intramuscular injection will not be absorbed until muscle perfusion is restored. Delayed absorption will have two consequences. First, the drug will not be effective within the expected time, which may lead to further doses being given. Second, if perfusion is then restored, plasma levels may suddenly rise into the toxic range. For these reasons, the intravenous route is preferred if there is any doubt as to the adequacy of perfusion.

Not all drugs can be given i.m., for example, phenytoin. Intramuscular injections may be painful (e.g. cyclizine) and may cause a local abscess or haematoma, so should be avoided in the coagulopathic patient. There is also the risk of inadvertent intravenous injection of drug intended for the intramuscular route.

Subcutaneous

Certain drugs are well absorbed from the subcutaneous tissues and this is the favoured route for low-dose heparin therapy. A further indication for this route is where patient compliance is a problem and depot preparations may be useful. Antipsychotic medication and some contraceptive formulations have been used in this way. Co-preparation of insulin with zinc or protamine can produce a slow absorption profile lasting several hours after subcutaneous administration.

As with the intramuscular route, the kinetics of absorption is dependent on local and regional blood flow, and may be markedly reduced in shock. Again, this has the dual effect of rendering the (non-absorbed) drug initially ineffective, and then subjecting the patient to a bolus once the perfusion is restored.

Transdermal

Drugs may be applied to the skin either for local topical effect, such as steroids, but also may be used to avoid first-pass metabolism and improve bioavailability. Thus, fentanyl and nitrates may be given transdermally for their systemic effects. Factors favouring transdermal absorption are high lipid solubility and a good regional blood supply to the site of application (therefore, the thorax and abdomen are preferred to limbs). Special transdermal formulations (patches) are used to ensure slow, constant release of drug for absorption and provide a smoother pharmacokinetic profile. Only small amounts of drug are released at a time, so potent drugs are better suited to this route of administration if systemic effects are required.

Local anaesthetics may be applied topically to anaesthetize the skin before venepuncture, skin grafts or minor surgical procedures. The two most common preparations are topical EMLA and topical amethocaine. The first is a eutectic mixture (each agent lowers the boiling point of the other forming a gel-phase) of lidocaine and prilocaine. Amethocaine is an ester-linked local anaesthetic, which may cause mild, local histamine release producing local vasodilatation, in contrast to the vasoconstriction seen with eutectic mixture of local anaesthetic (EMLA). Venodilatation may be useful when anaesthetizing the skin prior to venepuncture.

Inhalation

Inhaled drugs may be intended for local or systemic action. The particle size and method of administration are significant factors in determining whether a drug reaches the alveolus and, therefore, the systemic circulation, or whether it only reaches the upper airways. Droplets of less than 1 micron diameter (which may be generated by an ultrasonic nebulizer) can reach the alveolus and hence the systemic circulation. However, a larger droplet or particle size reaches only airway mucosa from the larynx to the bronchioles (and often is swallowed from the pharynx) so that virtually none reaches the alveolus.

Local site of action

The bronchial airways are the intended site of action for inhaled or nebulized bronchodilators. However, drugs given for a local or topical effect may be absorbed resulting in unwanted systemic effects. Chronic use of inhaled steroids may lead to Cushingoid side effects, whereas high doses of inhaled β_2-agonists (e.g. salbutamol) may lead to tachycardia and hypokalaemia. Nebulized adrenaline, used for upper airway oedema causing stridor, may be absorbed and can lead to significant tachycardia, arrhythmias and hypertension, although catecholamines are readily metabolized by lung tissue. Similarly, sufficient quantities of topical lidocaine applied prior to fibreoptic intubation may be absorbed and cause systemic toxicity.

Inhaled nitric oxide reaches the alveolus and dilates the pulmonary vasculature. It is absorbed into the pulmonary circulation but does not produce unwanted systemic effects as it has a short half-life, as a result of binding to haemoglobin.

Systemic site of action

The large surface area of the lungs (70 m^2 in an adult) available for absorption can lead to a rapid increase in systemic concentration and hence rapid onset of action at distant effect sites. Volatile anaesthetic agents are given by the inhalation route with their ultimate site of action the central nervous system.

The kinetics of the inhaled anaesthetics are covered in greater detail in Chapter 8.

Epidural

The epidural route is used to provide regional analgesia and anaesthesia. Epidural local anaesthetics, opioids, ketamine and clonidine have all been used to treat acute pain, whereas steroids are used for diagnostic and therapeutic purposes in patients with chronic pain. Drug may be given as a single bolus or, through a catheter placed in the epidural space, as a series of boluses or by infusion.

The speed of onset of block is determined by the proportion of unionized drug available to penetrate the cell membrane. Local anaesthetics are bases with pK_as greater than 7.4 so are predominantly ionized at physiological pH (see Chapter 1). Local anaesthetics with a low pK_a, such as lidocaine, will be less ionized and onset of the block will be faster than for bupivacaine, which has a higher pK_a. Thus lidocaine rather than bupivacaine is often used to 'top up' an existing epidural before surgery. Adding sodium bicarbonate to a local anaesthetic solution increases pH and the unionized fraction, further reducing the onset time. Duration of block depends on tissue binding; bupivacaine has a longer duration of action than lidocaine. The addition of a vasoconstrictor, such as adrenaline or felypressin, will also increase the duration of the block by reducing loss of local anaesthetic from the epidural space.

Significant amounts of drug may be absorbed from the epidural space into the systemic circulation especially during infusions. Local anaesthetics and opioids are both commonly administered via the epidural route and carry significant morbidity when toxic systemic levels are reached.

Intrathecal
Compared with the epidural route, the amount of drug required when given intrathecally is very small; little reaches the systemic circulation and this rarely causes unwanted systemic effects. The extent of spread of a subararachnoid block with local anaesthetic depends on volume and type of solution used. Appropriate positioning of the patient when using hyperbaric solutions, such as with 'heavy' bupivacaine, can limit the spread of block.

Distribution
Drug distribution depends on factors that influence the passage of drug across the cell membrane (see Chapter 1) and on regional blood flow. Physicochemical factors include: molecular size, lipid solubility, degree of ionization and protein binding. Drugs fall into one of three general groups:

- *Those confined to the plasma* – certain drugs (e.g. dextran 70) are too large to cross the vascular endothelium. Other drugs (e.g. warfarin) may be so intensely protein bound that the unbound fraction is tiny, so that the amount available to leave the circulation is immeasurably small.
- *Those with limited distribution* – the non-depolarizing muscle relaxants are polar, poorly lipid-soluble and bulky. Therefore, their distribution is limited to tissues supplied by capillaries with fenestrae (i.e. muscle) that allow their movement out of the plasma. They cannot cross cell membranes but work extracellularly.
- *Those with extensive distribution* – these drugs are often highly lipid-soluble. Providing their molecular size is relatively small, the extent of plasma protein binding does not restrict their distribution due to the weak nature of such interactions.

Other drugs are sequestered by tissues (amiodarone by fat; iodine by the thyroid; tetracyclines by bone), which effectively removes them from the circulation.

Those drugs that are not confined to the plasma are initially distributed to tissues with the highest blood flow (brain, lung, kidney, thyroid, adrenal) then to tissues with a moderate blood flow (muscle), and finally to tissues with a very low blood flow (fat). These three groups of tissues provide a useful model when explaining how plasma levels decline after drug administration.

Blood–brain barrier (BBB)

The BBB is an anatomical and functional barrier between the circulation and the central nervous system (see Chapter 1).

Active transport and facilitated diffusion are the predominant methods of molecular transfer, which in health is tightly controlled. Glucose and hormones, such as insulin, cross by active carrier transport, while only lipid-soluble, low molecular weight drugs can cross by simple diffusion. Thus inhaled and intravenous anaesthetics can cross readily whereas the larger, polar muscle relaxants cannot and have no central effect. Similarly, glycopyrrolate has a quaternary, charged nitrogen and does not cross the BBB readily. This is in contrast to atropine, a tertiary amine, which may cause centrally mediated effects such as confusion or paradoxical bradycardia.

As well as providing an anatomical barrier, the BBB contains enzymes such as monoamine oxidase. Therefore, monoamines are converted to non-active metabolites by passing through the BBB. Physical disruption of the BBB may lead to central neurotransmitters being released into the systemic circulation and may help explain the marked circulatory disturbance seen with head injury and subarachnoid haemorrhage.

In the healthy subject penicillin penetrates the BBB poorly. However, in meningitis, the nature of the BBB alters as it becomes inflamed, and permeability to penicillin (and other drugs) increases, so allowing therapeutic access.

Drug distribution to the fetus

The placental membrane that separates fetal and maternal blood is initially derived from adjacent placental syncytiotrophoblast and fetal capillary membranes, which subsequently fuse to form a single membrane. Being phospholipid in nature, the placental membrane is more readily crossed by lipid-soluble than polar molecules. It is much less selective than the BBB and even molecules with only moderate lipid solubility appear to cross with relative ease and significant quantities may appear in cord (fetal) blood. Placental blood flow and the free drug concentration gradient between maternal and fetal blood determine the rate at which drug equilibration takes place. The pH of fetal blood is lower than that of the mother and fetal plasma protein binding may therefore differ. High protein binding in the fetus increases drug transfer across the placenta since fetal free drug levels are low. In contrast, high protein binding in the mother reduces the rate of drug transfer since maternal free drug levels are low. The fetus also may metabolize some drugs; the rate of metabolism increases as the fetus matures.

The effects of maternal pharmacology on the fetus may be divided into those effects that occur in pregnancy, especially the early first trimester when organogenesis occurs, and at birth.

Drugs during pregnancy

The safety of any drug in pregnancy must be evaluated, but interspecies variation is great and animal models may not exclude the possibility of significant human teratogenicity. In addition, teratogenic effects may not be apparent for some years; stilboestrol taken during pregnancy predisposes female offspring to ovarian cancer at puberty. Wherever possible drug therapy should be avoided throughout pregnancy; if treatment is essential drugs with a long history of safety should be selected.

There are conditions, however, in which the risk of not taking medication outweighs the theoretical or actual risk of teratogenicity. Thus, in epilepsy the risk of hypoxic damage to the fetus secondary to fitting warrants the continuation of antiepileptic medication during pregnancy. Similarly, the presence of an artificial heart valve mandates the continuation of anticoagulation despite the attendant risks.

Drugs at the time of birth

The newborn may have anaesthetic or analgesic drugs in their circulation depending on the type of analgesia for labour and whether delivery was operative. Drugs with a low molecular weight that are lipid-soluble will be present in higher concentrations than large polar molecules.

Bupivacaine is the local anaesthetic most commonly used for epidural analgesia. It crosses the placenta less readily than does lidocaine as its higher pK_a makes it more ionized than lidocaine at physiological pH. However, the fetus is relatively acidic with respect to the mother, and if the fetal pH is reduced further due to placental insufficiency, the phenomenon of ion trapping may become significant. The fraction of ionized bupivacaine within the fetus increases as the fetal pH falls, its charge preventing it from leaving the fetal circulation, so that levels rise toward toxicity at birth.

Pethidine is commonly used for analgesia during labour. The high lipid solubility of pethidine enables significant amounts to cross the placenta and reach the fetus. It is metabolized to norpethidine, which is less lipid-soluble and can accumulate in the fetus, levels peaking about 4 hours after the initial maternal intramuscular dose. Owing to reduced fetal clearance the half-lives of both pethidine and norpethidine are prolonged up to three times.

Thiopental crosses the placenta rapidly, and experimentally it has been detected in the umbilical vein within 30 seconds of administration to the mother. Serial samples have shown that the peak umbilical artery (and hence fetal) levels occur within

3 minutes of maternal injection. There is no evidence that fetal outcome is affected with an 'injection to delivery' time of up to 20 minutes after injection of a sleep dose of thiopental to the mother.

The non-depolarizing muscle relaxants are large polar molecules and essentially do not cross the placenta. Therefore, the fetal neuromuscular junction is not affected. Only very small amounts of suxamethonium cross the placenta, though again this usually has little effect. However, if the mother has an inherited enzyme deficiency and cannot metabolize suxamethonium, then maternal levels may remain high and a significant degree of transfer may occur. This may be especially significant if the fetus has also inherited the enzyme defect, in which case there may be a degree of depolarizing blockade at the fetal neuromuscular junction.

Metabolism

While metabolism usually reduces the activity of a drug, activity may be designed to increase; a prodrug is defined as a drug that has no inherent activity before metabolism but that is converted by the body to an active moiety. Examples of prodrugs are enalapril (metabolized to enaloprilat), diamorphine (metabolized to 6-monoacylmorphine), and parecoxib (metabolized to valdecoxib). Metabolites also may have equivalent activity to the parent compound, in which case duration of action is not related to plasma levels of the parent drug.

In general, metabolism produces a more polar (water soluble) molecule that can be excreted in the bile or urine – the chief routes of drug excretion. There are two phases of metabolism, I and II.

Phase I (functionalization or non-synthetic)

- Oxidation
- Reduction
- Hydrolysis

Many phase I reactions, particularly oxidative pathways, occur in the liver due to a non-specific mixed-function oxidase system in the endoplasmic reticulum. These enzymes form the cytochrome P450 system, named after the wavelength (in nm) of their maximal absorption of light when the reduced state is combined with carbon monoxide. However, this cytochrome system is not unique to the liver; these enzymes are also found in gut mucosa, lung, brain and kidney. Methoxyflurane is metabolized by CYP2E1 in the kidney, generating a high local concentration of fluoride ions, which may cause renal failure (see sevoflurane metabolism, p. 123).

The enzymes of the cytochrome P450 system are classified into families and sub-families by their degree of shared amino acid sequences – families and subfamilies share 40% and 55% respectively of the amino acid sequence. In addition, the subfamilies are further divided into isoforms. Families are labelled CYP1, CYP2, and so on, the subfamilies CYP1A, CYP1B, and so on, and the isoforms CYP1A1, CYP1A2, and so on. Table 2.1 summarises isoenzymes of particular importance in the metabolism

Table 2.1. Metabolism of drugs by cytochrome P450 system.
CYP2C9 and CYP2D6 both demonstrate significant genetic polymorphism; other cytochromes also have variants, but these two are clinically important. Both losartan and parecoxib are prodrugs, so poor activity of CYP2C9 will limit active product availability.

CYP2B6	CYP2C9	CYP2C19	CYP2D6	CYP2E1	CYP3A4	CYP3A5
propofol	propofol	losartan	codeine	sevoflurane	diazepam	diazepam
	parecoxib	diazepam	flecainide	halothane	temazepam	
	losartan	phenytoin	metopropol	isoflurane	midazolam	
	S-warfarin	omeprazole		paracetamol	fentanyl	
					alfentanil	
					lidocaine	
					vecuronium	

of drugs relevant to the anaesthetist. Many drugs are metabolized by more than one isozyme (e.g. midazolam by CYP3A4 and CYP3A5). Genetic variants are also found, in particular CYP2D6 and CYP2C9; a variant of CYP2D6 is associated with defective metabolism of codeine.

The P450 system is not responsible for all phase I metabolism. The monoamines (adrenaline, noradrenaline, dopamine) are metabolized by the mitochondrial enzyme monoamine oxidase. Individual genetic variation, or the presence of exogenous inhibitors of this breakdown pathway, can result in high levels of monoamines in the circulation, with severe cardiovascular effects. Ethanol is metabolized by the cytoplasmic enzyme alcohol dehydrogenase to acetaldehyde, which is then further oxidized to acetic acid. This enzyme is one that is readily saturated, leading to a rapid increase in plasma ethanol if consumption continues. Esterases are also found in the cytoplasm of a variety of tissues, including liver and muscle, and are responsible for the metabolism of esters, such as etomidate, aspirin, atracurium and remifentanil. The lung also contains an angiotensin-converting enzyme that is responsible for AT1 to AT2 conversion; this enzyme is also able to break down bradykinin.

In addition, some metabolic processes take place in the plasma: cis-atracurium breaks down spontaneously in a pH- and temperature-dependent manner – Hofmann degradation – and suxamethonium is hydrolyzed by plasma cholinesterase.

Phase II (conjugation or synthetic)
- Glucuronidation (e.g. morphine, propofol)
- Sulphation (e.g. quinol metabolite of propofol)
- Acetylation (e.g. isoniazid, sulphonamides)
- Methylation (e.g. catechols, such as noradrenaline)

Although many drugs are initially metabolized by phase I processes followed by a phase II reaction, some drugs are modified by phase II reactions only. Phase II reactions increase the water solubility of the drug or metabolite to allow excretion into the bile or urine. They occur mainly in the hepatic endoplasmic reticulum but other sites, such as the lung, may also be involved. This is especially true in the case of acetylation, which also occurs in the lung and spleen.

In liver failure, phase I reactions are generally affected before phase II, so drugs with a predominantly phase II metabolism, such as lorazepam, are less affected.

Genetic polymorphism

There are inherited differences in enzyme structure that alter the way drugs are metabolized in the body. The genetic polymorphisms of particular relevance to anaesthesia are those of plasma cholinesterase, those involved in acetylation and the CYP2D6 variants mentioned above.

Suxamethonium is metabolized by hydrolysis in the plasma, a reaction that is catalysed by the relatively non-specific enzyme plasma cholinesterase. Certain individuals have an unusual variant of the enzyme and metabolize suxamethonium much more slowly. Several autosomal recessive genes have been identified, and these may be distinguished by the degree of enzyme inhibition demonstrated in vitro by substances such as fluoride and the local anaesthetic dibucaine. Muscle paralysis due to suxamethonium may be prolonged in individuals with an abnormal form of the enzyme. This is discussed in greater detail in Chapter 11.

Acetylation is a phase II metabolic pathway in the liver. Drugs metabolized by this route include hydralazine and isoniazid. There are genetically different isoenzymes that acetylate at a slow or fast rate. The pharmacokinetic and hence pharmacodynamic profile seen with these drugs depends on the acetylator status of the individual.

Enzyme inhibition and induction

Some drugs (Table 2.2) induce the activity of the hepatic microsomal enzymes. The rate of metabolism of the enzyme-inducing drug as well as other drugs is increased and may lead to reduced plasma levels. Other drugs, especially those with an imidazole structure (e.g. cimetidine), inhibit the activity of hepatic microsomal enzymes and may result in increased plasma levels.

Excretion

Elimination refers to the processes of removal of the drug from the plasma and includes distribution and metabolism, while excretion refers to the removal of drug from the body. The chief sites of excretion are in the urine and the bile (and hence the gastrointestinal tract), although traces of drug are also detectable in tears and breast milk. The chief route of excretion of the volatile anaesthetic agents is via the lungs; however, metabolites are detectable in urine, and indeed the metabolites of agents such as methoxyflurane may have a significant effect on renal function.

The relative contributions from different routes of excretion depend upon the structure and molecular weight of a drug. In general, high molecular weight

Table 2.2. Effects of various drugs on hepatic microsomal enzymes.

	Inducing	Inhibiting
Antibiotics	rifampicin	metronidazole, isoniazid, chloramphenicol acute use
Alcohol	chronic abuse	
Inhaled anaesthetics	enflurane, halothane	
Barbiturates	phenobarbital, thiopental	
Anti-convulsants	phenytoin, carbamazepine	
Hormones	glucocorticoids	
MAOIs		phenelzine, tranylcypromine
H$_2$ antagonists		cimetidine
Others	cigarette smoking	amiodarone, grapefruit juice

compounds (>30 000) are not filtered or secreted by the kidney and are therefore preferentially excreted in the bile. A significant fraction of a drug carrying a permanent charge, such as pancuronium, may be excreted unchanged in urine.

Renal excretion

Filtration at the glomerulus

Small, non-protein bound, poorly lipid-soluble but readily water-soluble drugs are excreted into the glomerular ultrafiltrate. Only free drug present in that fraction of plasma that is filtered is removed at the glomerulus. The remaining plasma will have the same concentration of free drug as that fraction filtered and so there is no change in the extent of plasma protein binding. Thus highly protein bound drugs are not extensively removed by filtration – but may be excreted by active secretory mechanisms in the tubule.

Secretion at the proximal tubules

There are active energy-requiring processes in the proximal convoluted tubules by which a wide variety of molecules may be secreted into the urine against their concentration gradients. Different carrier systems exist for acidic and basic drugs that are each capacity-limited for their respective drug type (i.e. maximal clearance of one acidic drug will result in a reduced clearance of another acidic drug but not of a basic drug). Drug secretion also may be inhibited, for example, probenecid blocks the secretion of penicillin.

Diffusion at the distal tubules

At the distal tubule, passive diffusion may occur down the concentration gradient. Acidic drugs are preferentially excreted in an alkaline urine as this increases the fraction present in the ionized form, which cannot be re-absorbed. Conversely, basic drugs are preferentially excreted in acidic urine where they are trapped as cations.

Biliary excretion

High molecular weight compounds, such as the steroid-based muscle relaxants, are excreted in bile. Secretion from the hepatocyte into the biliary canaliculus takes place against a concentration gradient, and is therefore active and energy-requiring, and subject to inhibition and competition for transport. Certain drugs are excreted unchanged in bile (e.g. rifampicin), while others are excreted after conjugation (e.g. morphine metabolites are excreted as glucuronides).

Enterohepatic circulation

Drugs excreted in the bile such as glucuronide conjugates may be hydrolyzed in the small bowel by glucuronidase secreted by bacteria. Lipid-soluble, active drug may result and be reabsorbed, passing into the portal circulation to the liver where the extracted fraction is reconjugated and re-excreted in the bile, and the rest passes into the systemic circulation. This process may continue many times. Failure of the oral contraceptive pill while taking broad-spectrum antibiotics has been blamed on a reduced intestinal bacterial flora causing a reduced enterohepatic circulation of oestrogen and progesterone.

Effect of disease

Renal disease

In the presence of renal disease, those drugs that are normally excreted via the renal tract may accumulate. This effect will vary according to the degree to which the drug is dependent upon renal excretion – in the case of a drug whose clearance is entirely renal a single dose may have a very prolonged effect. This was true of gallamine, a non-depolarizing muscle relaxant, which, if given in the context of renal failure, required dialysis or haemofiltration to reduce the plasma level and hence reverse the pharmacological effect.

If it is essential to give a drug that is highly dependent on renal excretion in the presence of renal impairment, a reduction in dose must be made. If the apparent volume of distribution remains the same, the loading dose also remains the same, but repeated doses may need to be reduced and dosing interval increased. However, due to fluid retention the volume of distribution is often increased in renal failure, so loading doses may be higher than in health.

Knowledge of a patient's creatinine clearance is very helpful in estimating the dose reduction required for a given degree of renal impairment. As an approximation, the dose, D, required in renal failure is given by:

$$D = \text{Usual dose} \times (\text{impaired clearance}/\text{normal clearance}).$$

Tables contained in the *British National Formulary* give an indication of the appropriate reductions in mild, moderate and severe renal impairment.

Liver disease

Hepatic impairment alters many aspects of the pharmacokinetic profile of a drug. Protein synthesis is decreased (hence decreased plasma protein levels and reduced protein binding). Both phase I and II reactions are affected, and thus the metabolism of drugs is reduced. The presence of ascites increases the volume of distribution and the presence of portocaval shunts increases bioavailability by reducing hepatic clearance of drugs.

There is no analogous measure of hepatic function compared with creatinine clearance for renal function. Liver function tests in common clinical use may be divided into those that measure the synthetic function of the liver – the international normalized ratio (INR) or prothrombin time and albumin – and those that measure inflammatory damage of the hepatocyte. It is possible to have a markedly inflamed liver with high transaminase levels, with retention of reasonable synthetic function. In illness, the profile of protein synthesis shifts toward acute phase proteins; albumin is not an acute phase protein so levels are reduced in any acute illness.

Patients with severe liver failure may suffer hepatic encephalopathy as a result of a failure to clear ammonia and other molecules. These patients are very susceptible to the effects of benzodiazepines and opioids, which should therefore be avoided if possible. For patients requiring strong analgesia in the peri-operative period a co-existing coagulopathy will often rule out a regional technique, leaving few other analgesic options other than careful intravenous titration of opioid analgesics, accepting the risk of precipitating encephalopathy.

The extremes of age

Neonate and infant

In the newborn and young, the pharmacokinetic profiles of drugs are different for a number of reasons. These are due to qualitative, as well as quantitative, differences in the neonatal anatomy and physiology.

Fluid compartments

The volume and nature of the pharmacokinetic compartments is different, with the newborn being relatively overhydrated and losing volume through diuresis in the hours and days after birth. As well as the absolute proportion of water being higher, the relative amount in the extracellular compartment is increased. The relative sizes of the organs and regional blood flows are also different from the adult; the neonatal liver is relatively larger than that of an adult although its metabolizing capacity is lower and may not be as efficient.

Distribution

Plasma protein levels and binding are less than in the adult. In addition, the pH of neonatal blood tends to be a lower value, which alters the relative proportions of ionized and unionized drug. Thus, both the composition and acid-base value of the blood affect plasma protein binding.

Metabolism and excretion

While the neonate is born with several of the enzyme systems functioning at adult levels, the majority of enzymes do not reach maturity for a number of months. Plasma levels of cholinesterase are reduced, and in the liver the activity of the cytochrome P450 family of enzymes is markedly reduced. Newborns have a reduced rate of excretion via the renal tract. The creatinine clearance is less than 10% of the adult rate per unit body weight, with nephron numbers and function not reaching maturity for some months after birth.

Though the implications of many of these differences may be predicted, the precise doses of drugs used in the newborn has largely been determined clinically. Preferred drugs should be those that have been used safely for a number of years, and in which the necessary dose adjustments have been derived empirically. In addition, there is wide variation between individuals of the same post-conceptual age.

Elderly

A number of factors contribute to pharmacokinetic differences observed in the elderly. The elderly have a relative reduction in muscle mass, with a consequent increase in the proportion of fat, altering volume of distribution. This loss of muscle mass is of great importance in determining the sensitivity of the elderly to remifentanil, which is significantly metabolized by muscle esterases. There is a reduction in the activity of hepatic enzymes with increasing age, leading to a relative decrease in hepatic drug clearance. Creatinine clearance diminishes steadily with age, reflecting reduced renal function.

As well as physiological changes with increasing age, the elderly are more likely to have multiple co-existing diseases. The implications of this are two-fold. First, the disease processes may directly alter drug pharmacokinetics and second, polypharmacy may produce drug interactions that alter both pharmacokinetics and pharmacodynamic response.

Drug action

Mechanisms of drug action

Drugs may act in a number of ways to exert their effect. These range from relatively simple non-specific actions that depend on the physicochemical properties of a drug to highly specific and stereoselective actions on proteins in the body, namely enzymes, voltage-gated ion channels and receptors.

Actions dependent on chemical properties

The antacids exert their effect by neutralizing gastric acid. The chelating agents are used to reduce the concentration of certain metallic ions within the body. Dicobalt edetate chelates cyanide ions and may be used in cyanide poisoning or following a potentially toxic dose of sodium nitroprusside. The new reversal agent, γ-cyclodextrin, selectively chelates rocuronium and reversal is possible from deeper levels of block than can be effected with the anticholinesterases.

Enzymes

Enzymes are biological catalysts, and most drugs that interact with enzymes are inhibitors. The results are twofold: the concentration of the substrate normally metabolized by the enzyme is increased and that of the product(s) of the reaction is decreased. Enzyme inhibition may be competitive (edrophonium for anticholinesterase), non-competitive or irreversible (aspirin for cyclo-oxygenase and omeprazole for the $Na^+/H^+ATPase$). Angiotensin-converting enzyme (ACE) inhibitors such as captopril prevent the conversion of angiotensin I to II and bradykinin to various inactive fragments. Although reduced levels of angiotensin II are responsible for the therapeutic effects when used in hypertension and heart failure, raised levels of bradykinin may cause an intractable cough.

Voltage-gated ion channels

Voltage-gated ion channels are involved in conduction of electrical impulses associated with excitable tissues in muscle and nerve. Several groups of drugs have specific blocking actions at these ion channels. Local anaesthetics act by inhibiting Na^+ channels in nerve membrane, several anticonvulsants block similar channels in the brain, calcium channel blocking agents act on vascular smooth muscle ion channels and antiarrhythmic agents block myocardial ion channels. These actions are described in the relevant chapters in Sections II and III.

Receptors

A receptor is a protein, often integral to a membrane, containing a region to which a natural ligand binds specifically to bring about a response. A drug acting at a receptor binds to a recognition site where it may elicit an effect (an agonist), prevent the action of a natural ligand (an inhibitor), or reduce a constitutive effect of a receptor (an inverse agonist). Natural ligands may also bind to more than one receptor and have a different mechanism of action at each (e.g. ionotropic and metabotropic actions of γ-aminobutyric acid (GABA) at $GABA_A$ and $GABA_B$ receptors).

Receptors are generally protein or glycoprotein in nature and may be associated with or span the cell membrane, be present in the membranes of intracellular organelles or be found in the cytosol or nucleus. Those in the membrane are generally for ligands that do not readily penetrate the cell, whereas those within the cell are for lipid-soluble ligands that can diffuse through the cell wall to their site of action, or for intermediary messengers generated within the cell itself.

Receptors may be grouped into three classes depending on their mechanism of action: (1) altered ion permeability; (2) production of intermediate messengers and (3) regulation of gene transcription.

1) Altered ion permeability: ion channels

Receptors of this type are part of a membrane-spanning complex of protein subunits that have the potential to form a channel through the membrane. When opened, such a channel allows the passage of ions down their concentration and electrical gradients. Here, ligand binding causes a conformational change in the structure of this membrane protein complex allowing the channel to open and so increasing the permeability of the membrane to certain ions (ionotropic). There are three important ligand-gated ion channel families: the pentameric, the ionotropic glutamate, and the ionotropic purinergic receptors.

The pentameric family

The pentameric family of receptors has five membrane-spanning subunits. The best-known example of this type of ion channel receptors is the nicotinic acetylcholine receptor at the neuromuscular junction. It consists of one β, one ϵ, one γ and two α subunits. Two acetylcholine molecules bind to the α subunits, resulting in a rapid increase in Na^+ flux through the ion channel formed, leading to membrane depolarization.

Another familiar member of this family is the $GABA_A$ receptor, in which GABA is the natural ligand. Conformational changes induced when the agonist binds causes a chloride-selective ion channel to form, leading to membrane hyperpolarization. The benzodiazepines (BDZs) can influence GABA activity at this receptor but augment chloride ion conductance by an allosteric mechanism (see below for explanation).

The 5-HT$_3$ receptor is also a member of this pentameric family; it is the only serotonin receptor to act through ion-channel opening.

Ionotropic glutamate

Glutamate is an excitatory neurotransmitter in the central nervous system (CNS) that works through several receptor types, of which NMDA, AMPA, and Kainate are ligand-gated ion channels. The NMDA receptors are comprised of two subunits, one pore-forming (NR1) and one regulatory that binds the co-activator, glycine (NR2). In vivo, it is thought that the receptors dimerize, forming a complex with four subunits. Each NR1 subunit has three membrane-spanning helices, two of which are separated by a re-entrant pore-forming loop. NMDA channels are equally permeable to Na$^+$ and K$^+$ but have a particularly high permeability to the divalent cation, Ca^{2+}. Ketamine, xenon and nitrous oxide are non-competitive antagonists at these receptors.

Ionotropic purinergic receptors

This family of receptors includes PX1 and PX2. Each has two membrane-spanning helices and no pore-forming loops. They form cationic channels that are equally permeable to Na$^+$ and K$^+$ but are also permeable to Ca^{2+}. These purinergic receptors are activated by ATP and are involved in mechanosensation and pain. These are not to be confused with the two G-protein coupled receptor forms of purinergic receptors, which are distinguished by selectivity for adenosine or ATP.

2) Production of intermediate messengers

There are several membrane-bound systems that transduce a ligand-generated signal presented on one side of the cell membrane into an intracellular signal transmitted by intermediate messangers. The most common is the G-protein coupled receptor system but there are others including the tyrosine kinase and guanylyl cyclase systems.

G-protein coupled receptors (GPCRs) and G-proteins

GPCRs are membrane-bound proteins with a serpentine structure consisting of seven helical regions that traverse the membrane. G-proteins are a group of heterotrimeric (three different subunits, α, β and γ) proteins associated with the inner leaflet of the cell membrane that act as universal transducers involved in bringing about an intracellular change from an extracellular stimulus. The GPCR binds a ligand on its extracellular side and the resultant conformational change increases the likelihood of coupling with a particular type of G-protein resulting in activation of intermediate messengers at the expense of GTP (guanylyl triphosphate) breakdown. This type of receptor interaction is sometimes known as **metabotropic** in contrast

3 Drug action

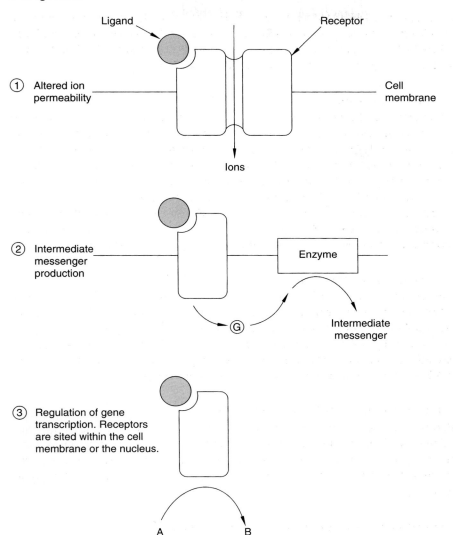

Figure 3.1. Mechanism of action of the three groups of receptors.

with ionotropic for ion-channel forming receptors. As well as transmitting a stimulus across the cell membrane the G-protein system produces signal amplification, whereby a modest stimulus may have a much greater intracellular response. This amplification occurs at two levels: a single activated GPCR can stimulate multiple G-proteins and each G-protein can activate several intermediate messengers.

G-proteins bind GDP and GTP, hence the name 'G-protein'. In the inactive form GDP is bound to the α subunit but on interaction with an activated GPCR GTP replaces GDP, giving a complex of α-GTP-$\beta\gamma$. The α-GTP subunit then dissociates from the $\beta\gamma$ dimer and activates or inhibits an effector protein, either an enzyme, such as **adenylyl cyclase** or **phospholipase C** (Figure 3.2) or an ion channel. For example, β-adrenergic agonists activate adenylyl cyclase and opioid receptor agonists, such as morphine, depress transmission of pain signals via inhibition of N-type Ca^{2+} channels through G-protein mechanisms. In some systems, the $\beta\gamma$ dimer can also activate intermediary mechanisms.

The α-subunit itself acts as a GTPase enzyme, splitting the GTP attached to it to regenerate an inactive α-GDP subunit. This then reforms the entire inactive G-protein complex by recombination with another $\beta\gamma$ dimer.

The α subunit of the G-proteins shows marked variability, with at least 17 molecular variants arranged into three main classes. G_s type G-proteins have α subunits that activate adenylyl cyclase, G_i have α subunits that inhibit adenylyl cyclase and G_q have α subunits that activate phospholipase C. Each GPCR will act via a specific type of G-protein complex and this determines the outcome from ligand-receptor coupling. It is known that the ratio of G-protein to GPCR is in favour of the G-proteins in the order of about 100 to 1, permitting signal amplification. Regulation of GPCR activity involves phosphorylation at the intracellular carboxyl-terminal that encourages binding of a protein, β-arrestin, which is the signal for removal of the receptor protein from the cell membrane. The binding of an agonist may increase phosphorylation and so regulate its own effect, accounting for tachyphylaxis seen with β-andrenergic agonists.

Adenylyl cyclase catalyzes the formation of cAMP, which acts as a final common pathway for a number of extracellular stimuli. All β-adrenergic effects are mediated through G_s and opiate effects through G_i. The cAMP so formed acts by stimulating protein kinase A, which has two regulatory (R) and two catalytic (C) units. cAMP binds to the R unit, revealing the active C unit, which is responsible for the biochemical effect, and it may cause either protein synthesis, gene activation or changes in ionic permeability.

cAMP formed under the regulation of the G-proteins is broken down by the action of the phosphodiesterases (PDEs). The PDEs are a family of five isoenzymes, of which PDE III is the most important in heart muscle. PDE inhibitors, such as theophylline and enoximone, prevent the breakdown of cAMP so that intracellular levels rise.

Therefore, in the heart, positive inotropy is possible by either increasing cAMP levels (with a β-andrenergic agonist or a non-adrenergic inotrope such as glucagon), or by reducing the breakdown of cAMP (with a PDE III inhibitor such as milrinone).

Phospholipase C is also under the control of the G-proteins, but the α subunit is of the G_q type. Activation of the G_q-proteins by formation of an active ligand-receptor complex promotes the action of phospholipase C. This breaks down a membrane

(a)

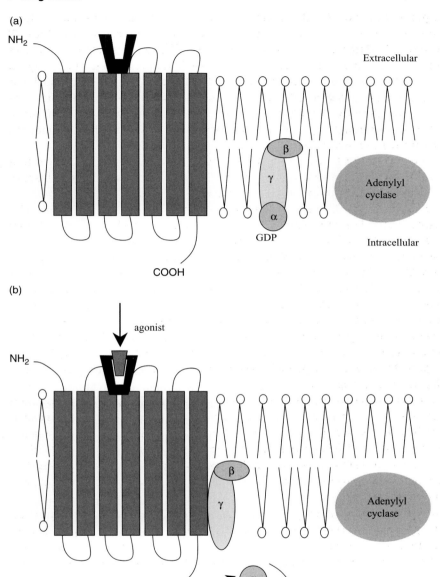

Figure 3.2. Effect of ligand-binding to G-protein Coupled Receptor (GPCR). Ligand binding to the 7-TMD GPCR favours association with the G-Protein, which allows GTP to replace GDP. The α unit then dissociates from the G-protein complex to mediate enzyme and ion-channel activation/inhibition.

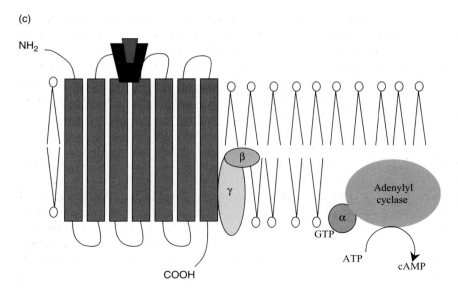

(c)

NH₂

β

γ

Adenylyl
cyclase

α

GTP

ATP

cAMP

COOH

Figure 3.2. (*Cont.*)

lipid, phosphatidylinositol 4,5-bisphosphate (PIP_2), to form inositol triphosphate (IP_3) and diacylglycerol (DAG).

The two molecules formed have specific actions; IP_3 causes calcium release in the endoplasmic reticulum, and DAG causes activation of protein kinase C, with a variety of biochemical effects specific to the nature of the cell in question. Increased calcium levels act as a trigger to many intracellular events, including enzyme action and hyperpolarization. Again, the common messenger will cause specific effects according to the nature of the receiving cellular subcomponent.

α_1-Adrenoceptors, the muscarinic cholinergic types 1, 3 and 5 as well as angiotensin II type 1 receptors exert their effects by activation of the G_q-proteins.

Membrane guanylyl cyclase. Some hormones such as atrial natriuretic peptide mediate their actions via membrane-bound receptors with intrinsic guanylyl cyclase activity. As a result cGMP levels increase and it acts as secondary messenger by phosphorylation of intracellular enzymes.

Nitric oxide exerts its effects by increasing the levels of intracellular cGMP by stimulating a cytosolic guanylyl cyclase rather than a membrane-bound enzyme.

Membrane tyrosine kinase. Insulin and growth factor act through the tyrosine kinase system, which is contained within the cell membrane, resulting in a wide range of physiological effects. Insulin, epidermal growth factor and platelet-derived growth factor all activate such tyrosine kinase-linked receptors.

The insulin receptor consists of two α and two β-subunits, the latter span the cell membrane. When a ligand binds to the α-subunits, intracellular tyrosine residues on its β-subunits are phosphorylated, so activating their tyrosine kinase activity. The activated enzyme catalyzes phosphorylation of other protein targets, which generate the many effects of insulin. These effects include the intracellular metabolic effects, the insertion of glucose transport protein into the cell membrane as well as those actions involving gene transcription.

3) Regulation of gene transcription

Steroids and thyroid hormones act through intracellular receptors to alter the expression of DNA and RNA. They indirectly alter the production of cellular proteins so their effects are necessarily slow. These cytoplasmic receptors act as ligand-regulated transcription factors; they are normally held in an inactive form by association with inhibitory proteins. The binding of an appropriate hormone induces a conformational change that activates the receptor and permits translation to the nucleolus, which leads to association with specific DNA promotor sequences and production of mRNA.

Adrenosteroid hormones

There are two types of corticosteroid receptor: the mineralocorticoid receptor, MR, and the glucocorticoid receptor, GR. The GR receptor is wide spread in cells, including the liver where corticosteroids alter the hepatic production of proteins during stress to favour the so-called acute-phase reaction proteins. The MR is restricted to epithelial tissue such as renal collecting tubules and colon, although these cells also contain GR receptors. Selective MR receptor activation occurs due to the presence of 11-beta hydroxysteroid dehydrogenase, which converts cortisol to cortisone: cortisone is inactive at the GR receptor.

Other nuclear receptors

The new antidiabetic drug rosiglitazone is an agonist at a nuclear receptor, peroxisome proliferator-activated receptor, which controls protein transcription associated with increased sensitivity to insulin in adipose tissue.

Dynamics of drug–receptor binding

The binding of a ligand (L) to its receptor (R) is represented by the equation:

$L + R \leftrightarrow LR$.

This reaction is reversible. The law of mass action states that the rate of a reaction is proportional to the concentrations of the reacting components. Thus, the velocity of the forward reaction is given by:

$V_1 = k_1 \cdot [L] \cdot [R]$,

where k_1 is the rate constant for the forward reaction (square brackets indicate concentration).

The velocity of the reverse reaction is given by:

$$V_2 = k_2 \cdot [LR],$$

where k_2 is the rate constant for the reverse reaction.

At equilibrium, the reaction occurs at the same rate in both directions ($V_1 = V_2$), and the equilibrium dissociation constant, K_D, is given by the equation:

$$K_D = [L] \cdot [R]/[LR] = k_2/k_1.$$

Its reciprocal, K_A, is the equilibrium association constant and is a reflection of the strength of binding between the ligand and receptor. Note that these constants do not have the same units; the units for K_D are $mmol.l^{-1}$ whereas those for K_A are $l.mmol^{-1}$ (when reading pharmacology texts take careful note of which of these two constants are being described). It was Ariens who first suggested that response is proportional to receptor occupancy and this was the basis of pharmacodynamic modelling. However, the situation is not as straightforward as this may imply and we need to explain the existence of partial agonists and inverse agonists as well as the phenomenon of spare receptors.

Receptor proteins can exist in a number of conformations that are in equilibrium, in particular the active and inactive forms; in the absence of an agonist the equilibrium favours the inactive form. Antagonists bind equally to both forms of the receptor and do not alter the equilibrium. Agonists bind to the receptor and push this equilibrium toward the active conformation. The active conformation then triggers the series of molecular events that result in the observed effect.

Types of drug-receptor interaction

The two properties of a drug that determine the nature of its pharmacological effect are affinity and intrinsic activity.

- Affinity refers to how well or avidly a drug binds to its receptor – in the analogy of the lock and key, this is how well the key fits the lock. The avidity of binding is determined by the K_D or K_A of the drug.
- Intrinsic activity (IA) or efficacy refers to the magnitude of effect the drug has once bound; IA takes a value between 0 and 1, although inverse agonists can have an IA between -1 and 0.

It is important to distinguish these properties. A drug may have a high affinity, but no activity, and thus binding will produce no pharmacological response. If such a drug prevents the binding of a more active ligand, this ligand will be unable to exert its effect – so the drug is demonstrating receptor antagonism. However, if a drug binds well but only induces a fractional response, never a full response, then the maximum possible response can never be achieved. This is the situation with partial agonists. Therefore:

- An agonist has significant receptor affinity *and* full intrinsic activity (IA = 1).
- An antagonist has significant receptor affinity but no intrinsic activity (IA = 0).
- A partial agonist has significant receptor affinity but only fractional intrinsic activity (0 < IA <1).
- An inverse agonist can be full or partial with $-1 \leq$ IA < 0.

Receptor agonism

Full agonists

Full agonists are drugs able to generate a maximal response from a receptor. Not only do they have a high affinity for the receptor, but also they have a high intrinsic activity. In clinical terms, the potency of the drug is determined by its K_D; the lower the K_D the higher the potency. For many drugs, the ED_{50} (the dose producing 50% of the maximum response) corresponds to the K_D.

Partial agonists

If an agonist drug has an intrinsic activity less than 1, such that it occupies receptors, but produces a submaximal effect compared with the full agonist, it is termed a partial agonist. The distinguishing feature of partial agonists is that they fail to achieve a maximal effect even in very high dose (i.e. with full receptor occupancy) (Figure 3.3(c)C). An example of a partial agonist is buprenorphine acting at the μ-opioid receptor. Partial agonists may act as either agonists or antagonists depending on circumstances. If used alone, they are agonists. When combined with a full agonist they produce additive effects at low doses of the full agonist, but this switches to competitive antagonism as the dose of full agonist increases; the full agonist needs to displace the partial agonist in order to restore maximum effect. In the case of partial agonists the equilibrium between active and inactive forms can never be entirely in favour of the active conformation, so the link between activation of receptor and effect is only a fraction of that seen with full agonists.

Inverse agonists

It is possible for a drug to bind and exert an effect opposite to that of the endogenous agonist. Such a drug is termed an inverse agonist and may have high or moderate affinity. The mechanism of inverse agonism is related to a constitutive action of receptors; some receptors can show a low level of activity even in the absence of a ligand, since the probability of taking up an active conformation is small but measurable. Inverse agonists bind to these receptors and greatly reduce the incidence of the active conformation responsible for this constitutive activity, as a result inverse agonists appear to exert an opposite effect to the agonist. The difference between

(a)

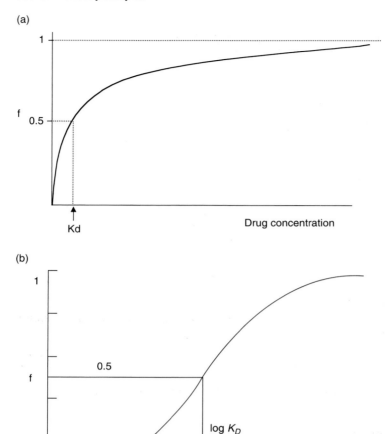

(b)

Figure 3.3. Dose–response curves. (a) Normal agonist dose–response curve, which is hyperbolic. (b) This curve is plotted using a log scale for dose and produces the classical sigmoid shape. (c) A and B are full agonists; B is less potent than A; C is a partial agonist that is unable to elicit a maximal response.

an inverse agonist and a competitive antagonist is important – an inverse agonist will favour a shift of equilibrium toward inactive receptors whereas a competitive antagonist binds equally to active and inactive receptors and simply prevents the agonist from binding. Inverse agonism was first described at benzodiazepine binding sites, but such convulsant agents have no clinical relevance, however ketanserin is an inverse agonist at $5HT_{2c}$ receptors.

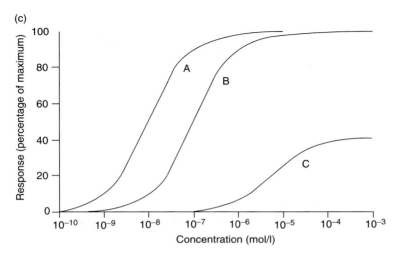

Figure 3.3. (*Cont.*)

Receptor antagonism

Antagonists exhibit affinity but no intrinsic activity. Their binding may be either reversible or irreversible.

Reversible

Reversible antagonists may either be competitive or non-competitive.

Competitive antagonists

For competitive antagonists the effect of the antagonist may be overcome by increasing the concentration of the agonist – the two molecules are competing for the same receptor and the relative amounts of each (combined with receptor affinity) determine the ratios of receptor occupation. In the presence of a competitive inhibitor the log[dose] versus response curve is shifted to the right along the x-axis; the extent of this shift is known as the dose-ratio (Figure 3.4(a)). It defines the factor by which agonist concentration must be increased in order to produce equivalent responses in the presence and absence of a competitive inhibitor. The pA_2 value, the negative logarithm of the concentration of antagonist required to produce a dose-ratio of 2, is used to compare the efficiency of competitive antagonism for different antagonists at a given receptor.

Examples of competitive inhibition include the non-depolarizing muscle relaxants competing with acetylcholine for cholinergic binding sites at the nicotinic receptor of the neuromuscular junction and β-blockers competing with noradrenaline at β-adrenergic receptor sites in the heart.

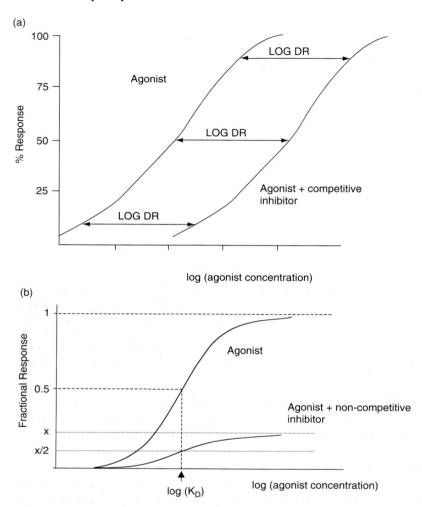

Figure 3.4. *Reversible antagonists.* (a) **competitive inhibition**. Note the parallel shift to the right in the presence of competitive inhibitor, with preservation of maximum response. DR represents dose-ratio (see text). (b) **non-competitive inhibition**. This time maximum possible response is given as a fraction. In the presence of the non-competitive inhibitor the curve is not shifted to the right, but the maximum obtainable response is reduced. K_D is the dissociation constant and is unaltered by the inhibitor.

As a general principle, first postulated by Bowman, weaker antagonists at the neuromuscular junction have a more rapid onset of action. This is because they are given in a higher dose for the same maximal effect so that more molecules are available to occupy receptors, and the receptor occupancy required for full effect is achieved more rapidly. Rocuronium, a non-depolarizing muscle relaxant, has only

(c)

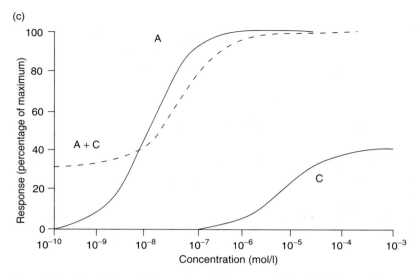

Figure 3.4. (*Cont.*) (c) **partial agonist acting as competitive inhibitor.** In this scenario A is a full agonist; C is a partial agonist. The dotted line, A + C, shows the dose-response curve for A in the presence of a sub-maximal dose of C. At low concentration of A the combination results in a greater effect than with A alone but as the dose of A is increased there comes a point at which the effect of A + C is less than with A alone. This is because at the crossover point the only way A can increase the response is by competing for receptors occupied by C. C therefore appears to act as a competitive inhibitor.

one-fifth of the potency of vecuronium, and therefore is given at five times the dose for the same effect. The relative flooding of the receptors means that the threshold receptor occupancy is achieved more rapidly, with a clear clinical benefit.

Non-competitive antagonists
Non-competitive antagonists do not bind to the same site as the agonist, and classically they do not alter the binding of the agonist. Their antagonism results from preventing receptor activation through conformational distortion. Their action cannot be overcome by increasing the concentration of an agonist present. An example is the non-competitive antagonism of ketamine with glutamate at NMDA receptors in the CNS. Recent classification of antagonists now groups non-competitive inhibitors and negative allosteric modulators (see later) together. This is because most non-competitive inhibitors, when investigated carefully, do alter agonist binding.

Allosteric modulation of receptor binding
Not all drugs with reversible activity will produce effects that fit neatly into either the competitive or non-competitive category. Some drugs can bind to sites distant from the agonist receptor site, yet still alter the binding characteristics of the agonist.

Such drugs are called allosteric modulators and may either reduce (negative allosteric modulators) or enhance (positive allosteric modulators) the activity of a given dose of agonist without having any discernible effects of their own. An example of a positive allosteric modulator is the effect of benzodiazepines on the activity of GABA at the $GABA_A$ receptor complex.

Irreversible

Irreversible antagonists may either bind irreversibly to the same site as the agonist or at a distant site. Whatever the nature of the binding site, increasing agonist concentration will not overcome the blockade. A clinical example is that of phenoxybenzamine that irreversibly binds to and antagonizes the effects of catecholamines at α-adrenoceptors. Aspirin is also an irreversible inhibitor; it causes cross-linking of the COX-1 enzyme in platelets rendering it inactive for the lifetime of the platelet. A single 75 mg dose is sufficient to block all platelet COX-1 and so return of normal function requires new platelet formation. This is why aspirin should be stopped 7–10 days before surgery where surgical bleeding must be minimized.

Spare receptors

The neuromuscular junction contains ACh receptors, which when occupied by ACh cause depolarization of the motor end plate. However, only a fraction of these receptors needs to be occupied to produce a maximal pharmacological effect. Occupancy of only a small proportion of the receptors ensures that a small quantity of ACh produces a maximal response. As a result there are 'spare receptors', which provide some protection against failure of transmission in the presence of toxins. This can be demonstrated as follows: if a small dose of an irreversible inhibitor is given then a proportion of the receptors are bound by the inhibitor and rendered unavailable so the log[dose] versus response curve for acetylcholine is shifted to the right because a higher fraction of the remaining receptors must be occupied to produce the original response. If a further irreversible antagonist is used more receptors are made unavailable and results in a further right-shift of the log[dose] versus response curve. When more than three-quarters of the receptors are occupied by irreversible antagonist then whatever the dose of ACh, a maximum response cannot occur and the shape of the curve changes so that both the maximum response and the slope is reduced.

Tachyphylaxis, desensitization and tolerance

Repeated doses of a drug may lead to a change in the pharmacological response, which may be increased or decreased for the same dose.

Tachyphylaxis

Tachyphylaxis is defined as a rapid decrease in response to repeated doses over a short time period. The most common mechanism is the decrease of stores of a transmitter before resynthesis can take place. An example is the diminishing response to repeated doses of ephedrine, an indirectly acting sympathomimetic amine, caused by the depletion of noradrenaline.

Desensitization

Desensitization refers to a chronic loss of response over a longer period and may be caused by a structural change in receptor morphology or by an absolute loss of receptor numbers. The term is often used synonymously with tachyphylaxis. An example is the loss of β-adrenergic receptors from the myocardial cell surface in the continued presence of adrenaline and dobutamine.

Tolerance

Tolerance refers to the phenomenon whereby larger doses are required to produce the same pharmacological effect, such as occurs in chronic opioid use or abuse. This reflects an altered sensitivity of the receptors of the central nervous system to opioids – the mechanism may be a reduction of receptor density or a reduction of receptor affinity. Tolerance occurs if nitrates are given by continuous infusion for prolonged periods as the sulphydryl groups on vascular smooth muscle become depleted. A drug holiday of a few hours overnight when the need for vasodilatation is likely to be at its lowest allows replenishment of the sulphydryl groups and restoration of the pharmacological effect.

Drug interaction

Interactions occur when one drug modifies the action of another. This interaction may either increase or decrease the second drug's action. Sometimes these interactions result in unwanted effects, but some interactions are beneficial and can be exploited therapeutically.

Drug interaction can be described as physicochemical, relating to the properties of the drug or its pharmaceutical preparation, pharmacokinetic due to alterations in the way the body handles the drug or pharmacodynamic where the activity of one drug is affected. The chance of a significant interaction increases markedly with the number of drugs used and the effects of any interaction are often exaggerated in the presence of disease or coexisting morbidity.

About one in six inpatient drug charts contain a significant drug interaction, one-third of which are potentially serious. An uncomplicated general anaesthetic for a relatively routine case may use ten or more different agents that may interact with one another or, more commonly, with the patient's concurrent medication.

Pharmaceutical

These interactions occur because of a chemical or physical incompatibility between the preparations being used. Sodium bicarbonate and calcium will precipitate out of solution as calcium carbonate when co-administered in the same giving set. However, one agent may inactivate another without such an overt indication to the observer; insulin may be denatured if prepared in solutions of dextrose and may, therefore, lose its pharmacological effect. Drugs also may react with the giving set or syringe and therefore need special equipment for delivery, such as a glass syringe for paraldehyde administration. Glyceryl trinitrate is absorbed by polyvinyl chloride; therefore, special polyethylene administration sets are preferred.

Pharmacokinetic

Absorption

In the case of drugs given orally, this occurs either as a result of one drug binding another in the lumen of the gastrointestinal tract or by altering the function of the gastrointestinal tract as a whole. Charcoal can adsorb drugs in the stomach, preventing absorption through the gastrointestinal tract (charcoal is activated by steam to cause fissuring, thereby greatly increasing the surface area for adsorption).

Metoclopramide when given as an adjunct for the treatment of migraines reduces gastrointestinal stasis, which is a feature of the disease, and speeds the absorption of co-administered analgesics. This is an example of a favourable interaction.

Distribution

Drugs that decrease cardiac output (such as β-blockers) reduce the flow of blood carrying absorbed drug to its site of action. The predominant factor influencing the time to onset of fasciculation following the administration of suxamethonium is cardiac output, which may be reduced by the prior administration of β-blockers. In addition, drugs that alter cardiac output may have a differential effect on regional blood flow and may cause a relatively greater reduction in hepatic blood flow, so slowing drug elimination.

Chelating agents are used therapeutically in both the treatment of overdose and of iron overload in conditions such as haemochromatosis. The act of chelation combines the drug with the toxic element and prevents tissue damage. Sodium calcium edetate chelates the heavy metal lead and is used as a slow intravenous infusion in the treatment of lead poisoning. Dicobalt edetate chelates cyanide ions and is used in the treatment of cyanide poisoning, which may occur following the prolonged infusion of sodium nitroprusside.

Competition for binding sites to plasma proteins has been suggested to account for many important drug interactions. This is not generally true; it is of importance only for highly protein bound drugs when enzyme systems are close to saturation at therapeutic levels. One possible exception is the displacement of phenytoin, which is 90% protein bound, from binding sites by a co-administered drug when therapeutic levels are already at the upper end of normal. In this case a 10% reduction in binding, to 81%, almost doubles the free phenytion level. Although hepatocytes will increase their metabolism as a result, the enzyme system is readily saturated and this leads to zero-order kinetics and the plasma level remains high instead of re-equilibrating. Most so-called 'protein binding' interactions are actually due to an alteration in metabolic capacity of one drug by the other. The commonest example seen in practice is the administration of amiodarone to a patient taking warfarin. Amiodarone inhibits the metabolism of S-warfarin by CYP2C9, which can significantly increase plasma levels of the active form of warfarin and produce iatrogenic coagulopathy. A similar interaction occurs with the NSAID phenylbutazone.

Metabolism

Enzyme induction will increase the breakdown of drugs metabolized by the cytochrome P450 family. Anticonvulsants and dexamethasone reduce the duration of action of vecuronium by inducing CYP3A4. Rifampicin can induce a number of the isoenzymes including 2B6, 2C9, 2D6 and 3A4. Conversely, drugs may inhibit enzyme activity, leading to a decrease in metabolism and an increase in plasma levels (see Table 2.1); cimetidine is much more potent than ranitidine at inhibiting 1A2, 2D6 and 3A4. Food and drink can also influence the activity of the cytochrome system; grapefruit juice inhibits CYP3A4, broccoli induces 1A2 and ethanol induces 2E1.

Excretion

Sodium bicarbonate will make the urine more alkaline, which enhances the excretion of weak acids such as aspirin or barbiturates. Thus, aspirin overdose has been treated with infusions of fluid to produce a diuresis, together with sodium bicarbonate, to alkalinize the urine and to promote its renal excretion.

Pharmacodynamic

Pharmacodynamic interactions may be direct (same receptor system) or indirect (different mechanisms, same end-effect).

Direct interactions

Flumazenil is used therapeutically to reverse the effects of benzodiazepines and naloxone to reverse the effects of opioids. This competitive antagonism is useful in treating drug overdose from these agents.

Indirect interactions

The use of neostigmine in the presence of non-depolarizing muscle relaxants (NDMRs) is an example of an indirect interaction that is used therapeutically. Neostigmine inhibits acetylcholinesterase and so increases acetylcholine concentration in the synaptic cleft that can then compete for nicotinic receptors and displace the NDMR.

Both enoximone and adrenaline are positive inotropic agents with different mechanisms of action that can interact indirectly to improve contractility. Adrenaline works via a GPCR whereas enoximone acts intracellularly by inhibiting phosphodiesterase but both actions result in an increase in intracellular cAMP levels. Captopril and β-blockers act additively to lower blood pressure by an indirect interaction; one via the renin-angiotensin system and the other via adrenoceptors.

Diuretics through their action on the levels of potassium may indirectly cause digoxin toxicity.

Summation

Summation refers to the action of the two drugs being additive, with each drug having an independent action in the absence of the other. Therefore, the co-administration of midazolam and propofol at the induction of anaesthesia reduces the amount of propofol necessary for the same anaesthetic effect.

4 Drug interaction

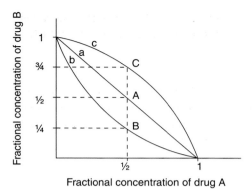

Figure 4.1. Isobolograms with lines of equal activity: (a) additive; (b) synergistic; (c) antagonistic (see text for explanation).

Potentiation

Potentiation results from an interaction between two drugs in which one drug has no independent action of its own, yet their combined effect is greater than that of the active drug alone. For example, probenecid reduces the renal excretion of penicillin, such that the effect of a dose of penicillin is enhanced without itself having antibiotic activity.

Synergism

Synergy occurs when the combined action of two drugs is greater than would be expected from purely an additive effect. Often this is because the drugs exert similar effects, but through different mechanisms. Propofol and remifentanil act synergistically when used to maintain anaesthesia.

Isobologram

The nature of interactions between different agents may be studied by use of an isobologram (Greek *isos*, equal; *bolus*, effect). An isobologram describes the combined effect of two different drugs. Consider two drugs A and B, each of which individually produce the required effect at concentrations a and b mmol.l^{-1}, respectively. A curve may be constructed from the fractional concentrations of each, plotted on the x- and y-axes, that produce the target effect. A straight line from 1 on the x-axis (drug A) to 1 on the y-axis (drug B) describes a purely additive effect where half the concentrations of each drug combine to produce the original target effect. When the resultant curve is not linear, some interaction between the drugs is occurring. Consider what happens when we have a concentration a/2 of drug A. If we can combine it with a concentration b/2 of drug B and the result is the same as with either drug alone, then the point A $(\frac{1}{2}, \frac{1}{2})$ can be marked, and there is a straight line indicating additivity. If however we need to combine a concentration a/2 of drug A with only a concentration b/4 of drug B to elicit the same response, the point $(\frac{1}{2}, \frac{1}{4})$ can be marked, which describes a curve that is concave, suggesting synergism between drugs A and B. Similarly, if we needed a concentration greater than b/2 of drug B the curve would be convex, indicating some antagonistic interaction between the two drugs point C $(\frac{1}{2}, \frac{3}{4})$ (Figure 4.1).

Isomerism

Isomerism is the phenomenon by which molecules with the same atomic formulae have different structural arrangements – the component atoms of the molecule are the same, but they are arranged in a different configuration. There are two broad classes of isomerism:
- **Structural isomerism**
- **Stereoisomerism**

Structural isomerism

Molecules that are structural isomers have identical chemical formulae, but the order of atomic bonds differs. Depending on the degree of structural similarity between the isomers, comparative pharmacological effects may range from identical to markedly different. Isoflurane and enflurane are both volatile anaesthetic agents; prednisolone and aldosterone have significantly different activities, with the former having glucocorticoid and mineralocorticoid actions but the latter being predominantly a mineralocorticoid. Isoprenaline and methoxamine have different cardiovascular effects, with methoxamine acting predominantly via α-adrenoceptors and isoprenaline acting via β-adrenoceptors. Dihydrocodeine and dobutamine are structural isomers with very different pharmacological effects; it is little more than coincidence that their chemical formulae are identical (Figure 5.1).

Tautomerism

Tautomerism refers to the dynamic interchange between two forms of a molecular structure, often precipitated by a change in the physical environment. For example, midazolam, which is ionized in solution at pH 4, changes structure by forming a seven-membered unionized ring at physiological pH 7.4, rendering it lipid-soluble, which favours passage through the blood–brain barrier and increases speed of access to its active sites in the central nervous system (see Figure 17.1). Another common form of isomerism is the keto-enol transformation seen in both morphine and thiopental.

Stereoisomerism

Stereoisomers have both the same chemical constituents and bond structure as each other but a different three-dimensional configuration. There are two forms of stereoisomerism:

(a) $C_{18}H_{23}NO_3$

Dihydrocodeine

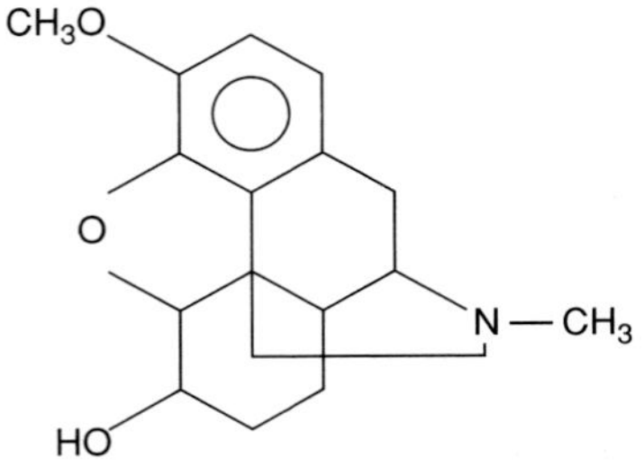

Dobutamine

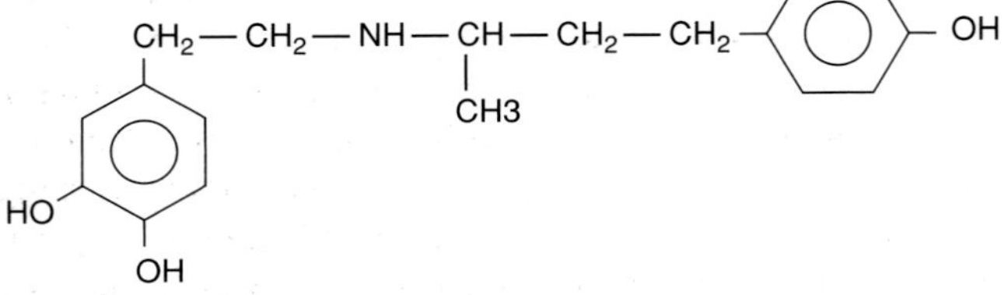

(b) $C_3H_2ClF_5O$

Isoflurane

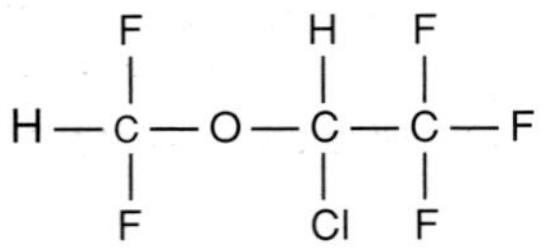

Enflurane

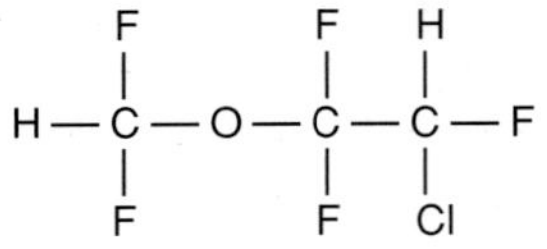

Figure 5.1. Structural isomers: (a) $C_{18}H_{23}NO_3$; (b) $C_3H_2ClF_5O$.

- **Geometric**
- **Optical**

Geometric isomerism

This exists when a molecule has dissimilar groups attached to two atoms (often carbon) linked either by a double bond or in a ring structure. The free rotation of groups is restricted and so the groups may either be on the same side of the

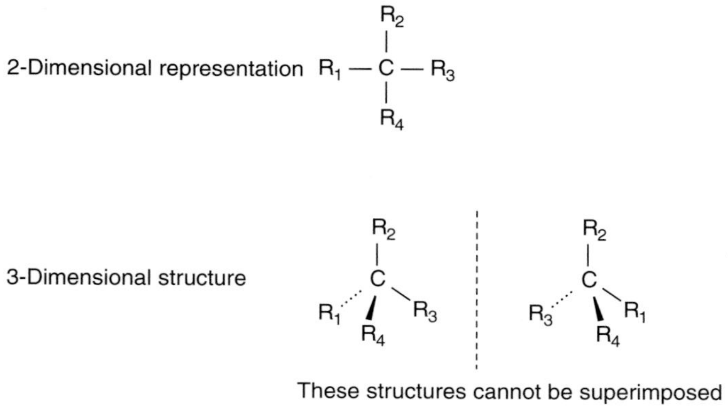

$$R_1 — \underset{\underset{R_4}{|}}{\overset{\overset{R_2}{|}}{C}} — R_3$$

2-Dimensional representation

3-Dimensional structure

These structures cannot be superimposed

Figure 5.2. Chiral centres.

plane of the double bond or ring, or on opposite sides. If the groups are on the same side the conformation is called cis- and if on opposite sides trans-. The bis-benzylisoquinolinium muscle relaxants, such as mivacuium, have two identical heterocyclic groups linked through an ester-containing carbon chain. Each of the heterocyclic groups contains a planar ring with groups that may either be arranged in the cis- or trans-conformation. So each of these compounds needs two prefixes describing their geometrical conformation, one for each heterocyclic group, hence cis-cis- in cis-atracurium. Mivacurium contains three such geometric isomers, trans-trans- (58%), cis-trans- (36%) and cis-cis (6%).

Optical stereoisomers

Optical stereoisomers may have one or more chiral centres. A chiral centre is a carbon atom or a quaternary nitrogen surrounded by four different chemical groups. The bonds are so arranged that in three dimensions they point to the vertices of a tetrahedron; thus, there are two mirror image conformations that could occur but which cannot be superimposed.

A single chiral centre

The absolute spatial arrangement of the four groups around a single chiral centre (Figure 5.2), either carbon or quaternary nitrogen, is now used to distinguish isomers as it unambiguously defines these spatial relationships. In the past the two isomers were distinguished by the direction in which they rotated plane polarized light (dextro− and laevo, d− and l−, + and −), but now their absolute configurations are designated R or S. This is determined by the absolute arrangement of the atoms of the four substituent groups directly attached to the chiral atom. First, the atom of lowest atomic number is identified and the observer imagines this group lying behind the plane of the page. The other three atoms now lie in this plane and their atomic numbers are identified; if their atomic numbers descend in a clockwise fashion then this is the R (rectus) form, if anticlockwise it is the S (sinister) form. The R and S structures are mirror images of each other and they are referred to as **enantiomers**. There is no link between the R and S classification and the laevo and dextro classification, and an S structure may be laevo or dextro-rotatory to plane polarized light.

In general, the three-dimensional conformation of a drug determines its pharmacodynamic actions at a molecular level. If the drug acts via a receptor, then conformation is of importance and there may be a marked difference in activity between enantiomers. However, if drug activity depends upon a physicochemical property then enantiomers would be expected to show similar activity.

Diastereoisomers

When more than one chiral centre is present there are multiple possible stereoisomers. These are not all mirror images of each other, so they cannot be called enantiomers, instead the term diastereoisomers is used.

More than one chiral centre. If a molecule contains more than one chiral atom, then with n such chiral centres n^2 stereoisomers are possible. Although the maximum number of possible isomers is n^2, if the molecule exhibits internal symmetry some of the possible configurations are duplicates. For example, atracurium has four chiral centres (two carbon atoms, two quaternary nitrogen atoms) with 16 theoretically possible isomers, but it is a symmetric molecule, so only ten distinct three-dimensional structures actually exist.

Some anaesthetic drugs are presented as a mixture of isomers (e.g. halothane, isoflurane) others have no chiral centre (e.g. sevoflurane, propofol). One recent development in the pharmaceutical industry is to identify the most active or least toxic isomer and produce the drug as a single isomer (e.g. ropivacaine). Such preparations, where just a single enantiomer is present, are called enantiopure (see below). In nature, molecules with chiral centres normally exist as single isomers (e.g. D-glucose) as enzymes selectively produce just one conformation. If natural agents are used for medicinal purposes, the purification process often results in racemization so both isomers will be present in the pharmaceutical preparation (e.g. atropine).

Racemic mixtures

These are mixtures of different enantiomers in equal proportions. Examples include the volatile agents (except sevoflurane), racemic bupivacaine and atropine. While the mixture may contain equal amounts of the two isomers, the contribution to activity, both pharmacodynamic and pharmacokinetic, may be very different and, indeed, one may be responsible for undesirable toxicity or side effects.

Enantiopure preparations

There may be advantages in selecting the more desirable moiety from a racemic mixture and producing it as a single isomer, known as an enantiopure preparation. The amide local anaesthetics of the mepivacaine series have enantiomeric forms. The R-form has a more toxic profile than the S-form so that both ropivacaine and bupivacaine are now available as enantiopure preparations – S-ropivacaine and S-bupivacaine. Other enantiopure preparations such as S-ketamine, dexketoprofen and dexmedetomidine are also available.

6

Mathematics and pharmacokinetics

Pharmacokinetics is the study of the way in which the body handles administered drugs. The use of mathematical models allows us to predict how plasma concentration changes with time when the dose and interval between doses are changed, or when infusions of a drug are used. Because there is an association between plasma concentration of a drug and its pharmacodynamic effect, models allow us to predict the extent and duration of clinical effects. Mathematical models may therefore be used to program computers to deliver a variable rate infusion to achieve a predetermined plasma level and hence a desired therapeutic effect.

It should be remembered that these pharmacokinetic models make a number of assumptions. Compartmental models make general assumptions based on virtual volumes without attempting to model 'real-life' volumes such as plasma or extracellular fluid volumes. Therefore, although convenient and useful to associate the virtual compartments with various tissue groups such as 'well perfused' or 'poorly perfused', this remains only an approximation of the physiological state.

Mathematics

Compartmental models are mathematical equations used to predict plasma concentrations of drugs based on experimental observations. Mathematical functions of importance in the understanding of these models are linear, logarithmic and exponential functions. Predicted behaviour and calculation of the parameters that define the model require manipulation of exponential functions, the logarithmic function and calculus. The following sections will cover all these concepts, starting with functions, particularly the exponential function, logarithms and finally calculus. In each section we will relate these to their use in pharmacokinetics, particularly the simple one-compartment model.

Functions

A function defines a unique value for y given a value for x. We write this as:

$$y = f(x).$$

For pharmacokinetics, we are interested in drug concentration (C) as a function of time (t). We can write:

$$C = f(t).$$

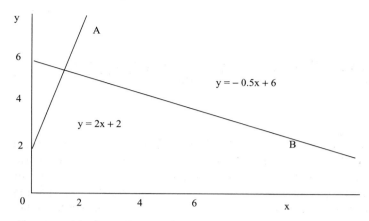

Figure 6.1. *The linear function.* Line A has a positive gradient of 2 and an intercept on the y axis of 2; line B has a negative gradient of 0.5 with an intercept on the y axis of 6. The equation for line B can also be written $2y = 12 - x$ by multiplying through by 2 and rearranging the terms on the right side of the equation.

For a one-compartment model the function is:

$$C = C_0 e^{-kt}.$$

Plasma concentration, C, depends on time, so t is the independent variable and plasma concentration, which is measured at a series of time-points, is the dependent variable. The relationship in this case is described by an exponential function.

The linear function

The equation for a straight line with a gradient of m is given by:

$$y = mx + c.$$

The constant, c, tells us the intercept on the y-axis and allows us to position the straight line in relation to the axes. If we knew only the gradient, we couldn't draw the line; we need at least one point to fix the exact place to draw it. Thus we need two pieces of information to draw a particular straight line: its gradient and its intercept on the y-axis. If m is negative the slope of the line is downward, if m is positive then the slope is upward (Figure 6.1). In a later section we meet differentiation; for a straight line the differential equation simply gives a constant, the value of the gradient, m. We meet a straight line in pharmacokinetics when taking a semi-logarithmic plot of the concentration–time curve for a simple one-compartmental model. The expression may look more complicated than the one above:

$$\ln(C) = \ln(C_0) - kt.$$

In this case we think of the y-axis as being $\ln(C)$ and the x-axis as being t. If we then compare this expression with $y = mx + c$ it should be clear that $-k$ is like m and represents the gradient and $\ln(C_0)$ represents the intercept on the y-axis.

The exponential function

An exponential function takes the form:

$$y = An^{ax}.$$

In this relationship n is the *base* and x the *exponent*; A and a are constants. Although it is possible to use any base for our exponential function, the natural number e is chosen for its mathematical properties. The exponential function, $y = e^x$, is the only function that integrates and differentiates to itself, making manipulation of relationships involving exponentials much easier than if another base were chosen. The number e is irrational, it cannot be expressed as a fraction, and takes the value 2.716 . . . where there is an infinite number of digits following the decimal point. Exponentials are positive if the *rate* of change of y increases or negative if the *rate* of change decreases as x increases; in the example above 'a' is positive for a positive exponential and negative for a negative exponential. Bacterial cell growth is an example of a positive exponential relationship between the number of bacteria and time; compound interest is a further example relating to the growth of an investment with time. For a negative exponential we write:

$$y = Be^{-bx}.$$

For the two examples above, A and B are constants that relate to the intercept on the y-axis and a and b are rate constants that determine how steep the exponential curve is. In pharmacokinetics, we consider time, t, to be our independent variable (equivalent to x) and plasma concentration, C, to be the dependent variable (equivalent to y). The simple wash-out curve (where plasma concentration declines and approaches zero) describes a negative exponential. This equation was given above:

$$C = C_0 e^{-kt}.$$

The 'steepness' of the wash-out curve depends on the rate constant, k. If k is halved and everything else remained constant, then the plasma concentration would take twice as long to reach any given level; if k is doubled then the time for the plasma concentration to reach a given level would halve. The wash-in curve also describes a negative exponential; although plasma concentration increases with time, the *rate* at which it approaches its maximum value is decreasing with time, making it a negative exponential (Figure 6.2).

Asymptote. Theoretically, a negative exponential process approaches its steady-state value evermore closely without actually reaching it. This steady-state value is termed the asymptote. For the wash-out curve this asymptote is zero; for the wash-in curve during a constant infusion it is the steady-state concentration reached, which is determined by the infusion rate and the clearance of the drug (Figure 6.2). If we consider the wash-out curve, after one half-life plasma concentration has fallen by 50%, after two half-lives it has fallen another (50/2)%, that is, a further 25% and after five half-lives the process will be $50 + 25 + 12.5 + 6.25 + 3.125 = 96.875\%$ complete, thus in practice five half-lives represents the approximate time needed to

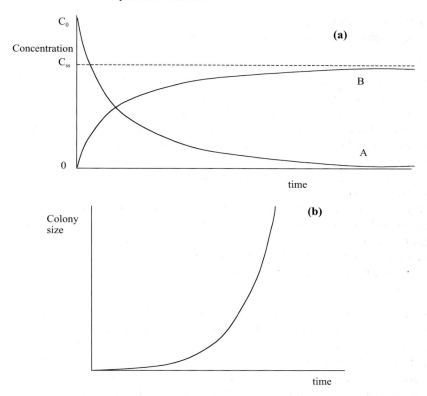

Figure 6.2. *The exponential function.* (a) Negative exponential function. Curve A is a simple wash-out curve for drug elimination, for example after a single bolus dose; the equation is $C = C_0 e^{-kt}$, the asymptote is zero and the starting point on the concentration-axis is defined as C_0. Curve B is a simple wash-in curve such as is seen when a constant rate infusion is used. The starting point on both axes is now zero and the asymptote is the concentration at steady-state C_{ss}. The equation is $C_{ss}(1 - e^{-kt})$. In both cases the rate constant for elimination is k. (b) Positive exponential function. This represents the exponential growth in a bacterial colony starting from a single organism. This organism divided; the two resultant organisms both divide and so on. There is a regular doubling of the number of bacteria so the equation is $N = 2^{t/d}$, where N is the number of organisms at time t and d is the time between consecutive cell divisions.

achieve steady-state. Because the time constant is longer than the half-life, it will take fewer time constants than half-lives to reach an approximate steady-state. After one time constant it will have fallen by 63.21%, and an approximate steady-state value is reached in three time constants.

The characteristic of an exponential relationship is that the *rate* at which the dependent variable changes is dependent on the *value* of that variable. We shall see later that this implies that when an exponential function is differentiated, the resulting expression must be related to the original function by a constant of proportionality. Experimentally we know that the rate of decline of plasma concentration with time in a wash-out curve is dependent on the plasma concentration. The constant of proportionality is k, defined as the rate constant for elimination:

$$dC/dt \propto C \quad \text{or} \quad dC/dt = -kC.$$

As we commented above, the only function that differentiates to itself is the exponential function, $y = e^x$, that is to say $dy/dx = e^x = y$. From the differential equation given above for the wash-out relationship we therefore know that the relationship between concentration and time will be exponential and take the form: $C = Be^{-bt}$. The rate constant, b, will be k (the rate constant for elimination). We define the concentration at time $t = 0$ to be C_0 so substituting these values in the equation the constant B must take the value C_0 (because $e^0 = 1$) giving the familiar equation $C = C_0e^{-kt}$.

The hyperbolic function

The simple rectangular hyperbolic function is:

$$y = 1/x.$$

It has asymptotes at $x = 0$ and $y = 0$, being symmetrical about the line $y = x$ (Figure 6.3). We are usually interested in the positive range of the function, that is, for $x > 0$. In pharmacokinetics, we need to know that integration of this function gives the natural logarithmic function (see below). The hyperbolic function is important in pharmacodynamics, where the relationship between dose and response is hyperbolic. The function relating fractional response (R/R_{max}) and dose (D) is:

$$R/R_{max} = D/(D + K_D).$$

Here K_D is the dissociation constant for the interaction of drug with receptor. This is a hyperbolic relationship because the fractional response is proportional to $1/(D + K_D)$. Although the hyperbolic function is not of direct importance to pharmacokinetic modelling, many people confuse the shape of the hyperbolic and exponential functions, as both are curves with asymptotes (Figure 6.4).

Logarithms and the logarithmic function

Most people are familiar with the idea that any number can be expressed as a power of 10; 1000 can be written 10^3, 0.01 as 10^{-2} and 5 as $10^{0.699}$. In these cases the *exponent* (or power) is defined as the logarithm to the base 10 (simply written as log) of each number. Thus the log of 1000 is 3, which can be written $\log(1000) = 3$, with $\log(0.01) = -2$ and $\log(5) = 0.699$. Note that $\log(10) = 1$ because $10^1 = 10$ and that $\log(1) = 0$ because $10^0 = 1$. Any number can be written in this way so that for any positive value of x

$$x = 10^{\log(x)}.$$

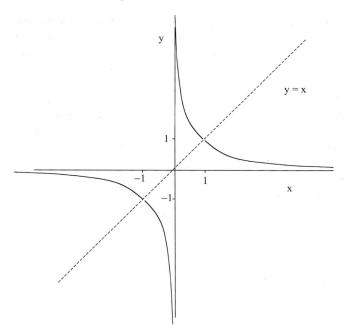

Figure 6.3. *The rectangular hyperbola.* In general, we are only concerned with the positive part of this curve. Any function where y is proportional to $1/(x + c)$, where c is a constant, will be a rectangular hyperbola.

For any number expressed this way, the *base* is 10 and the logarithm is the *exponent*. This describes a logarithmic function, where $y = \log(x)$; the scale is such that the integer values on the y-axis $-2, -1, 0, 1, 2, 3, \ldots$ correspond to 0.01, 0.1, 1, 10, 100, 1000, ... on the x-axis – there is no such thing as the logarithm of a negative number (Figure 6.5). If we multiply two numbers, w and z, together we can express each as an exponent of 10:

$$w = 10^x \quad \text{and} \quad z = 10^y,$$

so that:

$$w \times z = 10^x \times 10^y.$$

When we multiply two numbers that are expressed as powers of 10 together we *add* their exponents so we can rewrite this multiplication as:

$$w \times z = 10^x \times 10^y = 10^{(x+y)}.$$

We have now reduced multiplication to addition and in order to find the result of our calculation we can convert back using log tables, which was extremely useful in the days before cheap hand-held calculators were available. What we are adding are the logarithms of each number, $\log(w) = x$ and $\log(z) = y$, so that $\log(w \times z) = x + y$. For a fully expanded example, see the appendix at the end of this chapter.

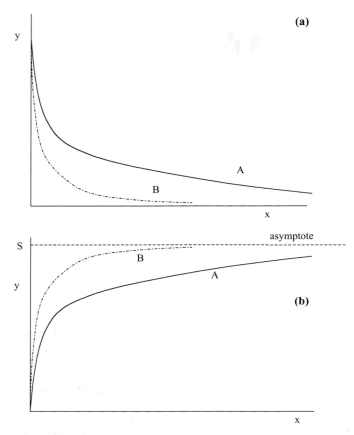

Figure 6.4. *Comparison of rectangular hyperbola and exponential curves.* (a) Curve A is a negative exponential ($y = Ae^{-ax}$), curve B is a positive rectangular hyperbola ($y = 1/x$). (b) Curve A is still a negative exponential ($y = S(1 - e^{-ax})$) but curve B is now a negative rectangular hyperbola ($y = S - 1/x$). Both graphs have effectively been reflected in the x-axis and moved upward in relation to the y-axis.

Furthermore, we can convert any expression such as $z = w10^y$ to its logarithmic equivalent. In this case:

$$\log(z) = \log(w10^y).$$

Because $w10^y = w \times 10^y$ and we add the logarithms of numbers that are multiplied together this can be written:

$$\log(z) = \log(w) + \log(10^y).$$

To find $\log(10^y)$ we need to remember that logarithms represent the power to which 10 is raised to give the required number. Thus, $1000 = 10^3 = 10 \times 10 \times 10$ and

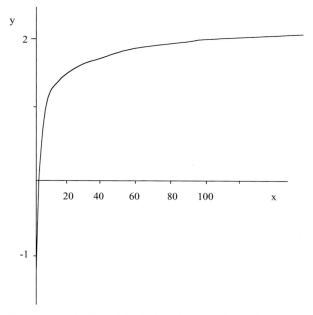

Figure 6.5. *The logarithmic function.* This shows the function $y = \log(x)$ for logarithms to the base 10. When $x = 1$ $y = 0$, which is a point common to all logarithmic relationships. Notice that unlike the exponential function, there is no asymptote corresponding to a maximum value for y. There is an asymptote on the x-axis, since the logarithm approaches negative infinity as x gets smaller and smaller and approaches 0; there is no such thing as a logarithm for a negative number.

$\log(10^3) = \log(10 \times 10 \times 10) = \log(10) + \log(10) + \log(10) = 3 \times \log(10) = 3$. So in our example expression:

$\log(z) = \log(w) + (y \times \log(10))$.

Because $\log(10) = 1$ this simplifies to:

$\log(z) = \log(w) + y$.

So far we have described the familiar situation where the *base* is 10 and the exponent is the logarithm to the base 10. We can actually write a number in terms of *any* base, not just 10, with a corresponding exponent as the logarithm to that base. In pharmacokinetics we are concerned with relationships involving the exponential function, $y = e^x$, so we use e as the base for all logarithmic transformations. If we write a number, say x, in terms of base e, then it is usual to write the logarithm of x to the base e as $\ln(x)$ rather than $\log(x)$ because the latter is often reserved for logarithms to the base of 10. Logarithms to base e are known as *natural* logarithms; for example 2 can be written $e^{0.693}$, so the natural logarithm of 2, $\ln(2)$, is 0.693 (this is a useful value to remember, as it is the factor that relates time constant to half-life).

We manipulate natural logarithms in the same way as we do logarithms to the base 10. In our pharmacokinetic models we come across the expression $C = C_0 e^{-kt}$ and we can convert this to its logarithmic equivalent. Because we have an expression involving e it makes sense to use natural logarithms rather than logarithms to the base 10. Using the same arguments as given earlier for logarithms to the base 10 we can rewrite this expression as:

$$\ln(C) = \ln(C_0 e^{-kt})$$
$$\ln(C) = \ln(C_0) + \ln(e^{-kt}).$$

In the same way that $\log(10^3) = 3 \times \log(10)$, $\ln(e^{-kt})$ can be written as $-kt \times \ln(e)$, so:

$$\ln(C) = \ln(C_0) + (-kt \times \ln(e)).$$

For the same reason that $\log(10) = 1$, $\ln(e) = 1$ (because $e = e^1$) and:

$$\ln(C) = \ln(C_0) - kt.$$

This gives the equation of the straight line we met above, with the gradient $-k$ and $\ln(C_0)$ the intercept on the $\ln(C)$ axis. Thus for a simple exponential relationship only two pieces of information are needed to draw both this line and the exponential it has been derived from, namely the rate constant for elimination and the intercept on the concentration axis, C_0 (Figure 6.6).

There is a simple relationship between logarithms to the base 10 and natural logarithms. For plasma concentration, C, we can write:

$$C = 10^{\log(C)} = e^{\ln(C)}.$$

Taking natural logarithms of both sides this can then be written:

$$\ln(C) = \ln(10^{\log(C)})$$
$$= \log(C) \times \ln(10).$$

Equally we could take log to the base 10 of each side and find that:

$$\log(C) = \log(e^{\ln(C)})$$
$$= \ln(C) \times \log(e).$$

So, if we know the natural logarithm of a number we can find its logarithm to base 10 simply by dividing by the natural logarithm of 10 (2.302); if we know the logarithm to base 10 we find its natural logarithm by dividing by the logarithm to the base 10 of e (0.434).

In pharmacokinetics we do a semi-log plot of concentration against time. It is easier to use natural logarithms for the concentration axis, because this gives a slope of $-k$ for the resultant straight line ($\ln(C) = \ln(C_0) - kt$). If logarithms to the base 10 are taken the equation of the straight line is $\log(C) = \log(C_0) - k\log(e)t$ so the slope will be different, by a factor of $\log(e)$. The other relationship that requires a natural logarithm as a factor is the relationship between time constant and half-life. Time constant (τ) is the inverse of the rate constant; it is the time taken for the

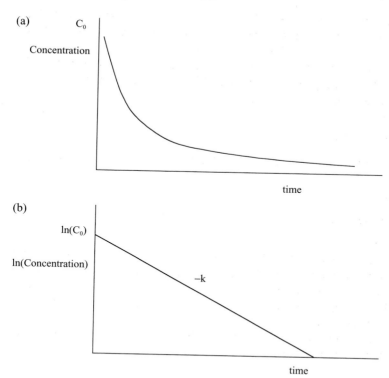

Figure 6.6. *Semilogarithmic transformation of the exponential wash-out curve.* (a) An exponential decrease in plasma concentration of drug against time after a bolus dose of a drug displaying single-compartment kinetics. (b) A natural logarithmic scale on the y-axis produces a straight line (C_0 is the plasma concentration at time, $t = 0$).

concentration to fall from C to C/e. Half-life ($t_{1/2}$) is similar in that it is the time taken for the plasma concentration to fall from C to C/2. If we think about the straight line relationship between ln(C) and time, then $(\ln(C) - \ln(C/2))/t_{1/2}$ will give the gradient of the line as does $(\ln(C) - \ln(C/e))/\tau$. Since $\ln(C) - \ln(C/2)$ is the same as $\ln(C \div C/2)$, i.e. ln(2) and $\ln(C) - \ln(C/e)$ is the same as ln $(C \div C/e)$, i.e. ln(e) or 1, this gives the relationship:

$$\ln(2)/t_{1/2} = 1/\tau$$
$$\ln(2) \cdot \tau = t_{1/2}.$$

We previously noted that ln(2) has a value of 0.693, so half-life is shorter than the time constant by a factor of 0.693. In one time constant the plasma concentration will have fallen to C/e or 0.37C, that is, 37% of its original value.

(a)

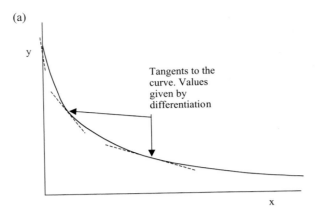

Tangents to the
curve. Values
given by
differentiation

(b)

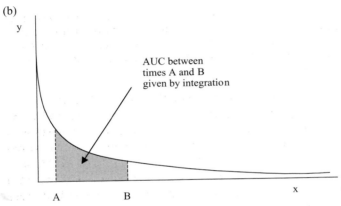

AUC between
times A and B
given by integration

Figure 6.7. Differentiation and integration. (a) Shows that when the equation for the curve
is differentiated it produces an expression that will give the value for the gradient of the
tangent to the curve at any selected point. (b) When finding the area under the curve (AUC),
it is essential to know the limiting values between which an area is defined. In the example
here, the upper limit is x = B and the lower limit x = A.

Differentiation

Differentiation is a mathematical process used to find an expression that gives the
rate at which the variable represented on the y-axis changes as x changes. When
evaluated, the expression gives the gradient of the tangent to the curve for each
value of x (Figure 6.7a). For the function $y = f(x)$ we indicate that differentiation is
needed by writing:

dy/dx.

Because differentiation only tells us about the *rate* at which a function is changing all
functions whose graphs have exactly the same shape, but only differ in their position

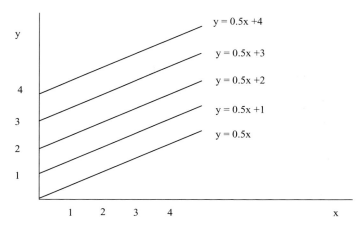

Figure 6.8. *A family of straight lines with the same gradient.* This family of straight lines, $y = 0.5x + c$, all have a gradient of 0.5; they differ only in their position with respect to the y-axis because they have different values for the constant c. Their gradients are the same so when we differentiate these equations they all differentiate to 0.5, the gradient of the line. Thus $dy/dx = 0.5$ for this family of curves.

with respect to the y-axis, will have the same differential equation. This is shown in Figure 6.8 for a family of simple linear equations where $y = mx + c$ each has the same gradient at any given time, so each will differentiate to the same expression – a constant in this case. This is because the value for c in each of these functions does not change as x changes, so when that part is differentiated it becomes zero. The idea that a family of curves differentiate to the same expression is important because the reverse of differentiation is integration – finding the area under the curve. In the case of integration the area under the curve clearly depends on the position of the graph with respect to the y-axis. If we have an expression for the rate at which y changes as x changes then we cannot give a single answer for reversing the process: we do not know the value for the constant c. It is therefore important to know at least one point on the curve – often the initial conditions when $x = 0$.

In pharmacokinetics, this gradient represents the rate at which plasma concentration is changing at a particular point in time. After a bolus dose of drug, we find that the rate at which plasma concentration changes falls as time passes; the rate of decline is dependent on the concentration itself. Differentiation defines how concentration changes with time and is indicated by:

dC/dt.

This can then be read as 'the rate of change of concentration with respect to time'. In a simple model we know that this is related to concentration itself. This can be written:

$dC/dt \propto C$.

By using a constant of proportionality (k) and observing that as time passes the concentration falls but more importantly the rate of change also falls, that is, the constant of proportionality must be negative, we can write:

$$dC/dt = -kC.$$

This describes a first-order differential equation, as it is dependent on C raised to the power one. If we now want an expression for C, we would need to integrate this expression. We saw earlier that this describes an exponential relationship. It can be shown that $dC/dt = -kC$ when integrated, gives the expression:

$$C = C_0 e^{-kt}.$$

To give the exact equation we use the condition that when $t = 0$, $C = C_0$. Note that a zero-order differential equation is dependent on C raised to the power zero, which is just one. A zero-order differential equation can therefore be written:

$$dC/dt = -k.$$

This tells us that the gradient is constant, which is true only for a straight line.

Integration

Integration can be thought of as a way in which we can find the area under a curve (AUC) if we know the equation that has been used to draw that curve. To find an area we need to define the starting and ending points of interest on the x-axis (Figure 6.7b). In pharmacokinetics the area we are interested in is that under the concentration, C (equivalent to the y-axis), against time, t (equivalent to the x-axis), curve. Usually we want to know the entire area under the curve, which starts at time $t = 0$ and runs to infinity; occasionally we choose other limits – for example between $t = 0$ and $t = t_{1/2}$ (where $t_{1/2}$ is the half-life). Although knowledge of *how* to integrate functions is not required, it is useful to know some important integrals related to pharmacokinetics.

Integration is indicated by the symbol $\int$ with the limiting values written above and below it. If no limits are given it is assumed that integration is taking place over the entire range possible. After the symbol for integration we write the function that is to be integrated together with an indication of the axis along which the limits have been given. For our concentration/time curve we integrate over time (rather than concentration) so we are integrating *with respect to* time, which is indicated using dt, just as for differentiation. So for a simple concentration against time curve modelled using one compartment we can write:

$$AUC = \int C_0 e^{-kt} dt.$$

This has omitted the limits, which are usually $t = 0$ and $t = $ infinity. Effectively we find the expression that gives the area under the curve, then evaluate it for the lower limit ($t = 0$) and subtract this from the value for the upper limit ($t = $ infinity); any constants will cancel out. We do not need to know how to do this particular integral, although we can note that it simplifies to:

$$AUC = C_0/k.$$

We mentioned in the previous section that integration can be thought of as the opposite of differentiation, but we need a little more information before integrating a differential equation back to the original relationship between variables. The information required is usually the initial conditions. For example, taking the differential equation we met previously:

$$dC/dt = -k \cdot C.$$

We can rearrange this and write:

$$(1/C) \cdot dC = -k \cdot dt.$$

If we then integrate both sides, knowing that the integral of $1/x = \ln(x)$ and the integral of the constant k is $kx + c$, where c is a different constant, we end up with an expression:

$$\ln(C) = -kt + c.$$

When $t = 0$, $C = C_0$ so putting in these initial conditions we find the value for c:

$$\ln(C_0) = c.$$

We can now substitute for c and write:

$$\ln(C) = -kt + \ln(C_0).$$

This is the linear relationship we have met before. We can now simplify this to get a relationship that does not involve logarithms; first re-arrange:

$$\ln(C) - \ln(C_0) = -kt.$$

We saw in a previous section that subtracting the logarithm of two numbers is the same as dividing one by the other, so we can write:

$$\ln(C/C_0) = -kt.$$

We can now convert back to the exponent form:

$$C/C_0 = e^{-kt}.$$

Re-arranging this now gives the familiar equation for the one-compartmental model:

$$C = C_0 e^{-kt}.$$

Pharmacokinetic models

Modelling involves fitting a mathematical equation to experimental observations of plasma concentration following drug administration to a group of volunteers or patients. These models can then be used to predict plasma concentration under a variety of conditions and because for many drugs there is a close relationship between plasma concentration and drug activity pharmacodynamic effects can also be predicted. There is a variety of models that can be used; most commonly we use compartmental models. In compartmental models we assume a single, central compartment is connected to one or two peripheral compartments. Drug is assumed to enter and leave only through the central compartment, although it can distribute to and re-distribute from the peripheral compartments. For each peripheral compartment we use an exponential term to model its volume and inter-compartmental clearance; the central compartment is also represented by an exponential term, but drug can be removed from the model entirely, so clearance from this compartment reflects removal from the body. There are also complex physiological models that can more closely predict drug concentrations in different organs as well as non-compartmental models based on the statistical concept of mean residence time. In this text we will concentrate on compartmental models.

Single bolus dose

The one-compartment model

The simplest model is that of a single, well-stirred, homogenous compartment. If a single dose of drug is given, then the model predicts that it instantaneously disperses evenly throughout this compartment and is eliminated in an exponential fashion with a single rate constant for elimination (Figure 6.9a). This is the one-compartment model that we have discussed in the mathematics section. Although such a model is not directly relevant to clinical practice, it is important to understand because it introduces the concepts that are further developed in more complex compartmental models. The pharmacokinetic parameters introduced are volume of distribution, clearance, rate constant for elimination, time constant and half-life. If we take C as drug concentration and t as time since administration of drug then this model is described by an equation with a single exponential term:

$$C = C_0 e^{-kt},$$

where C_0 is the concentration at time $t = 0$ and k is the rate constant for elimination. The volume of the single compartment is the volume of distribution, Vd, and the proportion of plasma from which drug is removed per minute is the rate constant for elimination, k. For example, if k is 0.1, then every minute a tenth of the compartment will have drug completely removed from it. The total volume cleared of drug every minute must therefore be the product of k and the compartment volume (k × Vd) (Figure 6.10). This is known as the clearance (Cl) of drug from the compartment; clearance has units of ml.min^{-1}:

$$Cl = k \times Vd.$$

Because the time constant τ is the inverse of the rate constant, clearance also can be expressed as the ratio of the volume of distribution and the time constant:

$$Cl = Vd/\tau.$$

(a) One-compartment model

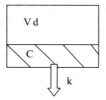

(b) Two-compartment model

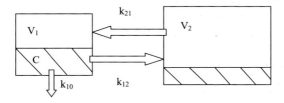

(c) Three-compartment model

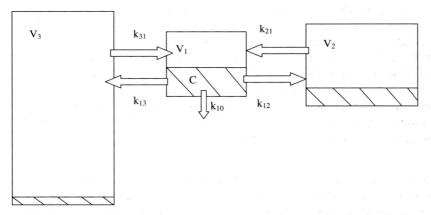

Figure 6.9. *Compartmental models.* (a) One-compartment model, volume of distribution Vd, rate constant for elimination k. (b) Two-compartment model, central compartment has volume V_1 and peripheral compartment has volume V_2. Rate constants for transfer between compartments are described in the text. The rate constant for elimination is k_{10}. (c) Three-compartment model. This is similar to the two-compartment model but with the addition of a second peripheral compartment, volume V_3, with slower kinetics.

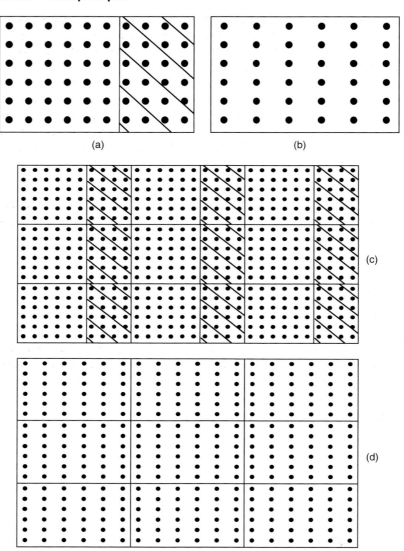

Figure 6.10. *Rate constant for elimination and clearance.* (a) This represents a unit of volume (e.g. one litre); if the rate constant for elimination (k) is 0.4 min^{-1} then 0.4 litres will have drug entirely removed from it every minute (2/5 of the volume, shaded area). (b) After 2/5 of the drug has been removed, the remaining drug is diluted into the full volume, so reducing its concentration. (c) This represents a drug with an apparent volume of distribution (Vd) of 9 litres, 2/5 of each of those litres will have drug removed every minute. Clearance is the product of Vd and k so the clearance in this example is 9 × 0.4 or 0.36 litres per minute. (d) In the case of our example the remaining drug disperses into the entire 9 litres and the concentration falls.

For any particular model k and Vd are constant, so clearance also must be a constant. Because clearance is the ratio of volume of distribution and time constant it is possible for drugs with very different values for Vd and τ to have the same clearance as long as the ratio of these two parameters is the same. So far we have considered the model in general, but we want to use the model to predict how the plasma concentration changes for a particular dose of drug. If a single bolus dose, X mg, of drug is given the concentration at time zero is defined as C_0; C_0 is X/Vd. If we then follow the amount of drug remaining in the body (X_t) it also declines in a negative exponential manner towards zero, as C is X_t/Vd. By substituting for C and C_0 this gives $X_t = Xe^{-kt}$ so the rate at which drug is eliminated (in mg per minute) is kX_t:

$$dX_t/dt = -kX_t.$$

We know that clearance is the product of k and Vd, so k is the ratio of clearance and Vd. If we put this into the expression above we can see that the rate at which drug is being eliminated is:

$$kX_t = (Cl/Vd)X_t$$
$$= Cl(X_t/Vd)$$
$$= Cl \times C$$

So, at a plasma concentration C, the drug is eliminated at a rate of $C \times Cl$ mg.min^{-1}.

The time constant is often defined as the time it would have taken plasma concentration to fall to zero if the original rate of elimination had continued. But the time constant τ is the inverse of the rate constant for elimination so it also represents the time it takes for the plasma concentration to fall by a factor of e (Figure 6.11). Since

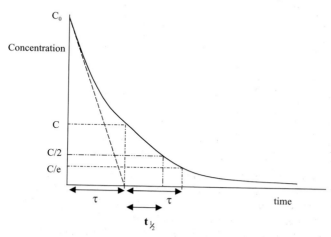

Figure 6.11. *Time constant.* The dashed line shows the tangent to the concentration–time curve at C_0; if this rate of decline had continued then the time it would have taken the concentration to reach zero is the time constant, τ. The time taken for the plasma concentration to fall from C to C/e, i.e. to 37% of C, is also one time constant.

τ has units of time, usually minutes, then k has units of time^{-1}, usually min^{-1}. In the section above we saw that the time constant τ is longer than the half-life; there is a simple inverse relationship between k and τ, whereas $k = \ln(2)/t_{1/2}$, so it is easier to use time constants rather than half-lives when discussing models.

Multi-compartment models

Multi-compartment models make allowance for the uptake of drug by different tissues within the body, and for the different blood flow rates to these tissues. Different tissues that share pharmacokinetic properties form compartments. Convenient labels include 'vessel rich' and 'vessel poor' compartments. The number of theoretical compartments that may be included in any model is limitless, but more than three compartments become experimentally indistinguishable. In these models it is important to realize that elimination can occur only from the central compartment and that the 'effect compartment' is in equilibrium with the central compartment. The volume of this effect compartment is very small so it does not contribute to the total volume, but is useful for predicting the onset and offset of the response when the observed effect is proportional to effect site concentration. Models for individual drugs differ in the volume of compartments and in transfer rates between compartments; the values for these pharmacokinetic parameters can vary enormously and depend on the physicochemical properties of a drug as well as the site and rate of drug metabolism.

Two compartments

In the two-compartment model the central compartment connects with a second compartment; the volume of the central compartment is V_1 and that of the peripheral compartment V_2 (Figure 6.9b). The total volume of distribution is the sum of these two volumes. Unlike the single compartment model, there are now two pathways for drug elimination from plasma: an initial rapid transfer from the central to peripheral compartment and removal from the central compartment. The latter removes drug from the system, whereas after distribution to the second compartment, the drug can re-distribute to the central compartment when conditions allow. Inspection of the concentration–time curve shows that the initial rate of decline in plasma concentration is much faster than would be expected from a single compartment model; this represents rapid distribution to the second compartment. A semi-logarithmic plot of ln (C) against time is now a curve, rather than a straight line, which is the sum of two straight lines representing the exponential processes with rate constants α and β (Figure 6.12).

Transfer between compartments is assumed to occur in an exponential fashion at a rate depending on the concentration difference between compartments and the equilibrium constants for transfer. Rate constants for transfer in each direction are described: k_{12} is the rate constant for the transfer from the central to peripheral compartment and k_{21} is the rate constant for the transfer from the peripheral to central compartment. The rate constant for elimination from the central compartment is now referred to as k_{10}. Drug is given into the central compartment and there is a rapid initial decline in concentration due to distribution into the peripheral compartment together with a slower decline, the terminal elimination, which is due both to elimination from the body and re-distribution of drug to plasma from the second compartment.

Consider a dose X mg of drug given into the central compartment with X_1 and X_2 representing the amount of drug in the central and peripheral compartments respectively after time t. We know that movement of drug is an exponential process depending on the rate constant and the amount of drug present so the rate at which the amount of drug in the central compartment changes with time depends on three processes: (1) removal of drug from the central compartment by metabolism and excretion; (2) drug distribution to the second compartment, both of which are dependent on X_1; and (3) re-distribution from the second compartment, which is dependent on X_2 and the rate constant for transfer, k_{21}. We can therefore write a differential equation for the rate of change of the amount of drug in the central compartment:

$$dX_1/dt = -k_{10}X_1 - k_{12}X_1 + k_{21}X_2.$$

This is much more complicated than the simple single compartment model and requires a special form of integral calculus to solve (Laplace transforms). It can be shown that using the result from integral calculus for the amount of drug, and dividing X_1 by V_1 to give the concentration in the central compartment, C, we get the equation:

$$C = A \cdot e^{-\alpha t} + B \cdot e^{-\beta t}.$$

The semi-logarithmic plot of ln(C) against time is the sum of two straight lines representing the two exponential processes in the relationship above (Figure 6.12). The intercepts of these two straight lines on the ln(C) axis (i.e. when t = 0) allow the constants A and B to be found and C_0 is the sum of A and B. The rate constants, α and β are found from the gradients of these lines and the reciprocals of these rate constants give the time constants τ_α and τ_β, which are related to the half-lives $t_{1/2\alpha}$ and $t_{1/2\beta}$, respectively (see above for relationship between time constant and half-life). Neither of these rate constants equates to any specific rate constant in the model, but each is a complex combination of all three. The steepness of the initial decline is determined by the ratio k_{12}/k_{21}. If the ratio k_{12}/k_{21} is high then the initial phase will be very steep, for a lower ratio the initial phase is much less steep. For example, after a bolus dose of fentanyl, where the ratio of k_{12}/k_{21} is about 4:1; the plasma concentration falls very rapidly. For propofol the ratio is close to 2:1 and the initial phase is less steep than for fentanyl. The absolute values for k_{12} and k_{21} determine the relative contribution of distribution to the plasma-concentration curve; the higher their value, the faster distribution occurs and the smaller the contribution so that for very high distribution rates the closer the model approximates a single

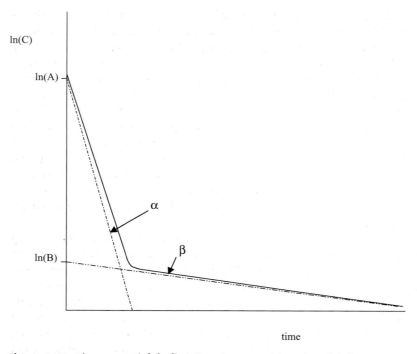

Figure 6.12. _Bi-exponential decline._ For a two-compartment model plasma concentration declines with a rapid exponential phase that has time constant α, this is due largely to distribution. Once distribution has occurred plasma concentration falls at a slower exponential rate – terminal elimination – with a time constant β. Neither α nor β equate to any one particular rate constant for the model.

compartment. This is clearly seen with remifentanil where k_{12} is 0.4 and k_{21} is 0.21; these are relatively large rate constants and so there is relatively little contribution from distribution and the behaviour of remifentanil is much closer to a one-compartment model than is that of fentanyl.

The volume of the central compartment is found by dividing the dose given, X, by C_0. As in the simple model, the central and peripheral compartments do not correspond to actual anatomical or physiological tissues. Thus, the central compartment is often larger than just the plasma volume, representing all tissues that, in pharmacokinetic terms, behave like plasma.

Three compartments

Modelling drug behaviour using three compartments requires three exponential processes. The equation for the plasma concentration (C) is now given by:

$$C = A \cdot e^{-\alpha t} + B \cdot e^{-\beta t} + G \cdot e^{-\gamma t}.$$

This is similar to the relationship for the two-compartment model, but with the addition of a third exponential process resulting from the presence of an additional compartment; the kinetic constants G and γ describe that additional process. The model consists of a central compartment into which a drug is infused and from which excretion can occur, together with two peripheral compartments with which drug can be exchanged (Figure 6.9c). These may typically represent well-perfused (the second compartment) and poorly perfused (the third compartment) tissues, respectively, with the central compartment representing plasma. Distribution into the second compartment is always faster than into the third compartment. This is a reasonable model for the majority of anaesthetic agents, where drug reaches the plasma and is distributed to muscle and fat. The volume of distribution at steady-state is the sum of the volumes of the three compartments. The mathematics is similar to that for two compartments, but more complicated as transfer into and out of the third compartment also must be taken into account.

As in the two-compartment model, there is final phase that can be described by a single exponential and the half-life associated with this phase is known as the **terminal elimination half-life**, which reflects both elimination from the body and re-distribution from the peripheral compartments. The rate constant for elimination is therefore *not* the inverse of the terminal elimination time constant; it can be calculated once the model parameters have been found. Clearance of drug out of the body is still defined as the product of V_1 and the rate constant for elimination; as discussed below clearance is usually found using a non-compartmental method and calculating the ratio of dose to the AUC.

Non-compartmental models

Non-compartmental models make no assumptions about specific volumes but use information from the AUC, as this reflects the removal of drug from plasma. The area under the concentration–time curve can be used to find clearance because AUC is the ratio of dose to clearance. Clearance (Cl) is therefore:

Cl = dose/AUC.

If we plot the *product* of concentration and time on the y-axis against time we produce what is known as the first moment curve. The area under this curve (AUMC) can be used to find a parameter known as mean residence time (MRT). Mean residence time is a measure of how long the drug stays in the body and is similar to a time constant in the compartmental models.

MRT = AUMC/AUC.

The product of clearance and MRT is the steady-state volume of distribution (V_{ss}) according to this model. So volume of distribution is:

V_{ss} = Cl $\times$ MRT.

Definition and measurement of pharmacokinetic parameters

The parameters described in the compartmental models are useful for comparing the persistence of different drugs in the body namely: volume of distribution (Vd), clearance (Cl) and time constants (τ in the single compartment and α, β and γ in multi-compartment models). Half-lives ($t_{1/2}$) are related to their corresponding time constants by a factor of $\ln(2)$, which is 0.693.

Volume of distribution

Volume of distribution (Vd) is defined as the apparent volume into which a drug disperses in order to produce the observed plasma concentrations. It does not correspond to any particular physiological volume and can be much larger than total body water. The physicochemical properties of a drug including its molecular size, lipid solubility and charge characteristics all influence the volume of distribution. Propofol is a very lipid-soluble drug and has a large volume of distribution of about 250 litres; pancuronium is a highly charged molecule and has a relatively small volume of distribution of about 17.5 litres. Tissue binding of drug, particularly intracellular sequestration, can account for extremely high volumes of distribution; the antimalarial chloroquine has a volume of distribution in excess of 10,000 litres. Pathology also influences the kinetic parameters; in hepatic and renal disease volumes of distribution are increased as the relative volumes of body fluid compartments change.

In the simple one-compartmental model, Vd is a constant that relates dose administered to the plasma concentration at time zero. It has the units of volume (e.g. litres) but can be indexed to bodyweight and expressed as $litres.kg^{-1}$. In the simple model, Vd is the initial dose divided by the plasma concentration occurring immediately after administration:

$$Vd = dose/plasma\ concentration = X/C_0.$$

In the multi-compartment models, the central compartment volume is the initial volume into which the drug disperses (V_{intial}). The volume of this compartment depends partly on the degree of protein binding; a highly protein bound drug will have a larger central compartment volume than a drug that is poorly bound. Propofol is 98% protein bound and has a central compartment volume of about 16 litres, compared with an actual plasma volume of about 3 litres. The volume of this central compartment can be estimated from the rapid distribution phase; if the dose given was X and the intercept on the y-axis is A then:

$$V_{intial} = X/A.$$

The total volume of distribution is the sum of all the volumes that comprise the model. There are several methods available that attempt to estimate this volume: V_{extrap}, V_{area} and V_{ss}. The first of these simply ignores the contribution made by any volume apart from that associated with the terminal phase of elimination; the intercept of the line representing terminal elimination is extrapolated back to its intercept on the ln(concentration) axis (ln(B) for the two compartment model) this gives a concentration which, when divided into X (dose given), will give V_{extrap}:

$V_{extrap} = X/B$.

It greatly overestimates the total volume of distribution for many drugs, particularly when the distribution phase contributes significantly to drug dispersion. The second method, V_{area}, is of more use because it is related both to clearance and the terminal elimination constant. This uses the non-compartmental method of calculating clearance from AUC and assumes that an 'average' rate constant for removal of drug from plasma can be approximated by the inverse of the terminal elimination time constant (β for the two-compartment model):

$V_{area} = Clearance/\beta = X/(AUC \times \beta)$.

This gives a better estimate of volume of distribution than V_{extrap}, but is still an overestimate; using β as the 'average' rate constant is an underestimate, particularly if there is significant distribution and re-distribution to and from compartments. However, it has the advantage of being easily calculated from experimental data. The final method V_{ss} is entirely based on non-compartment models (see above) and is calculated from the product of clearance and mean residence time:

$V_{ss} = (dose/AUC) \times (AUMC/AUC) = dose \times AUMC/AUC^2$.

This gives an estimate of volume of distribution that is independent of elimination, which can be useful. The estimate of volume of distribution using this method is smaller than for either of the other methods, but is usually close to the area method:

$V_{extrap} > V_{area} > V_{ss}$.

Clearance

Clearance (Cl) is defined as that volume of plasma from which drug is completely removed per unit time – the usual units are $ml.min^{-1}$. For the one-compartment model we saw that clearance is related to the rate constant for elimination; a high rate constant reflects rapid removal of drug since a large fraction of the distribution volume is cleared of drug. Clearance is simply the product of this rate constant and the volume of distribution (Figure 6.10). Clearance relates plasma concentration of drug at a given time to the actual rate of drug elimination ($Rate_{el}$ in $mg.min^{-1}$) at that time:

$Rate_{el} = C \times Cl$.

As we saw above, for the one-compartment model the clearance (Cl) of drug from the compartment is the product of the rate constant for elimination, k, and Vd, the volume of distribution. We can find k from the slope of the linear ln(C)-time graph and Vd from C_0, the concentration at t = 0, since we know the dose of drug given.

In the multi-compartment model, we can talk about inter-compartmental clearances as well as a clearance that describes loss of drug from the model. Quoted values for clearance define the removal of drug from the body, which is the product of the rate constant for elimination k_{10} and V_1, the volume of distribution of the central compartment. For example, propofol has a k_{10} of approximately 0.12, so about 1/8 of the plasma-equivalent volume has drug removed by elimination in unit time. For propofol, V_1 is about 16 litres and k_{10} is approximately 0.12, so the clearance of propofol is 16 × 0.12, which is about 2 litres per minute. Remifentanil has a much smaller central compartment volume but a higher k_{10}, so the clearance of remifentanil is 5.1 × 0.5, which is 2.5 litres, quite similar to that of propofol. If we do not know V_1 we could use V_{intial} as an estimate but it is often inaccurate due to sampling artefacts at early times when mixing has not taken place. Instead, clearance is usually calculated from the area under the concentration–time curve:

Clearance = Dose/AUC.

Elimination of drug from the model represents both metabolism and excretion of unchanged drug. Metabolism may occur in many sites and be organ-dependent or independent; a clearance that is greater than hepatic blood flow suggests that hepatic elimination is not the only route of elimination – either there are other sites of metabolism or the drug is excreted unchanged, for example through renal or pulmonary routes. Remifentanil has a very high clearance because it is eliminated by non-specific esterase in both plasma and tissue.

Inter-compartmental clearance relates to the movement of drug between compartments; C_{12} and C_{13} define drug transfer between compartments 1 and 2 and 1 and 3, respectively. For drugs with comparable compartmental volumes, the higher the inter-compartmental clearance the more rapidly distribution and re-distribution takes place.

Time constant and half-life ($t_{1/2}$)

In the single-compartment model there is just a single exponential relationship between plasma concentration and time. The time constant defines how quickly the plasma concentration falls with time and is defined as the time it would have taken plasma concentration to fall to zero if the original rate of elimination had continued (Figure 6.11). Time constant τ has units of time, usually minutes. The half-life is the time taken for the plasma concentration to fall to 50% of its initial value. In the mathematics section we saw that half-life is related to time constant by a constant of proportionality and half-life is $\ln2.\tau$, that is, half-life is $0.693.\tau$; the half-life is shorter than the time constant. Note that either half-life or time constant may be used to represent the time dependency of an exponential process. In the multi-compartment models there are several hybrid time constants each of which relates to one of the distinct exponential phases of drug elimination. As mentioned above, these do not relate directly to any one of the individual rate constants in the model.

Relationship between constants

The rate constant for elimination (k_{el} or k_{10}), clearance (Cl) and volume of distribution of the central compartment (Vd for one-compartment and V_1 for two-and three-compartment models) are all constant values for any one model and are closely related:

$$k_{el} = Cl/V_1 \quad \text{or} \quad Cl = V_1 \cdot k_{el}.$$

In the one compartment model the time constant for elimination, τ, is given by:

$$\tau = 1/k_{el}.$$

The relationship between time constant and clearance is therefore:

$$\tau = V_1/Cl.$$

Clearance is determined both by V_1 and τ; drugs with the same clearance can have very different volumes of distribution and time constants, it is the ratio of the two that is important. In non-compartment models, the mean residence time is equivalent to time constant and clearance is the ratio of dose given to the area under the concentration time curve.

Multiple doses and infusions

Loading dose, infusion rate and dose interval

If the initial volume of distribution (V_1) and the required plasma concentration are known then the dose needed to give a particular plasma concentration can be calculated:

$$\text{Dose} = V_1 \times \text{required concentration.}$$

If we want to maintain this particular plasma level, this first dose is known as the loading dose; repeated doses must be then given or the drug can be given by a constant infusion. The frequency of drug dosing depends on the rate at which drug is removed from plasma either by distribution or elimination. After one half-life, the concentration will have fallen to half of the initial value. If this concentration is acceptable as the minimum therapeutic concentration, then the dose frequency is equal to one elimination half-life (Figure 6.13). If the rate of removal is high, then the dosing interval must be short and doses given frequently; if the rate of removal is slow, then the dosing interval can be longer and doses given less frequently. The frequency and size of dose at the start of treatment influences the rate at which a steady state can be reached; for certain drugs, such as amiodarone, frequent initial dosing is replaced by less frequent and lower doses as the peripheral compartments become saturated with drug. Although many drugs have a high therapeutic index and large doses are well tolerated, some drugs have a narrow therapeutic index and maximum dose is restricted by adverse side effects. Thus dosing schedules are determined both by the pharmacokinetics and the pharmacodynamics of a drug.

Concentration

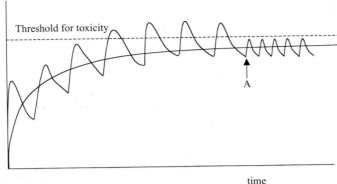

time

Figure 6.13. _Accumulation of a drug with intermittent boluses._ The dosing interval is equal to the half-life and after five doses this approaches a steady-state. This can be compared with an infusion designed to give the same steady-state concentration. This steady-state concentration is reached after approximately five half-lives. If the peak effect with bolus dosing exceeds the toxic threshold (dotted line) then doses should be reduced and dosing interval increased, as at point A.

Giving drug by repeated dose delivers a 'saw-tooth' pattern of plasma concentration. If we need to keep plasma concentration constant or within very narrow limits then an infusion may be appropriate. To do this we need to establish a steady-state where the rate of drug input ($Rate_{in}$) must equal the rate of drug output (i.e. rate of elimination):

$$Rate_{in} = Rate_{el}.$$

The rate of drug elimination is the product of clearance and plasma concentration, so to keep plasma concentration constant we must ensure that:

$$Rate_{in} = Cl \cdot C_p.$$

This last equation tells us how fast to run the drug infusion assuming we know its clearance. If no loading dose is given, and the infusion is started at a constant rate, steady-state will be reached after five half-lives or three time constants. The time to reach equilibrium is determined by the rate constant for elimination and the plasma level achieved at equilibrium is determined by the ratio of the infusion rate to the clearance. The delay in reaching equilibrium can be reduced either by giving a loading dose or by starting with a higher initial infusion rate that is reduced back to maintenance levels when the desired plasma concentration has been reached. The latter produces a smoother concentration profile than the former and is used in TCI (target-controlled infusion) pumps.

Context-sensitive half-times

The terminal elimination half-life is a value often cited for comparing the duration of action of different drugs, but this has little clinical relevance if pharmacokinetic behaviour follows a multi-compartmental model. Drug action is related to plasma concentration; in a three-compartment model after a single bolus dose initial distribution between compartments causes a rapid fall in plasma that limits the duration of pharmacological action more than does the elimination process; re-distribution will occur at a later stage, but the contribution from peripheral compartments in maintaining plasma levels is very small and is unlikely to prolong drug effects. On the other hand, if an infusion has been running for long enough to reach steady-state, the concentration in the peripheral compartments is the same as that in plasma. When the infusion is stopped plasma concentration will initially fall due to elimination, but this creates a concentration gradient between the central and peripheral compartments so drug in these compartments will be re-distributed to the central compartment so keeping the plasma concentration higher than would be seen after a bolus dose. For infusions of intermediate duration, concentration in plasma is still greater than that in the peripheral compartments so distribution will continue after stopping the infusion. However, the contribution of this initial distributive phase will be much smaller because concentration gradients between compartments are lower than at the start of the infusion. The rate at which re-distribution occurs depends on the inter-compartmental clearance. Fentanyl and propofol have similar compartmental volumes, but the inter-compartmental clearances for fentanyl are twice those for propofol; fentanyl re-distributes much more rapidly than propofol, which tends to maintain high plasma concentrations following a long infusion.

Thus the time course for the decline in plasma concentration at the end of an infusion depends on the duration of the infusion. The term **context-sensitive half-time** (CSHT) has been introduced to describe this variability; the term **context** refers to the duration of infusion. Context-sensitive half-time is defined as the time for the plasma concentration to fall to half of the value at the time of stopping an infusion. The longest possible context-sensitive half-time is seen when the infusion has reached steady state, when there is no transfer between compartments and input rate is the same as elimination rate. In general terms, the higher the ratio of distribution clearance to clearance due to elimination, the greater the range of context-sensitive half-time. Fentanyl re-distributes much more rapidly than propofol; in addition, its clearance due to elimination is about one-fifth that for distribution. As a consequence the CSHT for fentanyl increases rapidly with increasing duration of infusion. For propofol the clearance due to elimination is similar to that for distribution into compartment 2, so plasma concentration falls relatively rapidly after a propofol infusion due to elimination with a smaller contribution from distribution. The maximum possible context half-time for propofol is about 20 minutes, compared with 300 minutes for fentanyl based on current pharamacokinetic

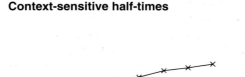

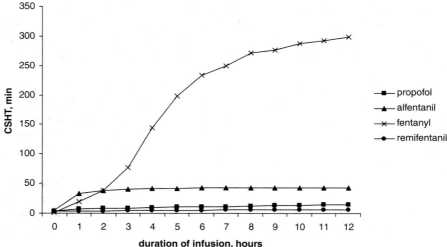

Figure 6.14. *Variation in contex-sensitive half-time (CSHT) with duration of infusion.*
This demonstrates the difference between propofol and fentanyl due to the more rapid
distribution and re-distribution kinetics of fentanyl and the more rapid elimination of propofol.
For short infusion times, fentanyl has a shorter CSHT than alfentanil, but after 2.5 hours,
alfentanil has a relatively constant CSHT compared with that for fentanyl, which continues to
increase.

models. For remifentanil, where this ratio is less than 1, the opposite is true; there is
very little variation in CSHT. Context-sensitive half-time is a more useful indicator of
a drug's behaviour in a given clinical setting. The variation of context-sensitive half-
time with duration of infusion for different intravenous agents is shown in Figure
6.14. It must be remembered that after one CSHT, the next period of time required
for plasma concentration to halve again will not be the same as the CSHT and is
likely to be much longer. This reflects the increasing importance of the slower re-
distribution and metabolism phases that predominate after re-distribution has taken
place. This explains the emphasis on half-*time* rather than half-*life*: half-lives are
constant whereas half-times are not.

Non-linear kinetics

So far we have considered models in which first-order kinetics determines elimination of drug from the body. Metabolic processes are usually first-order, as there
is a relative excess of enzyme over substrate, so enzyme activity is not rate limiting. However, in certain situations, some metabolic enzymes become saturated and
obey zero-order kinetics, in which the rate of change of plasma drug concentration is

constant rather than being dependent upon the concentration of drug. This is also known as saturation kinetics and indicates that enzyme activity is maximal, so cannot be influenced by increasing substrate concentration. An example is the metabolism of ethanol, which proceeds at a relatively constant rate after the ingestion of a moderate amount of alcohol. This is because the rate-limiting step in its metabolism by alcohol dehydrogenase is the presence of a co-factor for the reaction, which is present only in small quantities.

Certain processes obey first-order kinetics at low dose, but zero-order at higher doses. For example, the metabolism of phenytoin becomes saturable within the upper limit of the normal range, and the pharmacokinetics of thiopental obeys zero-order kinetics when used by infusion for prolonged periods, such as in the treatment of status epilepticus. There are two important implications of a process obeying zero-order kinetics within a normal dose range.

First, during zero-order kinetics a small increase in dose may cause a large increase in plasma level. If this occurs at a level near the upper limit of the therapeutic range, toxicity may be experienced after a modest dose increase. Checking plasma concentration is essential to avoid toxic levels when prescribing drugs where this is a problem, such as occurs with phenytoin.

Second, during zero-order kinetics there is no steady-state. If the rate of drug delivery exceeds the rate of drug excretion, plasma levels will continue to rise inexorably until ingestion stops or toxicity leads to death (Figure 6.15).

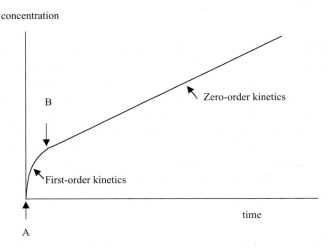

concentration

B

Zero-order kinetics

First-order kinetics

time

A

Figure 6.15. *Transition to non-linear (zero-order) kinetics.* If an infusion is started at a constant rate at point A, initially plasma concentration rises in a negative exponential fashion according to first-order kinetics. At point B the elimination process is overwhelmed and the plasma concentration continues to rise in a linear fashion, according to zero-order kinetics. This usually occurs because hepatic enzymes become saturated and work at maximum capacity.

Applied pharmacokinetics

Propofol

The intravenous anaesthetic propofol has become more popular than thiopental for induction of anaesthesia as many of its properties approximate to those of the ideal anaesthetic agent. It can be used both for induction and maintenance of anaesthesia, and it has become accepted as the anaesthetic agent of choice in daycase surgery due to its favourable 'wake up' profile. Although it is possible to give a bolus dose of propofol without understanding its pharmacokinetic properties, to use it sensibly by infusion requires some understanding of its disposition in the body.

Structure

Propofol is a sterically hindered phenol: the potentially active hydroxyl (-OH) group is shielded by the electron clouds surrounding the attached isopropyl ($(CH_3)_2CH-$) groups, which reduces its reactivity. So, unlike phenol, propofol is insoluble in water but highly soluble in fat and requires preparation as a lipid emulsion.

Pharmacokinetics

The usual induction dose of propofol is 1.5–2.5 mg.kg^{-1}, which when given intra-venously is extensively bound to plasma proteins (98% bound to albumin). Following an induction dose there is rapid loss of consciousness as the lipid tissue of the central nervous system (CNS) takes up the highly lipophilic drug. Over the next few minutes propofol then distributes to peripheral tissues and the concentration in the CNS falls, such that in the absence of further doses or another anaesthetic agent the patient will wake up. Its distribution half-life is 1–2 minutes (with distribution to the lipid tissues) and accounts for the rapid fall in plasma levels with a short duration of action. The terminal elimination half-life is very much longer (5–12 hours) and plays little or no role in offset of clinical action following a bolus dose.

Propofol causes peripheral vasodilatation, possibly through nitric oxide release in a similar manner to nitrates, so that when used in the elderly or hypovolaemic patient it may cause profound hypotension. This may be avoided by giving the drug as a slow infusion, however this results in the plasma concentration rising more slowly and onset of anaesthesia is delayed.

Context-sensitive half-time

Context-sensitive half-time is discussed above. When propofol is used by infusion it steadily loads the peripheral compartments; the longer the duration of the infusion, the more peripheral compartment loading will occur. Therefore, following a prolonged infusion, there will be more propofol to re-distribute from the peripheral compartments back into the central compartment, which will tend to maintain the plasma concentration and duration of action. In practice, the longer the duration of the infusion, the longer the time required before the plasma level falls below that required for anaesthesia. Although the CSHT has a maximum value of about 20 minutes, during long, stimulating surgery infusion rates will be high and the plasma concentration when wake-up occurs may be much less than half the plasma concentration at the end of the infusion. Thus time to awakening using propofol alone may be as long as 1 hour.

Remifentanil

Unlike most agents used in anaesthesia, remifentanil has a relatively constant context-sensitive half-time. Remifentanil is a fentanyl derivative that is a pure μ agonist. It has an ester linkage, which is very rapidly broken down by plasma and non-specific tissue esterases, particularly in muscle. The metabolites have minimal pharmacodynamic activity. With increasing age, muscle bulk decreases and this significantly influences the rate of remifentanil metabolism. The context-sensitive half-time of remifentanil is relatively constant over a wide range of contexts (infusion duration), from 3 to 8 minutes. Therefore a patient may be maintained on a remifentanil infusion for a long period, without significant drug accumulation as seen with other opioids. The advantage of this pharmacokinetic profile is that a patient may be given prolonged infusions of remifentanil for analgesia during surgery, with rapid offset of action when this is no longer required. The potential disadvantage is that analgesic effects wear off so rapidly that pain may be a significant problem immediately post-operatively. This must then be anticipated, either by using a regional technique or by the administration of a longer acting opioid shortly before the end of surgery.

Total intravenous anaesthesia (TIVA) and target-controlled infusion (TCI)

When using an infusion of propofol or remifentanil there is no 'point-of-delivery' measure of the target concentration comparable to the end-tidal monitoring of inhalational agents. A target-controlled infusion will display a *calculated* value for plasma concentration based upon the software model used and the information it has been given, usually patient weight and, for remifentanil, patient age.

TIVA: the Bristol model

The Bristol algorithm, based on a three-compartment model, provides a simple infusion scheme for propofol to achieve a target blood concentration of about 3 μg.ml^{-1} within 2 minutes and to maintain this level for the duration of surgery. This algorithm was based on plasma concentrations obtained from fit patients premedicated with temazepam and induced with fentanyl 3 μg.kg^{-1} followed by a propofol bolus of just 1 mg.kg^{-1}. Induction was followed by a variable-rate infusion of propofol at 10 mg.kg^{-1}.h^{-1} for 10 minutes, 8 mg.kg^{-1}.h^{-1} for 10 minutes then 6 mg.kg^{-1}.h^{-1} thereafter. This '10-8-6' infusion scheme was supplemented with nitrous oxide and patients were ventilated. The more usual induction dose of propofol is 2 mg.kg^{-1}, which is much higher than described in the Bristol regime and can produce adverse cardiovascular depression. This infusion regime may need adjusting according to the nature of the surgery either by giving boluses of propofol or by reducing or stopping the infusion altogether to allow the blood level of propofol to fall. Clearly, if higher plasma concentrations of propofol are needed to maintain adequate anaesthesia, then the 10-8-6 algorithm should be adjusted appropriately or an additional intravenous supplement used, such as a remifentanil infusion.

TCI

TCI is a technique that uses a microprocessor-controlled infusion pump programmed with a three-compartment model of propofol pharmacokinetics. There are two types of TCI: one that targets plasma concentration and, more recently introduced, one that targets the effect site. If the target concentration and the patient's weight are entered, the pump will infuse propofol at varying rates calculated to keep that target level constant. For remifentanil it is also important to enter the patient's age, since metabolism of remifentanil is significantly reduced in the elderly. There are also two different pharmacokinetic models for propofol infusion. The better known is the Marsh model, whereas the newer one is the Schnider model. They differ particularly in terms of the half-life reflecting equilibration with the effect compartment, known as the $t_{1/2keo}$. In the original pharmacokinetic model this constant was not defined, but experimentally it has been suggested that propofol has a $t_{1/2keo}$ of about 2.6 minutes; with the Schnider model, this has been reduced to about 1.5 minutes. The choice of model depends on the target chosen; in general the Schnider model is better where effect compartment is targeted whereas the Marsh model appears to perform better for targeting plasma concentration, particularly for longer procedures.

At induction, when the plasma concentration is the target, propofol is delivered at 1200 ml.h^{-1}, giving a bolus calculated to fill the central compartment. The infusion then continues at a diminishing rate, calculated to match the exponential transfer and uptake of drug to different compartments. If a higher blood level is required, for example to cover a highly stimulating point of surgery, the new target is entered and a small bolus is automatically delivered to reach the desired level. Similarly, if a lower level is required, the infusion automatically stops to allow a multi-exponential fall to the new level, at which point the infusion restarts at a lower rate.

The blood concentration targeted is titrated to clinical effect. For propofol the target concentration for an adult generally varies between 4 and 8 μg.ml^{-1}. In the unpremedicated patient an initial target of 5–6 μg.ml^{-1} can be used, whereas in the premedicated patient 3–4 μg.ml^{-1} may be more appropriate. These targets will be lower if remifentanil is co-infused, with propofol targets as low as 2–2.5 μg.ml^{-1} commonly used. The target for remifentanil is around 6–10 ng.ml^{-1} for induction, which can be reduced for maintenance to somewhere between 3 and 8 ng.ml^{-1}.

Again, it is important to realize that the actual blood level achieved by TCI pump in any individual patient is not necessarily the exact target level; there are pharmacokinetic variations between patients. In addition, this target level may or may not be appropriate for the stage of surgery. While a convenient aid to the anaesthetist, therefore, the infusion must be adjusted to effect, just as the vaporizer setting is adjusted during volatile anaesthesia.

Some TCI pumps have a **decrement time** displayed for propofol, which is a calculated value that is the predicted time for the plasma level to fall to a value of 1.2 μg.ml^{-1} (by default). At this level the patient is expected to awaken. However, there is a number of reasons why this time may be longer, particularly the use of hypnotics other than propofol (especially opioids).

Safety of TIVA and TCI in clinical practice

Delivering anaesthesia by the inhalational route to a spontaneously breathing patient has an inherent feedback that provides some degree of autoregulation for depth of anaesthesia. If the patient is too deep, the minute volume falls and delivery of the inhaled anaesthetic is reduced. Conversely, if the patient is too light, more volatile is inhaled and anaesthesia deepens. No such protection occurs during volatile anaesthesia in a paralyzed patient and this is also the situation for all patients anaesthetized with TIVA and TCI. Inadvertent discontinuation of the infusion will result in the patient waking up. This technique must therefore be used carefully to avoid awareness. Various measures may be taken to reduce this:

- The infusion should be either via a dedicated intravenous cannula or by a dedicated lumen of a multi-lumen central line, and it should be in view at all times so that a disconnection may be noticed. Ideally a non-refluxing valve should be used for each infusion.
- The use of midazolam in a small dose (2 mg) as an adjunct to anaesthesia reduces the incidence of awareness. Co-induction with propofol and midazolam allows a lower initial propofol target to be set for induction.
- Using oxygen in nitrous oxide rather than air to give an additional analgesic and anaesthetic effect (not strictly TIVA).

The pumps used for TCI infusions have two duplicate sets of circuitry to calculate the infusion rate and predicted effect site levels. If the two independent calculations do not agree, the pump will alarm. One advantage of using TIVA/TCI over conventional intravenous induction followed by volatile anaesthesia is that there is no 'twilight period' between the offset of intravenous anaesthetic effects and the onset of volatile anaesthesia. This period characteristically occurs at the time of intubation.

It should always be remembered that the effect site and/or plasma concentrations displayed on a TCI /TIVA pump remain a guide to the anaesthetist. More recent work has led to the development of a TCI pump for children and, as was mentioned above, a TCI pump that targets effect-site concentration rather than plasma concentration. Although targeting the effect site seems more appropriate, it is important to understand the different pharmacokinetic models available to choose one that suits the individual patient and their surgical intervention.

Appendix

Remember:

$$w \times z = 10^x \times 10^y = 10^{(x+y)}$$
$$w \div z = 10^x \div 10^y = 10^{(x-y)}.$$

• For example, multiply 13 by 257 using their logarithms:

[NB log(13) = 1.1139; i.e. $13 = 10^{1.1139}$ and log(257) = 2.4100; i.e. $257 = 10^{2.4100}$]

$$13 \times 257 = 10^{1.1139} \times 10^{2.4100}$$
$$= 10^{(1.1139+2.4100)}$$
$$= 10^{3.5239}.$$

To convert back to a numerical value we need to find the antilog of 3.5239 in the antilog table. However, only the numbers 0.0001 to 0.9999 are contained within antilog tables so we have to split the exponent into an integer part and a positive decimal part; for the example we used this gives $10^3 \times 10^{0.5239}$. We know this is 1000 × antilog(0.5239); we can look up 0.5239 in the body of the logarithm tables and find it corresponds to 3.341.

So the result of multiplying 13 by 257 is 1000 × 3.341, which is 3341.

• For example, divide 13 by 257 using their logarithms:

[NB log(13) = 1.1139; i.e. $13 = 10^{1.1139}$ and log(257) = 2.4100; i.e. $257 = 10^{2.4100}$]

$$13 \div 257 = 10^{1.1139} \div 10^{2.4100}$$
$$= 10^{(1.1139-2.4100)}$$
$$= 10^{(-1.2961)}.$$

Although this can be written $10^{-1} \times 10^{-0.2961}$, which is 0.1 × antilog(−0.2961), there are no tables of negative logarithms!

Therefore, we actually write it as $10^{-2} \times 10^{0.7039}$ because −2 + 0.7039 = −1.2961.

We now have 0.01 × antilog(0.7039) and the antilog of 0.7039 is 5.057, so the result of dividing 13 by 257 is 0.01 × 5.057, which is 0.05057.

Of course, this is a very old-fashioned way of finding logs and antilogs – a calculator can do both with much greater accuracy and without the need to change negative values to the sum of an integer part and a positive decimal part as we did in the second calculation. In fact, these days we would never dream of using logarithms for such calculations – that is what a calculator is for! However, it has introduced us to the idea of logarithms and shown that the logarithm to the base 10 of a number is the same as its exponent when it is written as a power of 10.

7

Medicinal chemistry

Structure-activity relationships (SAR) describe how the structure of related drugs influences their behaviour, for example whether they are agonists or antagonists. In order to understand how differences in drug structure can affect activity it is necessary to appreciate drug development methods and some basic organic chemistry. Once the properties of the contributing groups are understood, then it becomes easier to predict the likely behaviour of a drug molecule compared with the parent drug. In addition, knowledge of the structural properties of a drug may help us appreciate some of their physicochemical properties, such as their solubility in oil and water, their pKa values and whether they are weak acids or bases. These in turn help us understand the pharmacokinetic behaviour of a drug.

Drug design starts with a lead compound that has the required action in an animal model, but is not necessarily ideal; for example, the drug may resemble a neurotransmitter or be an enzyme inhibitor. By adding various functional groups to this compound it is possible to develop a more specific drug to target the required system. Once a compound with the most favourable pharmacodynamic effects is found, further modifications may be made to make the drug's pharmacokinetic behaviour more desirable.

In this chapter we will introduce some basic organic chemistry and identify the structures associated with drugs commonly used in anaesthesia. Those basic structures that should be readily identified are mentioned briefly below, together with diagrams of their structures and examples relevant to anaesthesia. These should be used in conjunction with a description of drug activity in Sections II–IV.

Organic chemistry is the study of carbon-based compounds. The position of carbon in the middle of the periodic table (Group 4) gives it an atomic structure that can form covalent bonds with elements from either end of the table. This contrasts with inorganic chemistry, where ionic bonds are most common. Covalent bonds are stronger than ionic bonds and do not interact readily with water, making many organic molecules insoluble in water. By the addition of functional groups (such as hydroxyl –OH or amine –NH$_2$) these organic compounds can become water-soluble. Organic molecules are the basis of life, from DNA to structural proteins and chemical messengers. Knowledge of these basic building blocks and signalling systems is crucial to an understanding of how therapeutic agents modify existing physiological processes at the molecular level.

Building blocks: amino acids, nucleic acids and sugars

Amino acids

The basic structure of an α-amino acid is a hydrocarbon group with both a carboxyl and amine group attached to the end carbon (the α-carbon). There are 20 commonly occurring α-amino acids that form the building blocks for protein synthesis (of which 5 cannot be synthesized – the essential amino acids). Not all amino acids form peptides and proteins; some amino acids are important precursors in neurotransmitter synthesis. For example phenylalanine can be metabolized to tyrosine which then enters adrenergic neurones as the substrate for catecholamine synthesis (see Chapter 12). Other α-amino acids are central neurotransmitters in their own right, for example, glycine and glutamate. Not all amino acids of importance are α-amino acids. GABA (γ-amino butyric acid), as its name suggests, is a γ-amino acid that has the carboxyl and amine groups on opposite ends of a butyl backbone; GABA is an important inhibitory neurotransmitter.

An α-amino acid   Phenylalanine   Glycine

GABA – γ-amino butyric acid

Nucleic acids, nucleosides and nucleotides

Nucleosides are formed from the combination of a nucleic acid with a sugar, usually ribose (e.g. adenosine, guanosine). Nucleotides are the building blocks of DNA/RNA and are formed from nucleosides linked to a phosphate group. The nucleic acids are either purines (adenine or guanine) or pyrimidines (cytosine, uracil or thymine). Many anti-cancer drugs are analogues of nucleic acids or nucleotides. Nucleosides are important intermediates in metabolic processes as they can combine with high-energy phosphate groups to act as co-factors in metabolic and catabolic processes within the cell.

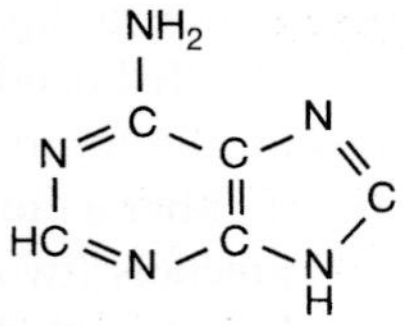

NH$_2$

Adenine

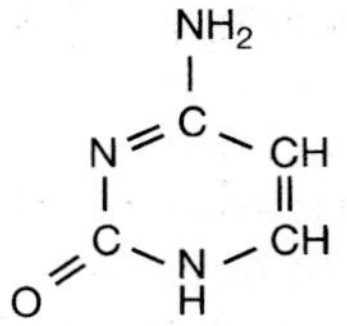

NH$_2$

Cytosine (4-amino 2-oxopyrimidine)

Sugars

These are carbohydrates with a chemical formula $(CH_2O)_n$, where n can be 3 (a triose, e.g. glyceraldehyde), 4 (a tetrose), 5 (a pentose, e.g. ribose) or 6 (a hexose, e.g. glucose). They are naturally occurring compounds and glucose is metabolized to carbon dioxide and water through oxidative tissue respiration. The pentoses and hexoses exist in cyclic forms in vivo.

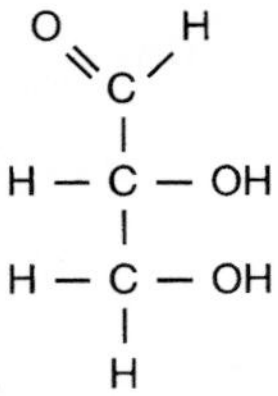

Glyceraldehyde (a triose)

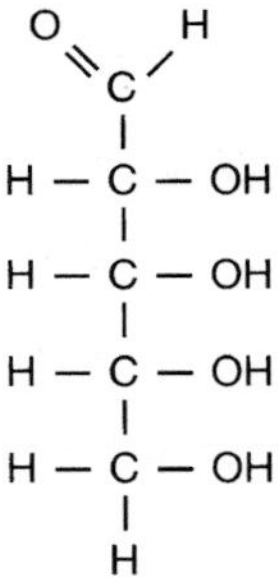

Ribose (a pentose)

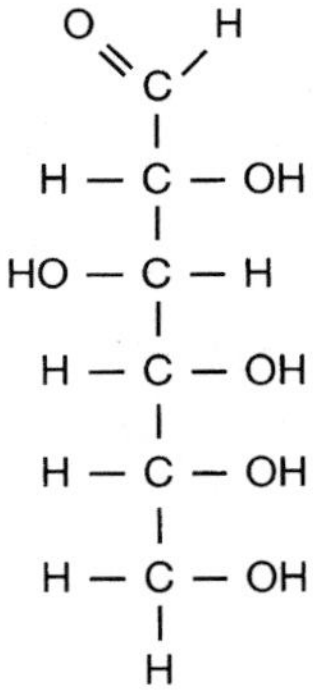

Glucose (a hexose)

Drugs and their structures

Many drugs are organic molecules and often derived from plant material. It is not possible here to describe all the molecular structures of groups of anaesthetically important drugs. In this section the following selected structures will be described: catecholamines, barbiturates, benzodiazepines, non-depolarizing muscle relaxants (bis-benzylisoquinoliniums and aminosteroids) and opioids.

Catecholamines and derivatives

These are derived from the amino acid tyrosine (see also Figure 12.3), which is hydroxylated (addition of an –OH group) and decarboxylated (removal of a –COOH group).

The side chain (ethylamine) consists of two carbons attached to an amine group. The α-carbon is bound to the amine group and the β-carbon is covalently linked to the catechol ring. The size and nature of the functional groups on the terminal amine and the α-carbon determine whether an agent is active at either α- or β-adrenoceptors or is an agonist or antagonist. In addition, only catechols (two adjacent –OH groups on the benzene ring) are metabolized by catechol-O-methyl transferase (COMT); derivatives without this feature may have a longer duration of action. Similarly, monoamine oxidase (MAO) will metabolize only drugs with a single amine group, preferably a primary amine, although adrenaline, a secondary amine (see mini-dictionary below), is a substrate (see Chapter 12).

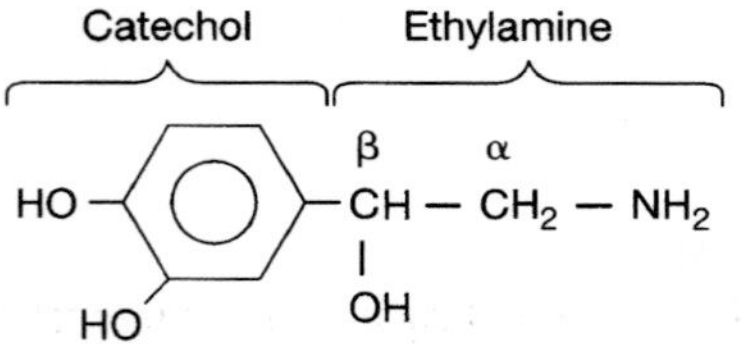

Noradrenaline

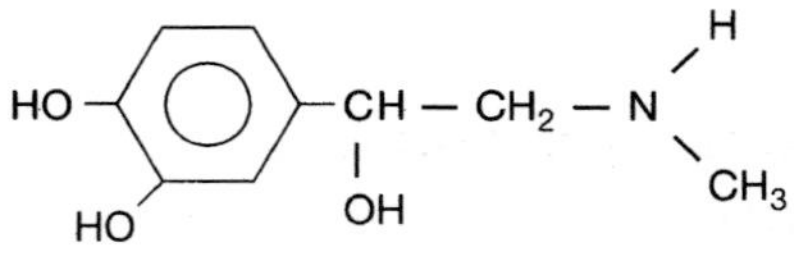

Adrenaline

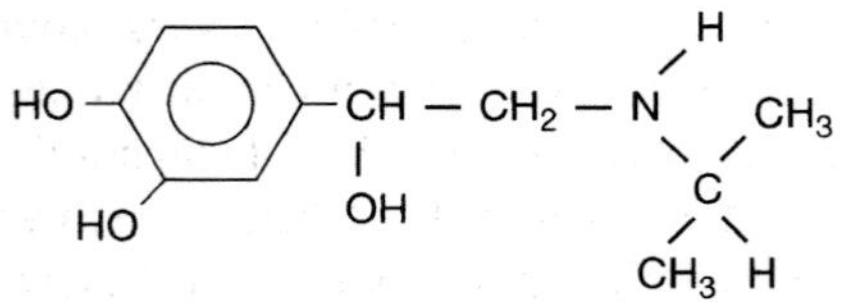

Isoprenaline
A β-selective agonist;
not a substrate for MAO,
a substrate for COMT.

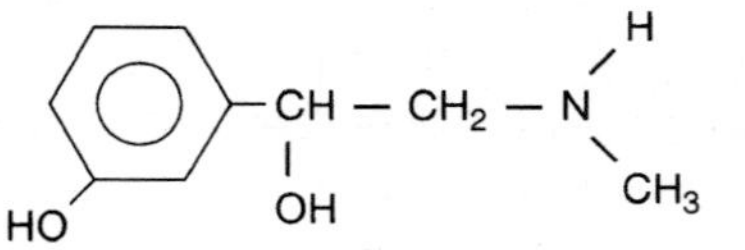

Phenylephrine
An α-selective agonist;
a substrate for MAO,
not a substrate for COMT.

Barbiturates

Barbiturates are derivatives of barbituric acid, which is formed by a condensation reaction (i.e. water is also formed) between malonic acid and urea. Barbiturates are weak acids, but also have imino groups present (see Figure 8.3). Thio barbiturates have, as their name suggests, a thio ($=S$) substitution for the keto group ($=O$). The types of hydrocarbon groups on the 5-carbon determine the duration of pharmacological action. Oxybarbiturates undergo less hepatic metabolism than the corresponding thiobarbiturate.

Barbituric acid

Barbiturates:

	R_1	R_2	R_3
Long acting Phenobarbitone	O	$- CH_2 CH_3$	—⟨benzene ring⟩
Intermediate acting Pentobarbitone	O	$- CH_2 CH_3$	$- \overset{\displaystyle |}{\underset{\displaystyle CH_3}{CH}} CH_2 CH_2 CH_3$
Short acting Thiopentone	S	$- CH_2 CH_3$	$- \overset{\displaystyle |}{\underset{\displaystyle CH_3}{CH}} CH_2 CH_2 CH_3$

Benzodiazepines (BDZ)

Members of this group of heterocyclic compounds are interesting in that structurally they have both six- and seven-membered rings, and some also have a five-membered ring. Their C-containing ring structures make benzodiazepines poorly water-soluble and diazepam requires a special lipid emulsion preparation (diazemuls) to be used intravenously. However, by altering the hydrocarbon groups and pH, an alternative tautomeric form without a closed seven-membered ring can be formed. Thus midazolam is presented in the ampoule as a water-soluble drug, but when it reaches the plasma it returns to the more lipid-soluble ring form (Figure 17.1). There are three groups of BDZs: 1,4 –benzodiazepines (diazepam, temazepam, lorazepam), heterocyclic benzodiazepines (midazolam) and 1,5-benzodiazepines (clobazam). Some of the 1,4-BDZs are metabolically related; diazepam is metabolized to oxazepam and temazepam.

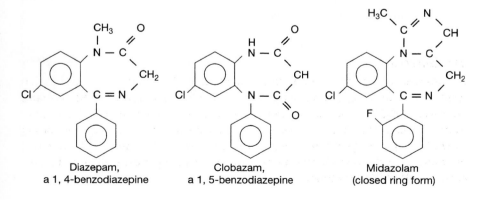

Diazepam,
a 1, 4-benzodiazepine

Clobazam,
a 1, 5-benzodiazepine

Midazolam
(closed ring form)

Non-depolarizing muscle relaxants

Bis-benzylisoquinoliniums

Bis-benzylisoquinoliniums is one of the two groups into which the non-depolarizing muscle relaxants can be divided, the other being the aminosteroids (see below). These are based on the structure of the naturally occurring drug tubocurarine. They are so named from their underlying structure of two (hence the bis-) isoquinolinium structures, linked through a carbon chain containing two ester linkages. The isoquinolinium structure is related to papaverine, which is a smooth muscle relaxant. Features of the moleculecular structure of atracurium are the distance between quaternary nitrogens (approximately 1 nm), the heterocyclic, bulky ring structures and the reverse orientation of the ester linkages that favours Hofmann degradation. In mivacurium the ester linkages are oriented the opposite way, which does not allow Hofmann degradation to occur. The nitrogen atom in each isoquinolinium group is quaternary, so the molecules are permanently charged and are presented as a salt. Multiple isomers exist, with differing activity (see Chapter 5).

Aminosteroids

The steroid nucleus is a complex polycyclic hydrocarbon structure. It is important to recognize that many hormones have this basic structure as well as many drugs. It has been popular as a drug skeleton because it is relatively inflexible. The aminosteroid non-depolarizing muscle relaxants are steroids, as is the intravenous agent althesin and the corticosteroid hormones. It is worth recognizing the numbering of the carbon atoms, since this will help identify metabolites and substitutions especially for muscle relaxants. Importantly, the steroid nucleus is not readily water-soluble; this requires hydrophilic substitution. In the aminosteroid family, not all are readily water-soluble and vecuronium has to be presented as a lyophilized preparation to ensure its stability (rapid freezing and dehydration of the frozen product under a high vacuum). Important features are the distance between nitrogen atoms, the acetyl groups ester linked to the 3 and 17 positions and the bis-quaternary structure of pancuronium but the monoquaternary structure of vecuronium and rocuronium with the N- in the 2 position protonated at pH 7.4.

Atracurium

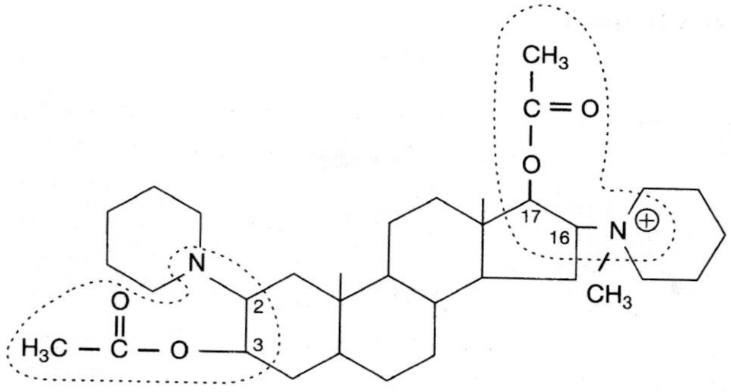

Vecuronium
The two acetylcholine-like moieties are outlined (dotted lines); loss of the
3- or 17-acetyl groups reduces potency.

Opioids

The parent compound is morphine, which has a complex ring structure. The important features include the phenolic hydroxyl (−OH) group in the 3 position, which is different from the cyclohexanol −OH group in the 6 position. The former is essential for activity in morphine-like opioids, but the latter is not; the 6-glucuronide metabolite of morphine is active, the 3- glucuronide is not. Modifications include acetylation at both the 3 and 6 positions to the pro-drug diamorphine; this increases lipid solubility and reduces onset time as only de-acetylation at the 3 position is essential for activity. Codeine is methylated through the 3 hydroxyl group increasing lipid solubility but reducing activity. The 6-keto derivatives are more active. The second important feature is the amine group, which is also necessary for receptor binding. Substitutions here can result in antagonists, such as naloxone. Not all rings are necessary for activity, with the phenolic ring being most important. Loss of various rings results in drugs such as fentanyl and its derivatives.

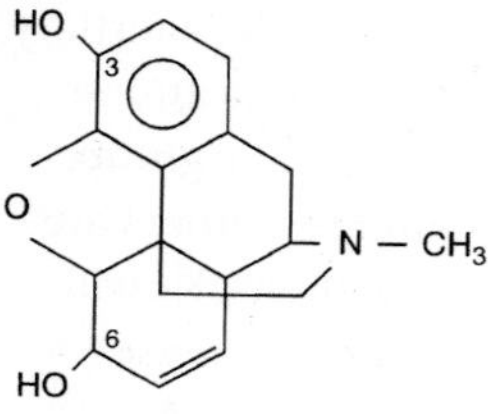

Morphine

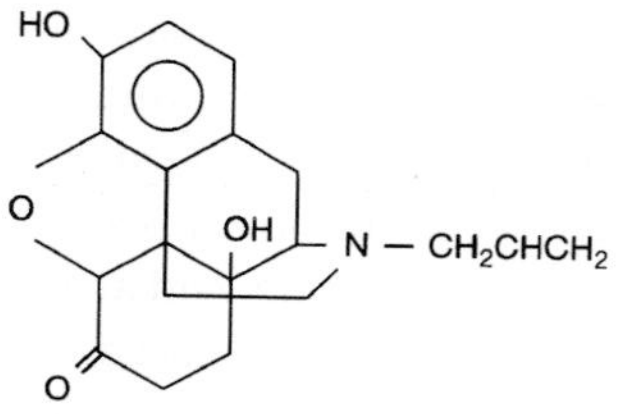

Naloxone

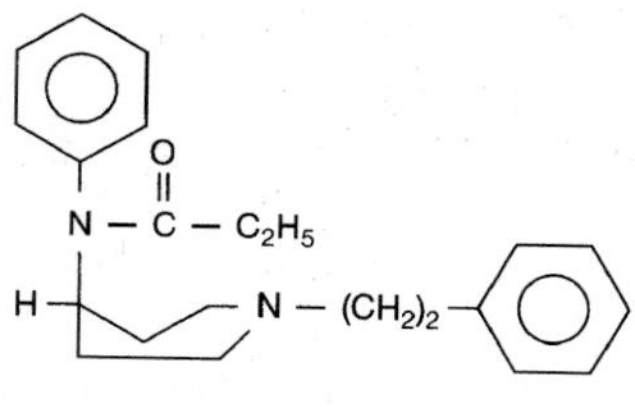

Fentanyl

Medicinal chemistry mini-dictionary

The following is not meant to be an exhaustive list of every possible chemical group or underlying drug structure. However, it covers terms encountered most commonly. It is designed as a quick reference to features of drug molecules.

Acetyl: Acetyl group CH_3COO-R (where R is a C-based group), acetic acid (= ethanoic acid) is CH_3COOH. A proton (H^+) donor group therefore acidic and hydrophilic. Aspirin is *acetyl*salicylic acid and some NSAIDs are phenyl*acetic acid* derivatives (e.g. diclofenac, ketoralac and indomethacin); present in the neurotransmitter *acetyl* choline.

$$H_2C - \overset{\overset{\displaystyle O}{\|}}{C} - O - CH_2 - CH_2 - \overset{\oplus}{N} (CH_3)_3$$

| Acetyl | Acetylcholine |

Alkane: A compound containing just carbon and hydrogen atoms (a hydrocarbon) forming a chain of carbon atoms with fully saturated bonds. The *normal* alkanes are unbranched and form a series starting with methane (CH_4), ethane (CH_3CH_3), propane ($CH_3CH_2CH_3$), and butane ($CH_3CH_2CH_2CH_3$). Lipid-soluble, short-chain alkanes are miscible with water.

Alkanol: Alkanes with one or more −OH substitutions. If one such substitution occurs on a terminal C, then this is an n-alkanol (or normal alkanol). If the substitution occurs on an inner C then this is an iso-alkanol. Presence of an −OH increases water solubility.

Alkyl: Indicates the presence of an alkane group. Naming depends on length of chain: 1 = methyl; 2 = ethyl; 3 = propyl; 4 = butyl; 5 = pentyl; 6 = hexyl; 7 = heptyl; 8 = octyl; 9 = nonyl; 10 = decyl; 11 = undecyl; 12 = duodecy. The longer the chain, the less water-soluble and more lipid-soluble. Compare the butyl- (bupivacaine) and propyl- (ropivacaine) substitutions in the mepivacaine local anaesthetic series.

Amide: This has an R-CO · NH_2 conformation. It is found in the chain linking the xylidine ring with the substituted amine in amide local anaesthetics (eg. lidocaine).

Amine: A primary amine group is R–NH_2. A secondary amine is R-NH-R′, a tertiary amine has all three H groups replaced. A monoamine contains just one amine group in its structure. Each amino acid has one terminal with an amine group, the other with a carboxyl group; some amino acids are monoamines, others are diamines. Amine groups are proton acceptors and at a pH above their pKa will become protonated and therefore carry a (+) charge. This can then increase water solubility. Conversely, below their pKa they are more lipid soluble. A quaternary nitrogen (sometimes misnamed a quaternary amine) is one where the N has four bonds and so is permanently charged. The non-depolarizing muscle relaxants have quaternary nitrogens (e.g. vecuronium, atracurium).

Benzyl: This group has an unsaturated (i.e. contains some double $C = C$ bonds) 6-carbon ring structure; benzene has the formula C_6H_6. It has a planar ring structure and is a solvent for lipids but is not water-soluble. It is a common group in drug molecules, for example, etomidate, and often substituted with a halogen as in ketamine (chlorine) and some benzodiazepines (chlorine).

Carbamyl: The group $-CONH_2$. The dimethyl derivative of this group is present and ester-linked in some of the anticholinesterase inhibitors, such as neostigmine (hence a carbamate ester). As a result of enzyme interaction the enzyme becomes carbamylated instead of acetylated with slower recovery of the esteratic site.

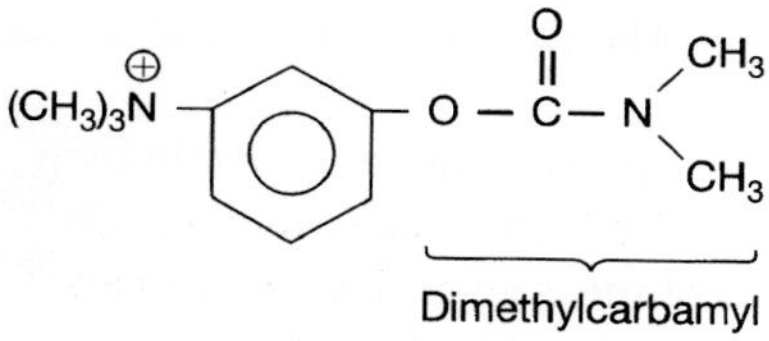

Dimethylcarbamyl

Neostigmine

Carboxylic acid: Generic term for acids derived from alkanols. The first two members of the series have special names: formic acid and acetic acid from methanol and ethanol. The others are named according to the alkanol, for example, propionic acid from n-propanol. Acids, therefore proton donors and water soluble.

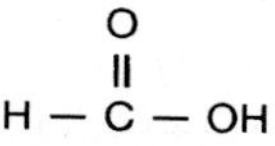

Formic acid 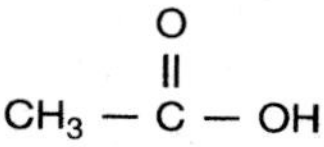   Acetic acid 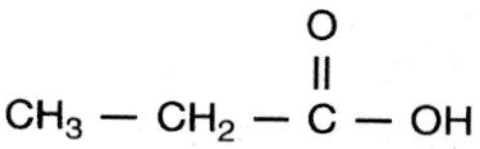   Propionic acid

Catechol: 1,2-hydroxybenzene. Both $-OH$ groups are required before a compound can be metabolized by COMT (catechol O-methyltransferase) when the $-OH$ group is methylated to $-OCH_3$. In noradrenaline, the main substituent on the benzyl ring is the ethylamine group, which is therefore numbered 1, so the two $-OH$ groups are renumbered as 3 and 4.

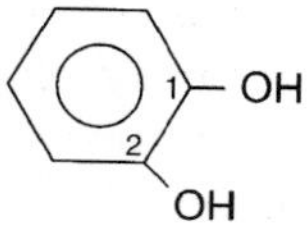

Catechol 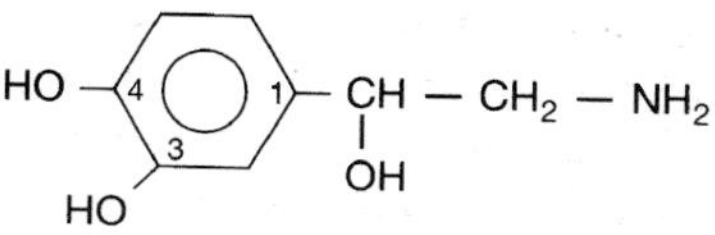   Noradrenaline

Choline: $CH_3N(CH_3)_3$, a precursor in acetylcholine synthesis.

Cyclohexanol: A cyclic alkanol with formula $C_6H_{11}OH$. It has very different properties from phenol the cyclic alcohol with a benzene ring structure. Tramadol is based on cyclohexanol.

Enol: The enol form in organic cyclic molecules is an −OH (hydroxyl) group adjacent to a C-C double bond, so allowing for tautomeric interconversion to the keto form =O with a single C-C bond. Seen in barbiturates.

Ester: A link formed by the interaction of a carboxylic acid with an alcohol, resulting in an ester and water, R–O–CO–R'. It is susceptible to hydrolysis, either by plasma or hepatic esterases. Many examples: aspirin, remifentanil, esmolol, mivacurium.

Ether: A link between two carbon-containing groups, R-O-R'. Important in structure of currently available volatile agents, all but halothane are ethers. Halothane is a halogen-substituted ethane (see **Alkane**). Not water-soluble, but lipid-soluble.

Glucuronide: A polar glucose group added during phase II hepatic metabolism, often through a hydroxy group (–OH). For example, benzodiazepines are glucuronidated after phase I metabolism, morphine is glucuronidated to an active (−6) and inactive (−3) glucuronide, propofol and its quinol derivative are also glucuronidated.

Glucuronidation of propofol

Halogen: A member of group VII of the periodic table. Includes fluorine, chlorine and bromine. Halogens are important substitutions on lead compounds in development of volatile anaesthetics. Fluorine is the most electronegative element and stabilizes the ethers, reducing the likelihood of metabolism.

Heterocyclic: A ring structure with at least one member of the ring *not* carbon.

Imidazole: Heterocyclic ring containing two N atoms and three C atoms. Part of the structures of etomidate, enoximone and phentolamine. These are weak bases, proton acceptors, so that pH will determine degree of ionization and hence water-solubility.

Imidazole (1,3 diazole)

Isoquinoline: A heterocyclic ring system, part of bis-benzylisoquinolinium structure of certain non-depolarizing blockers and found in papaverine.

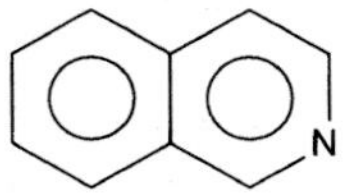

Isoquinoline

Keto: A keto group is the equivalent of an aldehyde group ($=O$) but in a ring structure. Under certain circumstances it exists in equilibrium with its enol form.

Laudanosine: One of the products of atracurium and cis-atracurium breakdown by Hofmann degradation. It is neurotoxic in certain non-primate species. The other product is an acrylate (CH_2CH-R).

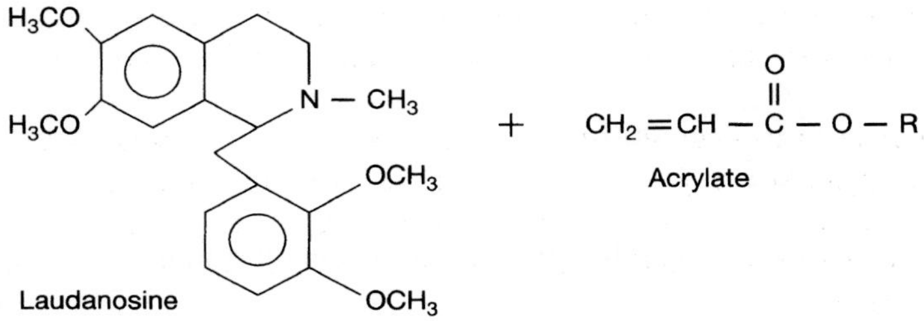

Laudanosine

Acrylate

Mandelic acid: Derivatives of mandelic acid are formed as a result of adrenaline and noradrenaline metabolism by MAO and COMT, e.g. 3-methoxy-4-hydroxymandelic acid.

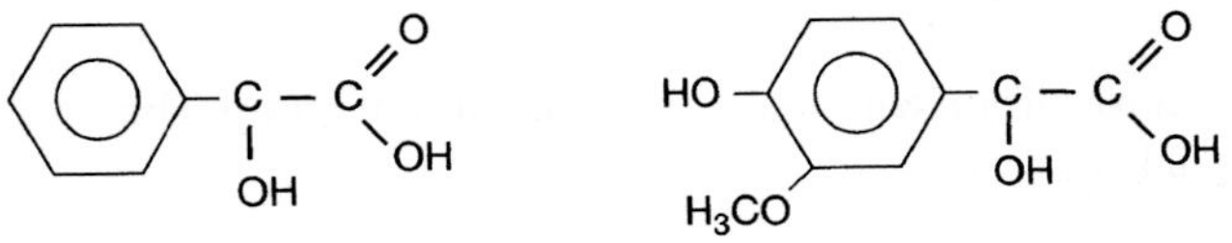

Mandelic acid   3-methoxy-4-hydroxy mandelic acid

Methoxy: $-OCH_3$ group, this has better lipid solubility than $-OH$. Codeine is 3-methoxymorphine. There are several methoxy- group substitutions in the benzylisoquinolinium non-depolarizing muscle relaxants which make them water-soluble.

Methyl: $-CH_3$ group (see **Alkyl**). Methylation and de-methylation are important routes of metabolism for many drugs, both in the liver and in other tissues. Nor-adrenaline is methylated to adrenaline in adrenal medullary cells whereas diazepam is de-methylated to nordiazepam and ketamine de-methylated to norketamine in the liver. Note that the prefix nor- and the prefix desmethyl- can both imply the removal of a methyl group from a parent structure.

Oxicam: Piroxicam and meloxicam are two examples of the NSAIDs with this underlying structure.

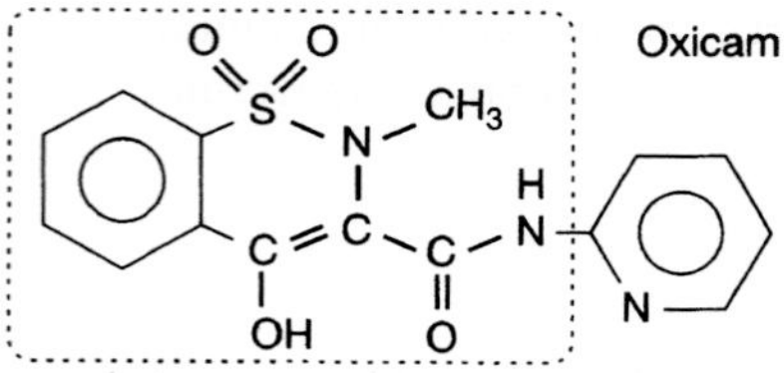

Oxicam

Piroxicam

Papaverine: Heterocyclic ring structure related to opioids and found with morphine in opium. Two papaverine-like ring structures are found in bis-benzylisoquiniliniums. Papaverine is a smooth muscle relaxant.

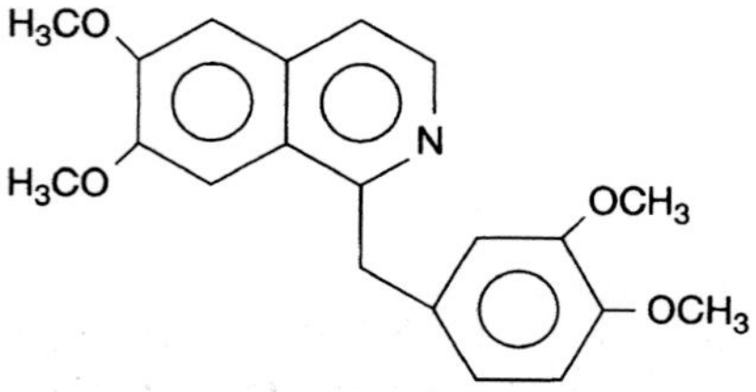

Papaverine

Phenanthrene: A polycyclic carbon ring structure related to morphine.

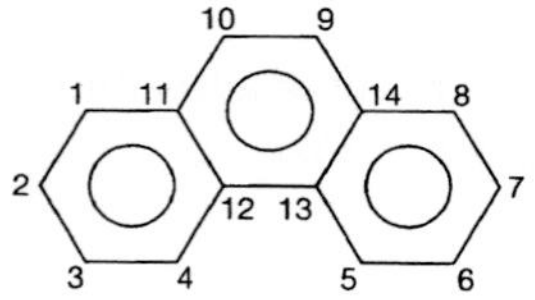

Phencyclidine: A cyclic hexacarbon with a phenolic substituent group. The underlying structure of ketamine.

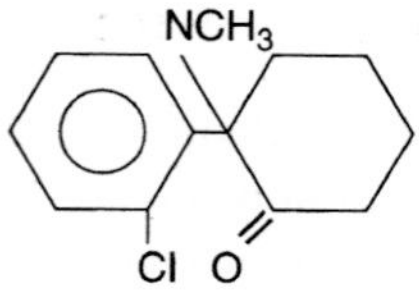

Ketamine

Phenyl: Phenol is hydroxylated benzene, C_6H_5OH. A phenyl group is $-C_6H_4OH$. Commonly part of drug structures, for example, paracetamol, propofol and edrophonium, and as a substituent, for example, in phentolamine and fentanyl. Phenol is water-soluble.

Piperazine: Heterocyclic ring containing two N atoms and 4 C atoms, $C_4H_{10}N_2$. The N atoms are in opposition, that is, in the 1 and 4 positions. The –NH- groups are bases, proton acceptors, so that pH and pKa will determine degree of ionization and hence water solubility.

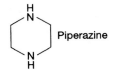

Piperazine

Piperidine: Heterocyclic ring containing one N atom and 5 C atoms, $C_5H_{11}N$. The NH group is a proton acceptor; pH and pKa determine degree of ionization. Piperidine rings are found in many drugs including fentanyl, alfentanil, remifentanil, bupivacaine and ropivacaine.

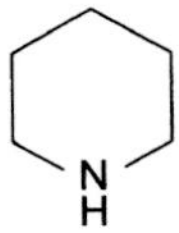

Piperidine

Propionic acid: Another of the chemical groups upon which NSAIDs are based, the underlying structure is the carboxylic acid of propanol, for example, ibuprofen.

Pyrazalones: Keto-modified pyrazole ring on which phenylbutazone and related NSAIDs are based.

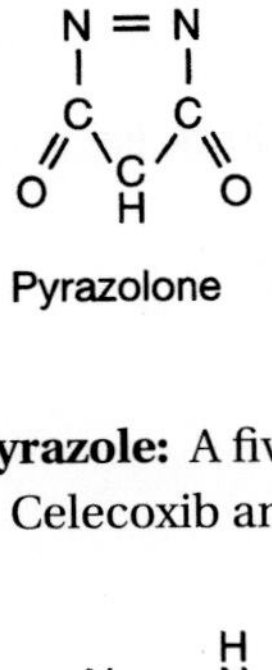

Pyrazolone

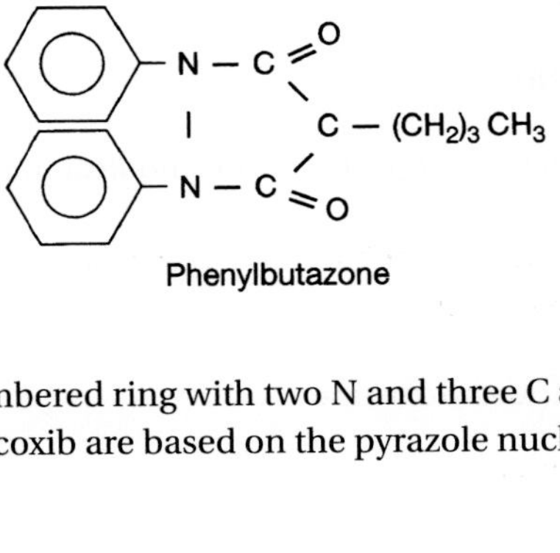

Phenylbutazone

Pyrazole: A five-membered ring with two N and three C atoms, $C_3H_3 \cdot N \cdot NH$. Celecoxib and rofecoxib are based on the pyrazole nucleus.

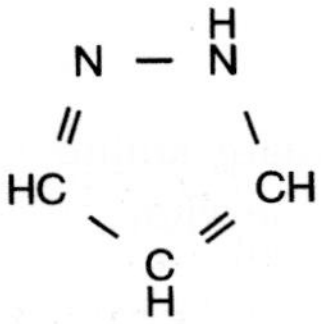

Pyrazole

Quinol: 1,4-dihydroxybenzene, also known as hydroquinone. One metabolite of propofol is the 4-glucuronide of 2,6-diisopropylquinol. The quinols are responsible for the green colour of urine in patients receiving propofol infusions.

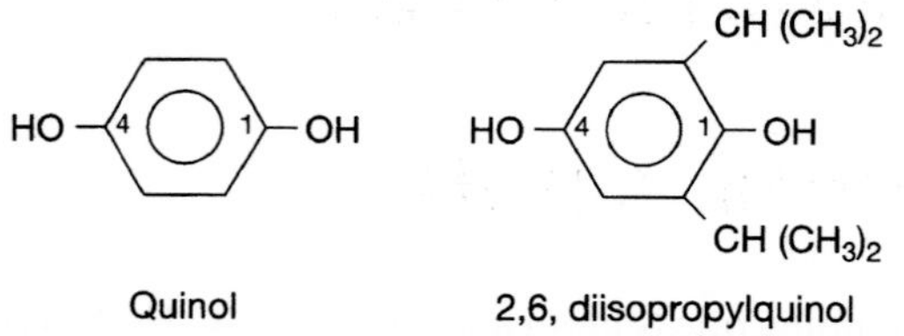

Quinol   2,6, diisopropylquinol

Salicylate: Aspirin is acetyl saliciylate and is metabolized to salicylic acid.

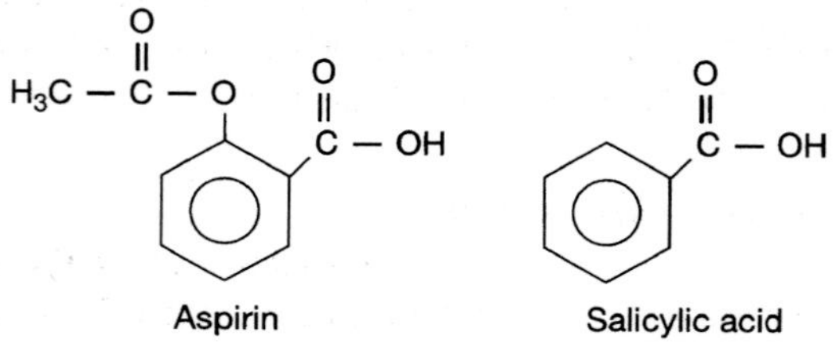

Aspirin   Salicylic acid

Thiazide: Sulphur containing heterocyclic ring, the structure of thiazide diuretics.

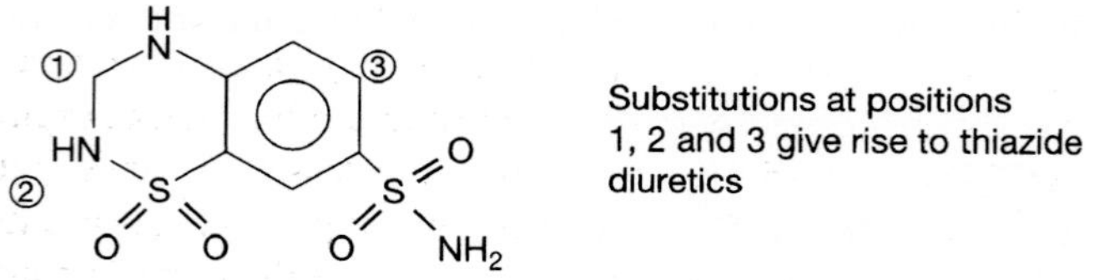

Substitutions at positions
1, 2 and 3 give rise to thiazide
diuretics

Xanthene: Methylxanthenes are important phosphodiesterase inhibitors, e.g. aminophylline.

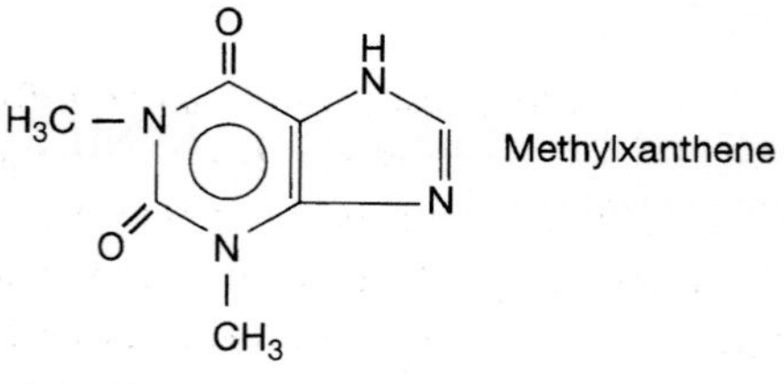

Methylxanthene

Xylidine: 2,6 bismethylaminobenzene. Xylides are metabolites of many amide anaesthetics. Lidocaine is metabolized to MEGX, monoethylglycinexylide.

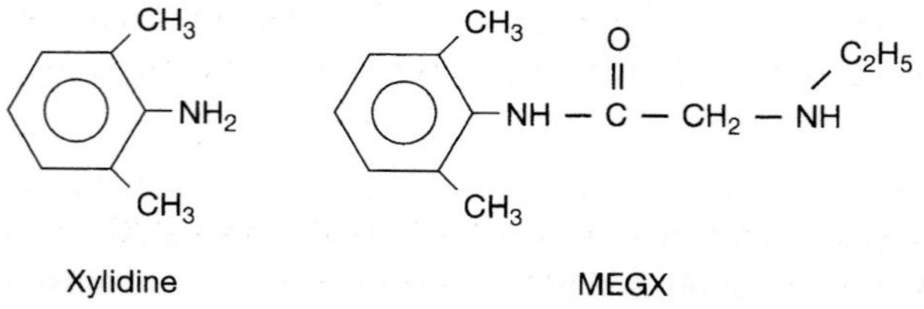

Xylidine   MEGX

General anaesthetic agents

Our understanding of the mechanisms involved in the action of general anaesthetics has increased considerably in recent times and is discussed below. This is followed by sections discussing intravenous and inhaled anaesthetic agents.

Mechanisms of general anaesthetic action

Any mechanism of general anaesthetic action must be able to explain: loss of conscious awareness, loss of response to noxious stimuli (anti-nociceptive effect) and perhaps most important of all, reversibility.

Anatomical sites of action

General anaesthetic agents affect both brain and spinal cord to account for physiological responses to nociception, loss of consciousness and inhibition of explicit memory. Auditory and sensory evoked potential data implicate the thalamus as the most likely primary target, but secondary sites such as the limbic system (associated with memory) and certain cortical areas are also important. Halogenated volatile anaesthetics appear to have a greater influence on spinal cord than do the intravenous agents.

Molecular theories

At the beginning of the 19th century, Overton and Meyer independently described the linear correlation between the lipid solubility of anaesthetic agents and their potency (Figure 8.1). This correlation was so impressive, given the great variation in structure of these agents, that it suggested a non-specific mechanism of action based on this physicochemical property. Later interpretation pointed out that any highly lipophilic area was a potential site of action, with cell membranes being the most likely contender given the high concentration of lipids. There are problems with a unified theory based on lipid interactions: some general anaesthetics, such as ketamine, are extreme outliers, and the stereoisomers R-etomidate and S-etomidate have identical lipid solubility but only R-etomidate has anaesthetic properties.

Membrane lipids

There are several potential lipophilic sites in cell membranes, including the lipid bilayer itself and the annular lipids surrounding ionic channels.

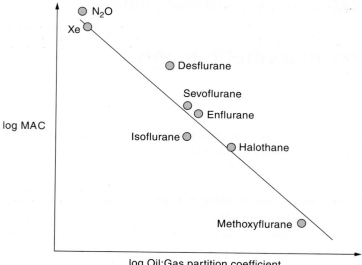

Figure 8.1. Straight line relationship between MAC and an index of lipid solubility (note: logarithmic scales).

Initially it was suggested that anaesthetic agents could penetrate the bilayer and alter the molecular arrangement of the phospholipids, which led to expansion of the membrane and disruption of the function of membrane-spanning ionic channels. Calculations identifying the volume of anaesthetic agent required to expand membranes led to a "critical volume hypothesis". Against such a theory, a 1°C rise in temperature increases membrane thickness to a similar extent as that seen with volatile agents, yet increased temperature does not enhance anaesthesia – the opposite is true.

A further theory suggested anaesthetic agents act at specific lipid site(s). The composition of phospholipids in the immediate vicinity of ion channels is different from that of the general lipid bilayer. This proposed disruption of annular lipids associated with specific ion-channels led to the perturbation theory.

A rapid advance in receptor protein identification within the central nervous system has led to newer theories based on interactions with specific proteins. It now seems likely that the correlation between potency and lipid solubility reflects the lipophilic nature of specific protein-based binding site(s).

Protein site(s) of action

Ligand-gated ionic channels are more sensitive to the action of general anaesthetics than are voltage-gated channels. The interaction at inhibitory (GABA$_A$ and glycine) and excitatory (neuronal nicotinic and NMDA) channels have all been studied. Table 8.1 summarizes the relative activity of a number of agents at these receptors.

100

Table 8.1. General anaesthetic effects at central receptors.

	Inhibitory Neurotransmitters		Excitatory Neurotransmitters	
	GABA$_A$	Glycine	NMDA	Neuronal nACh
propofol	++++	++	0	−
thiopental	+++++	++	0	−
R-etomidate	+++++	0	0	0
S-etomidate	0	0	0	0
Ketamine	0	0	−	0
Isoflurane	++++	+++	0	−
Nitrous Oxide	0	0	−	0
Xenon	0	0	−	0

+: enhances effect of neurotransmitter; −: reduces effect of neurotransmitter; 0: no effect on neuro-transmitter. nACh: central nicotinic acetylcholine receptor.

GABA$_A$ receptor

The GABA$_A$ receptor, like the nicotinic acetylcholine receptor, belongs to the pentameric family of ligand-gated ion-channel receptors. It has binding sites for GABA associated with α subunits and modulatory sites at the α/γ interface for benzodiazepines and on the β subunit for etomidate, barbiturates, propofol and volatile agents (Figure 8.2). The stereospecificity of the action of etomidate, presented as an

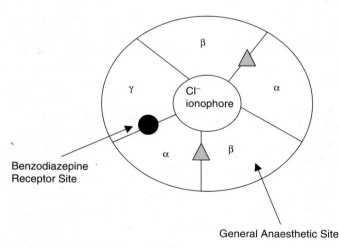

Figure 8.2. The GABA$_A$ receptor.
The GABA$_A$ Receptor Complex, from above. The grey triangles show the two agonist sites for gamma amino butyric acid (GABA). Diazepam, temazepam and midazolam are agonists and flumazenil is an antagonist at the benzodiazepine site. Propofol, etomidate, barbiturates and halogenated volatile agents are agonists at the general anaesthetic site. Both sites produce positive allosteric modulation.

enantiopure preparation of the R(+) isomer, supports the protein-based action of anaesthetics. The S(−) form of etomidate is clinically inactive and at the $GABA_A$ receptor there is a 30-fold difference in activity.

Anaesthetics increase channel opening time, so allowing for increased chloride entry resulting in hyperpolarisation. The effect is seen for etomidate, propofol and barbiturates, as well as halogenated volatiles. Etomidate is selective for the $GABA_A$ receptor but propofol will also increase glycine channel opening time and is inhibitory at neuronal nicotinic and $5HT_3$ receptors. The site(s) on the $GABA_A$ receptor associated with anaesthetic action are associated with the β subunit and are distinct from the benzodiazepine receptor site. There are at least 30 types of $GABA_A$ receptor, each with different subunit composition; β_2 and β_3 subunits are more sensitive to the effects of etomidate than is the β_1 subunit.

Glycine receptor

The major inhibitory transmitter in the spinal cord and brainstem is glycine, which is associated with a chloride channel similar to the $GABA_A$ receptor. The volatile anaesthetics all markedly potentiate the action of glycine, although there is no evidence of stereoselectivity. It has been suggested that the spinal cord is an important site of action for volatile rather than intravenous anaesthetic agents. Efficacy here correlates more with immobility than awareness.

NMDA receptor

Neuronal signalling may also be reduced by inhibition of excitatory pathways. The NMDA receptor is involved in long-term signal potentiation associated with learning and memory; it is activated by glutamate, modulated by magnesium and inhibited in a non-competitive manner by ketamine, nitrous oxide and xenon. This glutamate-mediated mechanism represents an additional pathway for anaesthesia. Other anaesthetic agents, such as barbiturates, can reduce the effectiveness of glutamate but at a lower potency than for inhibition of $GABA_A$ receptor function.

Intravenous anaesthetic agents

Intravenous anaesthetics have been defined as agents that will induce loss of consciousness in one arm–brain circulation time.

The introduction of barbiturates in the 1930s was a significant advance in anaesthesia. Their rapid onset and relatively short duration of action made them different from previously used agents. Hexobarbitone was introduced first, followed by thiopental and subsequently methohexitone. Phencyclidine (angel dust) was withdrawn due to serious psychotomimetic reactions, but the chemically related compound ketamine is still used. The imidazole ester, etomidate, is useful due to its cardiovascular stability but side-effects limit its use. The phenolic derivative propofol has become the most popular agent in recent years due to its ready-to-use formulation, favourable recovery profile and use in target-controlled anaesthesia. Steroidal compounds have also been used, however poor solubility (pregnalolone) together with an association with anaphylactic reactions (due to cremophor EL – used to solubalize the steroid althesin) has led to their demise.

The ideal intravenous anaesthetic agent

Were an ideal intravenous anaesthetic agent to exist, it should have the following properties:

- Rapid onset (mainly unionized at physiological pH)
- High lipid solubility
- Rapid recovery, no accumulation during prolonged infusion
- Analgesic at sub-anaesthetic concentrations
- Minimal cardiovascular and respiratory depression
- No emetic effects
- No pain on injection
- No excitation or emergence phenomena
- No interaction with other agents
- Safe following inadvertent intra-arterial injection
- No toxic effects
- No histamine release
- No hypersensitivity reactions
- Water-soluble formulation
- Long shelf-life at room temperature

The currently used agents are discussed below under the following headings:
- **Barbiturates (thiopental, methohexitone)**
- **Non-barbiturates (propofol, ketamine, etomidate)**

Barbiturates

All barbiturates are derived from barbituric acid, which is the condensation product of urea and malonic acid (Figure 8.3). When oxygen is exchanged for sulphur at the C2 position, oxybarbiturates become thiobarbiturates.

Barbiturates are not readily soluble in water at neutral pH. Their solubility depends on transformation from the keto to the enol form (tautomerism), which occurs most

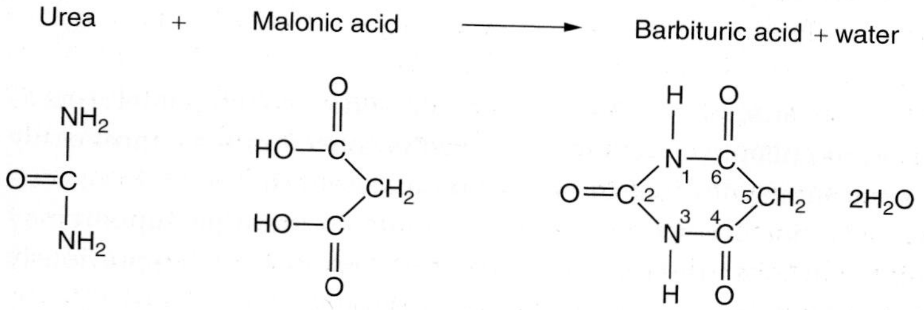

Figure 8.3. Formation of barbituric acid.

Table 8.2. Lipid solubility and protein binding of a few barbiturates.

	Type	Lipid solubility	Protein binding (%)
Thiopental	Thio	+++++	80
Pentobarbitone	Oxy	+++	40
Phenobarbitone	Oxy	+	10

readily in alkaline solutions (Figure 8.4). In general, thiobarbiturates are very lipid-soluble, highly protein bound and completely metabolized in the liver. In contrast, the oxybarbiturates are less lipid-soluble, less protein bound, and some are excreted almost entirely unchanged in the urine (Table 8.2).

Thiopental
Thiopental is the sulphur analogue of the oxybarbiturate pentobarbitone.

Presentation
Thiopental is formulated as the sodium salt and presented as a pale yellow powder. The vial contains sodium carbonate (Na_2CO_3, 6% by weight) and nitrogen in place of air. These two measures are designed to improve solubility of the solution by the following mechanisms:

1. Sodium carbonate reacts with water in the following manner

$$Na_2CO_3 + H_2O \rightarrow NaHCO_3 + Na^+ + OH^-$$

   The result is a strongly alkaline solution (pH 10.5) favouring the water-soluble enol form which is more desirable as a preparation.
2. Air contains small amounts of carbon dioxide. Were this to be present and react with water it would tend to release bicarbonate and hydrogen ions which in turn would result in a less alkaline solution. As a result thiopental would be in a less favourable solution in terms of water solubility. Nitrogen is used in place of air to prevent this occuring.

The 2.5% solution is stable for many days and should be bacteriostatic due to its alkaline pH.

Uses
Apart from induction of anaesthesia (3–7 mg.kg^{-1} intravenously) thiopental is occasionally used in status epilepticus. At sufficient plasma concentrations (most easily maintained by continuous infusion) thiopental produces an isoelectric EEG, confirming maximal reduction of cerebral oxygen requirements. Inotropic support may be required to maintain adequate cerebral perfusion at these doses. It has previously been used rectally, although it has a slow onset via this route.

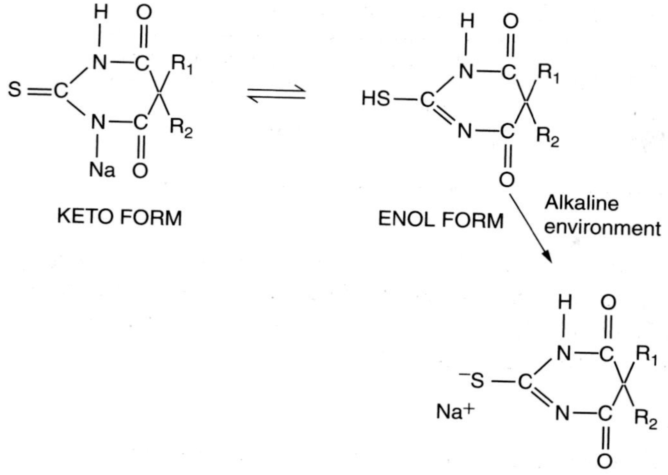

Figure 8.4. Keto-enol transformation of barbiturates – tautomerism. Alkaline solutions favour the water-soluble enol form.

Effects

- Cardiovascular – there is a dose-dependent reduction in cardiac output, stroke volume and systemic vascular resistance that may provoke a compensatory tachycardia. These effects are more common in patients that are hypovolaemic, acidotic and have reduced protein binding.
- Respiratory – respiratory depression is dose-dependent. It may produce a degree of laryngospasm and bronchospasm.
- Central nervous system – a single dose will rapidly induce general anaesthesia with a duration of about 5 to 10 minutes. There is a reduction in cerebral oxygen consumption, blood flow, blood volume and cerebrospinal fluid pressure. When used in very low doses it is antanalgesic.
- Renal – urine output may fall not only as a result of increased anti-diuretic hormone release secondary to central nervous system depression, but also as a result of a reduced cardiac output.
- Severe anaphylactic reactions – these are seen in approximately 1 in 20 000 administrations of thiopental.
- Porphyria – it may precipitate an acute porphyric crisis and is therefore absolutely contraindicated in patients with porphyria. The following drugs may also precipitate an acute porphyric crisis:
  - Other barbiturates
  - Etomidate
  - Enflurane

- Halothane
- Cocaine
- Lidocaine and prilocaine (bupivacaine safe)
- Clonidine
- Metoclopramide
- Hyoscine
- Diclofenac
- Ranitidine

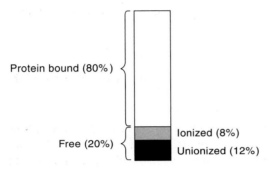

Protein bound (80%)

Free (20%)

Ionized (8%)

Unionized (12%)

Figure 8.5. Thiopental in plasma. Only 12% is immediately available as non-protein bound and unionized drug.

Kinetics

Thiopental has a pKa of 7.6, so that 60% is unionized at pH 7.4. However, as only 20% of administered thiopental is unbound, only 12% is *immediately* available in the unbound and unionized form (Figure 8.5). Its pKa of 7.6 means that 60% of free drug is unionized. Despite this it has a rapid onset due to its high lipid solubility and the large cardiac output that the brain receives. In addition, a dynamic equilibrium exists between protein bound and free drug. Critically ill patients tend to be acidotic and have reduced plasma protein-binding, resulting in a greater fraction of drug in the unionized form and fewer plasma protein-binding sites, so that significantly less thiopental is required to induce anaesthesia. Non-steroidal anti-inflammatory drugs may also reduce available protein-binding sites and increase the fraction of free drug.

Rapid emergence from a single bolus dose is due to rapid initial distribution into tissues, not metabolism. A tri-exponential decline is seen representing distribution to well-perfused regions (brain, liver) followed by muscle and skin. The final decline is due to hepatic oxidation mainly to inactive metabolites (although pentobarbitone is also a metabolite). When given as an infusion its metabolism may become linear (zero-order, cf. p. 78) due to saturation of hepatic enzymes. The hepatic mixed-function oxidase system (cytochrome P450) is induced after a single dose.

Intra-arterial injection

As 2.5% thiopental at pH 10.5 is injected into arterial blood with a pH of 7.4 the tautomeric equilibrium swings away from the enol towards the keto form resulting in a less water-soluble solution. This in turn leads to the precipitation of thiopental crystals which become wedged into small blood vessels leading to ischaemia and pain. Thiopental does not precipitate when injected intravenously as it is continually diluted by more venous blood. Treatment should begin immediately and may include intra-arterial injection of papaverine or procaine, analgesia, sympathetic block of the limb and anticoagulation.

Peri-vascular injection is painful and may cause serious tissue necrosis if large doses extravasate.

Methohexitone

Methohexitone is a methylated oxybarbiturate and is no longer available in the UK.

Presentation

Methohexitone was produced as the sodium salt with sodium carbonate (6% by weight) which was readily soluble in water forming an alkaline solution (pH 11.0). It had a pKa = 7.9 so that 75% of unbound drug was unionized at pH 7.4. However, 60% of an administered dose was protein bound. There are four optically active isomers but the preparation used clinically was a racemic mixture of α-D and α-L methohexitone.

Uses

Methohexitone was used as a 1% solution at 1–2 mg.kg^{-1} for the induction of anaesthesia where excitatory phenomena were of little concern (notably for electroconvulsive therapy).

Effects

Methohexitone has a similar pharmacological profile to thiopental, producing rapid loss of consciousness, rapid emergence due to distribution and exerts similar effects on the cardiovascular and hepatic systems. It may also precipitate a porphyric crisis.

Differences from thiopental

Methohexitone sometimes caused an excitatory phase before loss of consciousness, with muscle twitching, increased tone and hiccup. It occasionally precipitated convulsions in those with a history of epilepsy and its use in this setting was controversial. Recovery was more rapid after methohexitone due to a higher hepatic clearance. When injected intra-arterially or subcutaneously there were fewer vascular complications and there was less tissue damage. This was probably due to the lower concentrations used. Methohexitone was associated with a greater incidence of hypersensitivity reactions although these did not appear to be as severe. Its main metabolite hydroxymethohexitone had only limited hypnotic activity (Table 8.3).

Non-barbiturates

Propofol

Presentation
This phenolic derivative (2,6 diisopropylphenol) is highly lipid-soluble and is presented as a 1% or 2% lipid–water emulsion (containing soya bean oil and purified egg phosphatide) due to poor solubility in water. It is a weak organic acid with a pKa = 11 so that it is almost entirely unionized at pH 7.4.

Uses
Propofol is used for the induction and maintenance of general anaesthesia and for sedation of ventilated patients in intensive care. The induction dose is 1–2 mg.kg^{-1} while a plasma concentration of 4–8 μg.ml^{-1} will maintain anaesthesia.

Effects
- Cardiovascular – the systemic vascular resistance falls resulting in a drop in blood pressure. A reflex tachycardia is rare and propofol is usually associated with a bradycardia especially if administered with fentanyl or alfentanil. Sympathetic activity and myocardial contractility are also reduced.
- Respiratory – respiratory depression leading to apnoea is common. It is rare to observe cough or laryngospasm following its use and so it is often used in anaesthesia for ease of placement of a laryngeal mask.
- Central nervous system – excitatory effects have been associated with propofol in up to 10% of patients. They probably do not represent true cortical seizure activity; rather they are the manifestation of subcortical excitatory–inhibitory centre imbalance. The movements observed are dystonic with choreiform elements and opisthotonos. Propofol has been used to control status epilepticus.
- Gut – some evidence exists to suggest that propofol possesses anti-emetic properties following its use for induction, maintenance or in subhypnotic doses postoperatively. Antagonism of the dopamine D$_2$ receptor is a possible mechanism.
- Pain – injection into small veins is painful but may be reduced if lidocaine is mixed with propofol or if a larger vein is used.
- Metabolic – a fat overload syndrome, with hyperlipidaemia, and fatty infiltration of heart, liver, kidneys and lungs can follow prolonged infusion.
- Miscellaneous – it may turn urine and hair green.

Table 8.3. Pharmacokinetics of some intravenous anaesthetics.

	Dose (mg.kg^{-1})	Volume of distribution (l.kg^{-1})	Clearance (ml.kg^{-1}.min^{-1})	Elimination half-life (h)	Protein binding (%)	Metabolites
Thiopental	3–7	2.5	3.5	6–15	80	active
Methohexitone	1.0–1.5	2.0	11	3–5	60	minimal activity
Propofol	1–2	4.0	30–60	5–12	98	inactive
Ketamine	1–2	3.0	17	2	25	active
Etomidate	0.3	3.0	10–20	1–4	75	inactive

Kinetics

Propofol is 98% protein bound to albumin and has the largest volume of distribution of all the induction agents at 4 l.kg^{-1}. Following bolus administration, its duration of action is short due to the rapid decrease in plasma levels as it is distributed to well-perfused tissues.

Metabolism is largely hepatic; about 40% undergoing conjugation to a glucuronide and 60% metabolized to a quinol, which is excreted as a glucuronide and sulphate, all of which are inactive and excreted in the urine. Its clearance exceeds hepatic blood flow suggesting some extra-hepatic metabolism. Owing to this high clearance, plasma levels fall more rapidly than those of thiopental following the initial distribution phase. Its terminal elimination half-life is 5–12 hours although it has been suggested that when sampling is performed for longer than 24 hours the figure approaches 60 hours and may reflect the slow release of propofol from fat. During prolonged infusion its context-sensitive half-time increases, although where the infusion has been titrated carefully, waking may still be relatively rapid.

Toxicity

Propofol has been associated with the unexpected deaths of a small number of children being ventilated for respiratory tract infection in intensive care. Progressive metabolic acidosis and unresponsive bradycardia lead to death. The serum was noted to be lipaemic. While further small studies failed to demonstrate a worse outcome when propofol was used as sedation for critically ill children, a more recent study showed a higher overall death rate and the Committee on Safety of Medicines (CSM) has advised that propofol should be contraindicated for sedation in intensive care units in children 16 years and younger.

Patients allergic to eggs are usually allergic to egg protein or albumin. The egg component of the propofol preparation is lecethin, which is a phosphatide, therefore it is unlikely that allergic reactions are due to these components of its preparation. Propofol does not appear to be allergenic in patients who are sensitive to soya beans because all protein within the soya bean oil is removed.

It does not appear to cause any adverse effects when given intra-arterially, although onset of anaesthesia is delayed.

Ketamine

Ketamine is a phencyclidine derivative.

Presentation and uses

Ketamine is presented as a racemic mixture or as the single S(+) enantiomer, which is 2 to 3 times as potent as the R(–) enantiomer. It is soluble in water forming an acidic solution (pH 3.5–5.5). Three concentrations are available: 10, 50 and

100 mg.ml^{-1}, and it may be given intravenously (1–2 mg.kg^{-1}) or intramuscularly (5–10 mg.kg^{-1}) for induction of anaesthesia. Intravenous doses of 0.2–0.5 mg.kg^{-1} may be used to provide analgesia during vaginal delivery and to facilitate the positioning of patients with fractures before regional anaesthetic techniques are performed. It has been used via the oral and rectal route for sedation and also by intrathecal and epidural routes for analgesia. However, its use has been limited by unpleasant side effects.

Effects

- Cardiovascular – ketamine is unlike other induction agents in that it produces sympathetic nervous system stimulation, increasing circulating levels of adrenaline and noradrenaline. Consequently heart rate, cardiac output, blood pressure and myocardial oxygen requirements are all increased. However, it does not appear to precipitate arrhythmias. This indirect stimulation masks the mild direct myocardial depressant effects that racemic ketamine would otherwise exert on the heart. S(+) ketamine produces less direct cardiac depression in vitro compared with R(−) ketamine. In addition while racemic ketamine has been shown to block ATP-sensitive potassium channels (the key mechanism of ischaemic myocardial preconditioning), S(+) ketamine does not, which therefore must be considered advantageous for patients with ischaemic heart disease.
- Respiratory – the respiratory rate may be increased and the laryngeal reflexes relatively preserved. A patent airway is often, but not always, maintained, and increased muscle tone associated with the jaw may precipitate airway obstruction. It causes bronchodilation and may be useful for patients with asthma.
- Central nervous system – it produces a state of dissociative anaesthesia that is demonstrated on EEG by dissociation between the thalamocortical and limbic systems. In addition, intense analgesia and amnesia are produced. The α rhythm is replaced by θ and δ wave activity. Ketamine is different from other intravenous anaesthetics as it does not induce anaesthesia in one arm–brain circulation time – central effects becoming evident 90 seconds after an intravenous dose. Vivid and unpleasant dreams, hallucinations and delirium may follow its use. These emergence phenomena may be reduced by the concurrent use of benzodiazepines or opioids. S(+) ketamine produces less intense although no less frequent emergence phenomena. They are less common in the young and elderly and also in those left to recover undisturbed. Cerebral blood flow, oxygen consumption and intracranial pressure are all increased. Muscle tone is increased and there may be jerking movements of the limbs.
- Gut – nausea and vomiting occur more frequently than after propofol or thiopental. Salivation is increased requiring anticholinergic premedication.

Kinetics

Following an intravenous dose the plasma concentration falls in a bi-exponential fashion. The initial fall is due to distribution across lipid membranes while the slower phase is due to hepatic metabolism. Ketamine is the least protein bound (about 25%) of the intravenous anaesthetics and is demethylated to the active metabolite norketamine by hepatic P450 enzymes. Norketamine (which is 30% as potent as ketamine) is further metabolized to inactive glucuronide metabolites. The conjugated metabolites are excreted in the urine.

Etomidate

Etomidate is an imidazole derivative and an ester. While it continues to be used infrequently in the UK it has been withdrawn in North America and Australia.

Presentation

Etomidate is prepared as a 0.2% solution at pH of 4.1 and contains 35% v/v propylene glycol to improve stability and reduce its irritant properties on injection. A lipid formulation is now also available.

Uses

Etomidate is used for the induction of general anaesthesia at a dose of 0.3 mg.kg^{-1}.

Effects

At first glance etomidate would appear to have some desirable properties, but due to its side effects its place in anaesthesia has remained limited.

- Cardiovascular – of the commonly used intravenous anaesthetics it produces the least cardiovascular disturbance. The peripheral vascular resistance may fall slightly (but less so than with other induction agents), while myocardial oxygen supply, contractility and blood pressure remain largely unchanged. Hypersensitivity reactions are less common following etomidate and histamine release is rare.
- Metabolic – it suppresses adrenocortical function by inhibition of the enzymes 11β-hydroxylase and 17α-hydroxylase, resulting in inhibition of cortisol and aldosterone synthesis. It was associated with an increase in mortality when used as an infusion to sedate septic patients in intensive care. Single doses can influence adrenocortical function but are probably of little clinical significance in otherwise fit patients. However it is it unlikely to be used to induce elective patients. In other words the situation in which it has the best cardiovascular profile is the unwell patient in whom the consequences of steroid inhibition are likely to be the most detrimental.

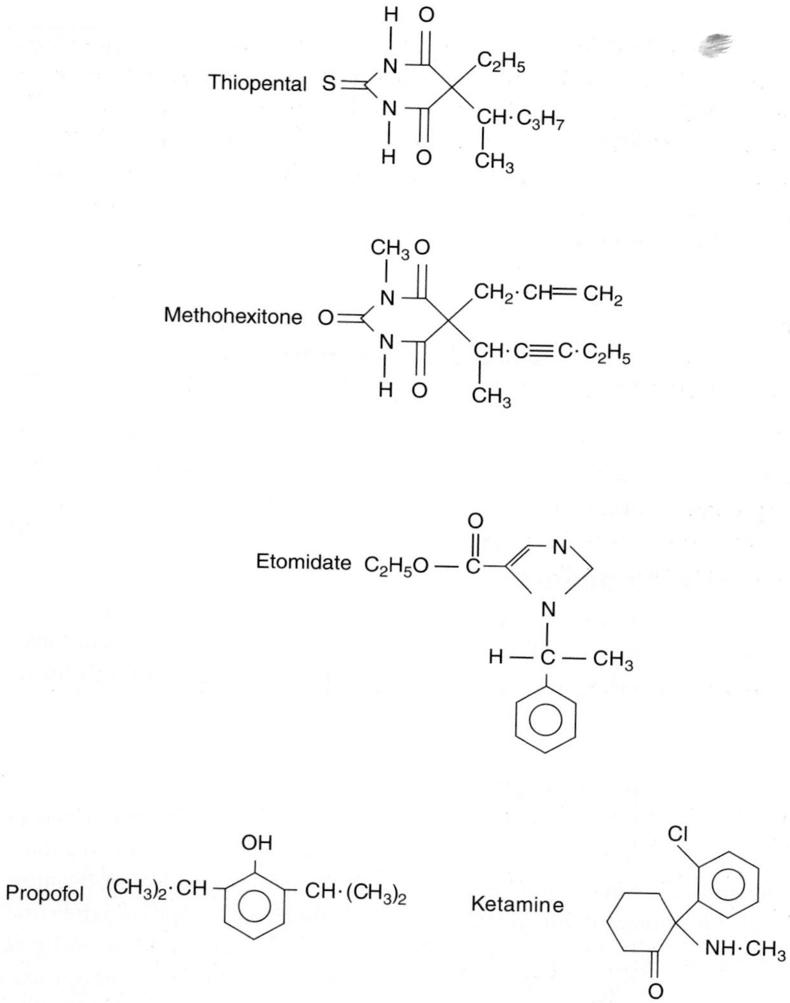

Figure 8.6. Chemical structure of some intravenous anaesthetics.

- Miscellaneous – unpleasant side effects relate to pain on injection in up to 25% of patients, excitatory movements and nausea and vomiting. It may also precipitate a porphyric crisis.

Kinetics

Etomidate is 75% bound to albumin. Its actions are terminated by rapid distribution into tissues, while its elimination from the body depends on hepatic metabolism and

Table 8.4. Pharmacological properties of some intravenous anaesthetics.

	Thiopental	Methohexitone	Propofol	Ketamine	Etomidate
BP	↓	↓	↓↓	↑	→
CO	↓	↓	↓↓	↑	→
HR	↑	↑	↓→	↑	→
SVR	↑↓	↑↓	↓↓	→	→
RR	↓	↓	↓	↑	↓
ICP	↓	↓	↓	↑	→
IOP	↓	↓	↓	↑	→
Pain on injection	no	yes	yes	no	yes
Nausea and vomiting	no	no	? reduced	yes	yes

renal excretion. Non-specific hepatic esterases and possibly plasma cholinesterase, hydrolyse etomidate to ethyl alcohol and its carboxylic acid metabolite. It may also inhibit plasma cholinesterase.

Inhaled anaesthetic agents

Inhaled anaesthetic agents in current use include nitrous oxide (N_2O) and the volatile liquids isoflurane, halothane, sevoflurane, desflurane and enflurane. Xenon has useful properties but is expensive to extract from the atmosphere, which currently limits its clinical use.

Minimum alveolar concentration

Minimum alveolar concentration (MAC) is a measure of potency and is defined as the minimum alveolar concentration at steady-state that prevents reaction to a standard surgical stimulus (skin incision) in 50% of subjects at one atmosphere. Because the majority of anaesthetics involving inhaled agents are given at approximately one atmosphere the indexing of MAC to atmosphereic pressure may be forgotten and lead the unwary to conclude that concentration is the key measure. However the key measure is the *partial pressure* of the agent. When measured using kPa the concentration and partial pressure are virtually the same as atmsopheric pressure approximates to 100 kPa.

MAC is altered by many physiological and pharmacological factors (Table 8.5) and is additive when agents are administered simultaneously.

The ideal inhaled anaesthetic agent

While the agents in use today demonstrate many favourable characteristics, no single agent has all the desirable properties listed below. 'Negative' characteristics (e.g. not epileptogenic) are simply a reflection of a currently used agent's side effect.

Table 8.5. Factors altering MAC.

Factors increasing MAC	Factors decreasing MAC
Infancy	During the neonatal period
	Increasing age
	Pregnancy
	Hypotension
Hyperthermia	Hypothermia
Hyperthyroidism	Hypothyroidism
Catecholamines and sympathomimetics	α_2-agonists
	Sedatives
Chronic opioid use	Acute opioid use
Chronic alcohol intake	Acute alcohol intake
Acute amphetamine intake	Chronic amphetamine intake
Hypernatraemia	Lithium

Physical
- Stable to light and heat
- Inert when in contact with metal, rubber and soda lime
- Preservative free
- Not flammable or explosive
- Pleasant odour
- Atmospherically friendly
- Cheap

Biochemical
- High oil:gas partition coefficient; low MAC
- Low blood:gas partition coefficient
- Not metabolized
- Non-toxic
- Only affects the CNS
- Not epileptogenic
- Some analgesic properties

Kinetics of inhaled anaesthetic agents

At steady-state, the partial pressure of inhaled anaesthetic within the alveoli (P_A) is in equilibrium with that in the arterial blood (P_a) and subsequently the brain (P_B). Therefore, P_A gives an indirect measure of P_B. However, for most inhaled anaesthetics steady-state is rarely achieved in the clinical setting as the process may take many hours (Figure 8.7).

Physiological and agent-specific factors influence the speed at which inhaled anaesthetics approach equilibrium.

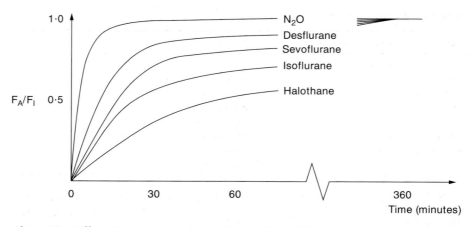

Figure 8.7. Different agents approach a F_A/F_I ratio of 1 at different rates. Agents with a low blood:gas partition coefficient reach equilibrium more rapidly. (F_A/F_I represents the ratio of alveolar concentration to inspired concentration.)

Alveolar ventilation

Increased alveolar ventilation results in a faster rise in P_A. Consequently, P_B increases more rapidly and so the onset of anaesthesia is faster. A large functional residual capacity (FRC) will effectively dilute the inspired concentration and so the onset of anaesthesia will be slow. Conversely, those patients with a small FRC have only a small volume with which to dilute the inspired gas and so P_A rises rapidly resulting in a fast onset of anaesthesia.

Inspired concentration

A high inspired concentration leads to a rapid rise in P_A and so onset of anaesthesia is also rapid.

Cardiac output

A high cardiac output will tend to maintain a concentration gradient between the alveolus and the pulmonary blood so that P_A rises slowly. Conversely, a low cardiac output favours a more rapid equilibration and so onset of anaesthesia will also be more rapid. However, modern anaesthetic agents, which are relatively insoluble in blood, are affected to a much lesser extent by cardiac output when compared with agents of greater blood solubility.

Blood:gas partition coefficient

The blood:gas partition coefficient is defined as the ratio of the amount of anaesthetic in blood and gas when the two phases are of equal volume and pressure and in equilibrium at 37°C.

Table 8.6. Metabolism of inhaled anaesthetic agents.

Agent	Percentage metabolized	Metabolites
N_2O	<0.01	(N_2)
Halothane	20	Trifluoroacetic acid, Cl^-, Br^-
Sevoflurane	3.5	Inorganic and organic fluorides
		Compound A in the presence of soda lime and heat (Compound B, C, D and E)
Enflurane	2	Inorganic and organic fluorides
Isoflurane	0.2	Trifluroacetic acid and F^-
Desflurane	0.02	Trifluroacetic acid

Although it might be expected that agents with a high blood:gas partition coefficient (i.e. high solubility) would have a rapid onset, this is not the case because these agents only exert a low partial pressure in blood, even when present in large amounts. It is the partial pressure of the agent in the blood and subsequently the brain that gives rise to anaesthesia and not the total amount present. Agents with a low blood:gas partition coefficient exert a high partial pressure and will, therefore, produce a more rapid onset and offset of action. Although a low blood:gas partition coefficient is important, MAC and respiratory irritability can also alter the speed of induction.

Concentration and second gas effect

These are described in the section on nitrous oxide.

Metabolism

Hepatic cytochrome P450 metabolizes the C-(halogen) bond to release halogen ions (F^-, Cl^- Br^-), which may cause hepatic or renal damage. The C–F bond is a stable one and is only minimally metabolized unlike C–Cl, C–Br and C–I which become progressively easy to metabolize (Table 8.6).

Pharmacology of inhaled anaesthetic agents

Nitrous oxide

Nitrous oxide (N_2O) is used widely alongside the volatile agents and in combination with oxygen (O_2) as entonox. Apart from a high MAC, it has favourable physical properties. However, during even relatively short exposure it interferes with DNA synthesis and increasing concern over this and other aspects of N_2O may limit its future use.

Manufacture

Nitrous oxide is manufactured by heating ammonium nitrate to 250°C.

$$NH_4NO_3 \rightarrow N_2O + 2H_2O$$

Unless the temperature is carefully controlled N_2O may contain the following contaminants: NH_3, N_2, NO, NO_2 and HNO_3. These impurities are actively removed by passage through scrubbers, water and caustic soda.

Storage

Nitrous oxide is stored as a liquid in French blue cylinders (C = 450 litres up to G = 9000 litres) with a gauge pressure of 51 bar at 20°C, which therefore bears no correlation to cylinder content until all remaining N_2O is in the gaseous phase. The filling ratio (mass of N_2O in cylinder/mass of water that the cylinder could hold) is 0.75 in temperate regions, but it needs to be reduced to 0.67 in tropical regions to avoid cylinder explosions. Its critical temperature is 36.5°C; its critical pressure is 72 bar.

Effects

- Respiratory – it causes a small fall in tidal volume that is offset by an increased respiratory rate so that minute volume and $PaCO_2$ remain unchanged.
- Cardiovascular – although N_2O has mild direct myocardial depressant effects, it also increases sympathetic activity by its central effects. Therefore, in health the circulatory system is changed very little. However, for patients with cardiac failure who are unable to increase their sympathetic drive the direct myocardial depressant effects may significantly reduce cardiac output. It does not sensitize the heart to catecholamines.
- Central nervous system – N_2O increases cerebral blood flow and is sometimes avoided in patients with a raised intracranial pressure. Despite a MAC of 105%, its potential to cause anaesthesia in certain patients should not be ignored.

Concentration effect, second gas effect and diffusion hypoxia

The concentration effect

The concentration effect is an observed phenomenon that describes the disproportionate rate of rise of the alveolar fraction compared with the inspired fraction when high concentrations of N_2O are inspired (Figure 8.8a). The rate of rise is disproportionate when compared with the situation where low concentrations of N_2O are inspired. The concentration effect only applies to N_2O because N_2O is the only agent used at sufficiently high concentration. Various models have been used to explain the phenomenon; all have limitations.

However, the fundermental driving force for the process is the large gradient which the high concentrations of N_2O generate. As a result large amounts of N_2O (50% is assumed in the model shown in Figure 8.8b) are absorbed into the pulmonary capillaries despite the fact that it is usually considered an insoluble agent (blood:gas solubility coefficient 0.47). In order for the alveolar volume to remain constant, gas

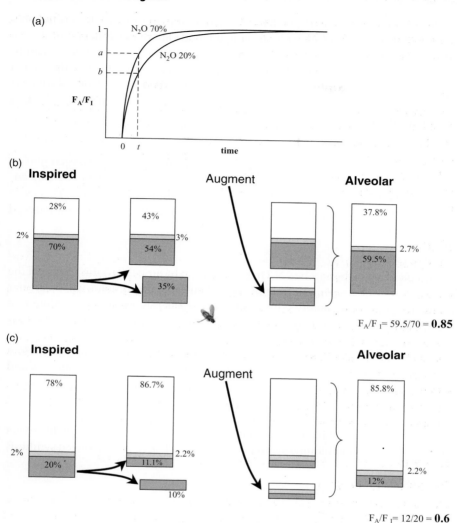

Figure 8.8. The concentration effect. See text for details.

that was in the conducting airways is drawn down into the alveoli so that the various alveolar concentrations change.

In the final analysis, when comparing two separate scenarios, the first using high concentrations of N_2O (Figure 8.8b) and the second using low concentrations of N_2O (Figure 8.8c), the F_A/F_I ratio is disproportionately high (point a at time t, Figure 8.8a) where large concentrations of N_2O are used, compared to the F_A/F_I ratio when lower concentrations of N_2O are used (point b at time t, Figure 8.8a).

The model described in Figure 8.8 is limited in numerous ways (N_2O is the only gas absorbed and the effects of N_2 leaving the body are not included), but it does serve to illustrate the mechanism by which the concentration effect is thought to occur. In addition it illustrates the second gas effect. It assumes that half the N_2O in the alveoli is absorbed into the pulmonary capillaries, the volume deficit of which is made good by augmented ventilation which has the same fractional composition as the initial alveolar gas.

The second gas effect

The second gas effect is a direct result of the concentration effect. Oxygen plus or minus volatile agents used alongside high concentrations of N_2O will be concentrated by the rapid uptake of N_2O and augmented alveolar ventilation. This leads to increased concentrations of oxygen and volatile agents resulting in a reduced induction time.

Diffusion hypoxia

At the end of anaesthesia when N_2O/O_2 is replaced by air (N_2/O_2) the reverse of the second gas effect is seen. The volume of N_2O entering the alveolus will be greater than the volume of N_2 entering the pulmonary capillaries resulting in a dilution of all alveolar gases. Most volatile anaesthetics end by changing N_2O/O_2 to 100% O_2 which prevents diffusion hypoxia.

In addition to the effects seen across the alveolar membrane, N_2O will cause a rapid expansion of any air filled space (pneumothorax, vascular air embolus and intestinal lumen).

Toxicity

The cobalt ion present in vitamin B_{12} is oxidized by N_2O so that it is unable to act as the cofactor for methionine synthase (Figure 8.9). The result is reduced synthesis

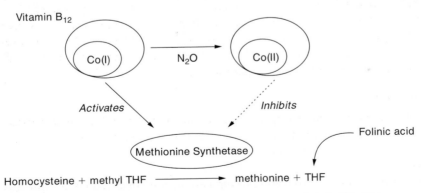

Figure 8.9. N_2O inhibits methionine synthetase by oxidizing cobalt (Co(I)). THF, tetrahydrofolate.

of methionine, thymidine, tetrahydrofolate and DNA. Methionine synthetase also appears to be directly inhibited by N_2O. Exposure of only a few hours may result in megaloblastic changes in bone marrow but more prolonged exposure (i.e. days) may result in agranulocytosis. Recovery is governed by synthesis (taking a few days) of new methionine synthase, but may be helped by the administration of folinic acid, which provides a different source of tetrahydrofolate.

In a properly scavenged environment where N_2O concentrations are less than 50 ppm there is no effect on DNA synthesis. However, in unscavenged dental surgeries where large amounts are used, chronic exposure may result in neurological syndromes that resemble subacute combined degeneration of the cord, as a result of chronic vitamin B_{12} inactivation.

In experimental conditions N_2O has been shown to be teratogenic to rats but this effect is prevented by folinic acid. While this has never been unequivocally demonstrated in humans, N_2O is often not used in the first trimester when anaesthesia is required.

Entonox

Entonox is a 50:50 mixture of N_2O and O_2. The two gases effectively dissolve into each other and do not behave in a way that would be predicted from their individual properties. This phenomenon is called the Poynting effect.

Uses
Entonox is widely used for analgesia during labour and other painful procedures.

Storage
Entonox is stored as a gas in French blue cylinders (G = 3200 litres; J = 6400 litres) with white and blue checked shoulders at 137 bar. It separates into its constituent parts below its pseudo-critical temperature, which is about $-7°C$ and is most likely to occur at 117 bar. Higher or lower pressures reduce the likelihood of separation. When delivered via pipeline at 4.1 bar the pseudo-critical temperature is less than $-30°C$. If a cylinder is used following separation, the inspired gas will initially produce little analgesia as it contains mainly O_2, but as the cylinder empties the mixture will become progressively potent and hypoxic as it approaches 100% N_2O.

Isoflurane

This halogenated ethyl methyl ether is a structural isomer of enflurane. It is widely used to maintain anaesthesia. Its physical properties are summarized in Table 8.7.

Effects
- Respiratory – isoflurane depresses ventilation more than halothane but less than enflurane. Minute volume is decreased while respiratory rate and $PaCO_2$ are increased. It is rarely used to induce anaesthesia due to its pungent smell,

which may cause upper airway irritability, coughing and breath-holding. However, despite its pungent smell it causes some bronchodilation.

- Cardiovascular – its main effect is to reduce systemic vascular resistance. The resulting reflex tachycardia suggests that the carotid sinus reflex is preserved. It causes only a small decrease in myocardial contractility and cardiac output. It has been suggested that isoflurane may cause coronary steal whereby normally responsive coronary arterioles are dilated and divert blood away from areas supplied by unresponsive diseased vessels, resulting in ischaemia. However more recent work has suggested that as long as coronary perfusion is maintained coronary steal does not occur. In addition isofluane may have myocardial protective properties via its effects on ATP-dependent potassium channels.
- Central nervous system – of all the volatile agents isoflurane produces the best balance of reduced cerebral oxygen requirement and minimal increase in cerebral blood flow. At concentrations up to 1 MAC cerebral autoregulation is preserved.

Metabolism

Only 0.2% is metabolized and none of the products has been linked to toxicity.

Toxicity

Owing to the presence of a $-CHF_2$ group in its structure it may react with dry soda lime (or baralyme) producing carbon monoxide. Reports of this relate to circle systems that have been left with dry gas circulating over a weekend so that subsequent use of isoflurane causes release of carbon monoxide. Enflurane and desflurane also possess $-CHF_2$ groups and may react in a similar manner.

Sevoflurane

Sevoflurane is a polyfluorinated isopropyl methyl ether and has the favourable combination of a relatively low blood:gas partition coefficient (0.7), pleasant odour and relatively low MAC (1.8). However during storage where the concentration of added water is below 100 ppm it is susceptible to attack by Lewis acids at its ether and halogen bonds, releasing the highly toxic hydrofluoric acid (HF). (A Lewis acid is defined as any substance that can accept an electron pair and includes many metal oxides but also H^+; glass is a source of Lewis acids.) Hydrofluoric acid corrodes glass exposing sevoflurane to further Lewis acids. As a result sevoflurane is formulated with 300 ppm of water, which acts as a Lewis acid inhibitor. In addition it is stored in polythylene napthalate bottles, rather than glass. A dry formulation containing less than 130 ppm water is now available and is presented in an aluminium bottle lined with an epoxyphenolic resin lacquer. Unlike the other volatile agents sevoflurane is achiral.

Manufacture

- The one pot method – all the ingredients are added together to produce sevoflurane and then water is added to 300 ppm.

- The chloro-fluoro method – here the basic molecular architecture is manufactured but with chlorine attached. This is then substituted with flourine to produce sevoflurane.

Effects

- Respiratory – sevoflurane is a useful agent for induction of anaesthesia due to its pleasant odour and favourable physical properties. It does, however, depress ventilation in a predictable fashion with a reduction in minute volume and a rise in $PaCO_2$.
- Cardiovascular – the systemic vascular resistance falls and, due to an unchanged heart rate, the blood pressure falls. Cardiac contractility is unaffected and the heart is not sensitized to catecholamines. Vascular resistance to both cerebral and coronary circulations is decreased.
- Central Nervous System – compared with halothane, there is evidence that children exhibit a higher incidence of post-operative agitation and delirium, which may extend beyond the initial recovery period.

Metabolism

Sevoflurane undergoes hepatic metabolism by cytochrome P450 (isoform 2E1) to a greater extent than all the other commonly used volatile agents except halothane (Table 8.6). Hexafluoroisopropanol and inorganic F^- (known to cause renal toxicity) are produced. The now obsolete volatile anaesthetic methoxyflurane was also metabolized by hepatic P450 releasing F^-, and when plasma levels rose above 50 μmol.l^{-1} renal toxicity was observed. However, renal toxicity is not observed following sevoflurane administration even when plasma levels reach 50 μmol.l^{-1}. A possible explanation lies in the additional metabolism of methoxyflurane by renal P450 to F^-, which generates a high local concentration while sevoflurane undergoes little or no renal metabolism.

Toxicity

Compounds A, B, C, D and E have all been identified when sevoflurane is used in the pressence of carbon dioxide absorbents. Only compounds A and B (which is less toxic) are present in sufficient amount to make analysis feasible. Their formation is favoured in the presence of potassium hydroxide rather than sodium hydroxide based absorbents particularly when dry. The reaction releases heat and consumes sevoflurane both of which are readily detectible.

The lethal concentration of compound A in 50% of rats is 300–400 ppm after 3 hours exposure. Extrapolation of these and other animal studies suggest a human nephrotoxic threshold of 150–200 ppm. Recent work suggests that even with flow rates of 0.25 l.min^{-1} for 5 hours the level of compound A peaks at less than 20 ppm and is not associated with abnormal tests of renal function.

Halothane

This halogenated hydrocarbon is unstable when exposed to light, and corrodes certain metals. It is stored with 0.01% thymol to prevent the liberation of free bromine. It dissolves into rubber and may leach out into breathing circuits after the vaporizer is turned off. Its physical properties are summarized in Table 8.7.

Effects

- Respiratory – the minute ventilation is depressed largely due to a decreased tidal volume. The normal responses to hypoxia and hypercarbia are also blunted and these effects are more pronounced above 1 MAC. Bronchiolar tone is reduced and it is useful in asthmatic patients. Owing to its sweet non-irritant odour it may be used to induce anaesthesia.
- Cardiovascular – halothane has significant effects on the heart. Bradycardia is produced by increased vagal tone, depressed sino-atrial and atrioventricular activity. It has direct myocardial depressant properties that reduce cardiac output. It sensitizes the heart to catecholamines, which may lead to arrhythmias (especially ventricular and bradyarrhythmias) and are more common than compared to other agents. Where adrenaline is infiltrated to improve the surgical field less than 100 μg per 10 minutes should be given. Drugs that specifically reduce atrioventricular conductivity (e.g. verapamil) should be used with caution alongside halothane. The systemic vascular resistance is reduced resulting in increased cutaneous blood flow. However, due to a reduced cardiac output blood flow to the liver and kidneys is reduced.
- Central nervous system – halothane increases cerebral blood flow more than any other volatile agent leading to significant increases in intracranial pressure above 0.6 MAC. Cerebral oxygen requirements are reduced.

Metabolism

Up to 25% of inhaled halothane undergoes oxidative metabolism by hepatic cytochrome P450 to produce trifluoroacetic acid, Br^- and Cl^-. However, reductive metabolism producing F^- and other reduced metabolites predominate when the liver becomes hypoxic. While these reduced metabolites are toxic it is thought that they are not involved in halothane hepatitis.

Toxicity

Hepatic damage may take one of two forms:

- A reversible form that is often subclinical and associated with a rise in hepatic transaminases. This is probably due to hepatic hypoxia.
- Fulminant hepatic necrosis (halothane hepatitis). Trifluoroacetyl chloride (an oxidative metabolite of halothane) may behave as a hapten, binding covalently with hepatic proteins, inducing antibody formation. The diagnosis of halothane

Table 8.7. Physiochemical properties of inhaled anaesthetics.

	Halothane	Isoflurane	Enflurane	Desflurane	Sevoflurane	N_2O	Xenon
MW	197.0	184.5	184.5	168.0	200.1	44.0	131.0
BP (°C)	50.2	48.5	56.5	23.5	58.5	−88.0	−108
SVP at 20°C (kPa)	32.3	33.2	23.3	89.2	22.7	5200	
MAC (%)	0.75	1.17	1.68	6.60	1.80	105	71.0
Blood:gas partition coefficient	2.40	1.40	1.80	0.42	0.70	0.47	0.14
Oil:gas partition coefficient	224	98	98	29	80	1.4	1.9
Odour	non-irritant, sweet	irritant	non-irritant	pungent	non-irritant	odourless	odourless

hepatitis is based on the exclusion of all other forms of liver damage. The incidence in children is between 1 in 80 000–200 000 while in the adult it is 1 in 2500–35 000. The following are risk factors: multiple exposures, obesity, middle age and female sex. The mortality rate is 50–75%.

Halothane should be avoided if administered within the previous 3 months, there is a history of a previous adverse reaction to halothane or pre-existing liver disease.

Enflurane has also been reported to cause hepatic necrosis. Its incidence is much lower due to its lower rate of metabolism. In theory the other volatile agents may cause a similar reaction but due to their even lower rates of metabolism this becomes increasingly unlikely.

Enflurane

This halogenated ethyl methyl ether is a structural isomer of isoflurane. Its use is decreasing due to newer agents with more favourable profiles.

Effects

- Respiratory – enflurane causes more depression of ventilation than the other agents. The minute volume decreases and the $PaCO_2$ will rise. The ventilatory response to hypoxia and hypercarbia are also blunted.
- Cardiovascular – while the heart rate increases, cardiac output, contractility and blood pressure fall along with a small fall in systemic vascular resistance. The heart is not sensitized to catecholamines, and arrhythmias are relatively uncommon.
- Central nervous system – high concentrations of enflurane in the presence of hypocarbia produce a 3 Hz spike and wave pattern on the EEG consistent with grand mal activity. While there is no evidence that these changes are seen more frequently in epileptics, enflurane is usually avoided in this group of patients. The increase in cerebral blood flow and accompanying increase in intracranial pressure lie between those observed with halothane and isoflurane.

Metabolism

Only 2% is metabolized by hepatic cytochrome P450. F^- ions are produced but rarely reach the levels (>40 μmol.l^{-1}) known to produce reversible nephropathy. It is usually avoided in patients with renal impairment.

Toxicity

Hepatic damage may occur (cf. halothane metabolism).

Desflurane

Desflurane (a fluorinated ethyl methyl ether) was slow to be introduced into anaesthetic practice due to difficulties in preparation and administration. It has a boiling point of 23.5°C, which renders it extremely volatile and, therefore, dangerous to administer via a conventional vaporizer. It is, therefore, administered via the electronic Tec 6 vaporizer that heats desflurane to 39°C at 2 atmospheres. Its low blood: gas partition coefficient (0.42) ensures a rapid onset and offset, but high concentrations are required due to its MAC of 6.6%.

Effects

- Respiratory – desflurane shows similar respiratory effects to the other agents, being more potent than halothane but less potent than isoflurane and enflurane. $PaCO_2$ rises and minute ventilation falls with increasing concentrations. Desflurane has a pungent odour that causes coughing and breath-holding. It is not suitable for induction of anaesthesia.
- Cardiovascular – these may be thought of as similar to isoflurane. However, in patients with ischaemic heart disease particular care is required as concentrations above 1 MAC may produce cardiovascular stimulation (tachycardia and hypertension). It does not sensitize the heart to catecholamines. Vascular resistance to both cerebral and coronary circulations is decreased.

Metabolism

Only 0.02% is metabolized and so its potential to produce toxic effects is minimal.

Xenon

Xenon (Xe) is an inert, odourless gas with no occupational or environmental hazards and makes up 0.0000087% of the atmosphere. It has a MAC = 71% and a very low blood:gas partition coefficient (0.14). Consequently, its onset and offset of action are faster than both desflurane and N_2O.

Manufacture

Xenon is produced by the fractional distillation of air, at about 2000 times the cost of producing N_2O.

Effects

- Respiratory – in contrast to other inhaled anaesthetic agents xenon slows the respiratory rate, while the tidal volume is increased so that the minute volume remains constant. Compared with N_2O, xenon has a higher density ($\times 3$) and viscosity ($\times 1.5$), which might be expected to increase airway resistance when used in high concentrations. However, its clinical significance is probably minimal. Despite its use at high concentrations it does not appear to result in diffusion hypoxia in a manner similar to that seen with N_2O.
- Cardiovascular – xenon does not alter myocardial contractility but may result in a small decrease in heart rate.
- Central nervous system – xenon may be used to enhance CT images of the brain while [133]xenon may be used to measure cerebral blood flow. However, in humans

Table 8.8. Cardiovascular effects of inhaled anaesthetics.

	Halothane	Isoflurane	Enflurane	Desflurane	Sevoflurane
Contractility	↓↓↓	↓	↓↓	minimal	↓
Heart rate	↓↓	↑↑	↑	↑ (↑↑ > 1.5 MAC)	nil
Systemic vascular resistance	↓	↓↓	↓	↓↓	↓
Blood pressure	↓↓	↓↓	↓↓	↓↓	↓
Coronary steal syndrome	no	possibly	no	no	no
Splanchnic blood flow	↓	unchanged	↓	unchanged	unchanged
Sensitization to catecholamines	↑↑↑	nil	↑	nil	nil

Table 8.9. Respiratory effects of inhaled anaesthetics.

	Halothane	Isoflurane	Enflurane	Desflurane	Sevoflurane
Respiratory Rate	↑	↑↑	↑↑	↑↑	↑↑
Tidal volume	↓	↓↓	↓↓↓	↓↓	↓
$PaCO_2$	unchanged	↑↑	↑↑↑	↑↑	↑

it appears to increase the cerebral blood flow in a variable manner, and its use in anaesthesia for neurosurgery is not recommended.

- Analgesia – it has significant analgesic properties.

Elimination

Xenon is not metabolized in the body, rather it is eliminated via the lungs.

Non-anaesthetic medical gases

Oxygen

Manufacture and storage

Oxygen (O_2) is manufactured by the fractional distillation of air or by means of an oxygen concentrator in which a zeolite mesh adsorbs N_2 so that the remaining gas is about 97% O_2. It is stored as a gas in black cylinders with white shoulders at 137 bar and as a liquid in a vacuum insulated evaporator (VIE) at 10 bar and $-180°C$, which must be located outside. The VIE rests on three legs; two are hinged while the third serves as a weighing device, enabling its contents to be displayed on a dial.

Physiochemical properties

- Boiling point $-182°C$
- Critical temperature $-119°C$
- Critical pressure 50 bar

Table 8.10. Other effects of inhaled anaesthetics.

	Halothane	Isoflurane	Enflurane	Desflurane	Sevoflurane
Cerebral blood flow	↑↑	↑ (nil if <1 MAC)	↑	↑	↑
Cerebral O_2 requirement	→	→	→	→	→
EEG	burst suppression	burst suppression	epileptiform activity (3 Hz spike and wave)	burst suppression	burst suppression
Effect on uterus	some relaxation	some relaxation	some relaxation	some relaxation	some relaxation
Potentiation of muscle relaxation	some	significant	significant	significant	significant
Analgesia	none	some	some	some	some

Uses

It is used to prevent hypoxaemia.

Measurement

Depending on the sample type, various means are used to measure O_2. In a mixture of gases a mass spectrometer, paramagnetic analyzer or fuel cell may be used; when dissolved in blood a Clarke electrode, transcutaneous electrode or pulse oximetry may be used; in vitro blood samples may be analyzed by bench or co-oximetry.

Effects

- Cardiovascular – if O_2 is being used to correct hypoxaemia then an improvement in all cardiovascular parameters will be seen. However, prolonged administration of 100% O_2 will directly reduce cardiac output slightly and cause coronary artery vasoconstriction. It causes a fall in pulmonary vascular resistance and pulmonary artery pressure.
- Respiratory – in healthy subjects, a high concentration causes mild respiratory depression. However, in those patients who are truly dependent on a hypoxic drive to maintain respiration, even a modest concentration of O_2 may prove fatal.

Toxicity

O_2 toxicity is caused by free radicals. They affect the CNS resulting in anxiety, nausea and seizures when the partial pressure exceeds 200 kPa. The alveolar capillary membrane undergoes lipid peroxidation and regions of lung may collapse. Neonates are susceptible to retrolental fibroplasia, which may be a result of vasoconstriction of developing retinal vessels during development.

Nitric oxide

Nitric oxide (NO) is an endogenous molecule but it is potentially a contaminant in nitrous oxide cylinders. It was formerly known as endothelium-derived relaxing factor (EDRF).

Synthesis

Nitric oxide is synthesized from one of the terminal guanidino nitrogen atoms of L-arginine in a process catalyzed by nitric oxide synthase (NOS), which is present in two forms:

- Constitutive – which is normally present in endothelial, neuronal, skeletal muscle, cardiac tissue and platelets. Here NOS is Ca^{2+}/calmodulin-dependent and is stimulated by cGMP.
- Inducible – which is seen only after exposure to endotoxin or certain cytokines in endothelium, vascular smooth muscle, myocytes, macrophages and neutrophils.

Following induction large quantities of NO are produced, which may be cytotoxic. In addition, it may form radicals leading to cellular damage and capillary leakage.

Effects

- Cardiovascular – vasodilator tone in small arteries and arterioles is dependent on a continuous supply of locally synthesized NO. Shear stresses in these vessels increase NO production and may account for flow-dependent vasodilatation. Nitric oxide derived from the endothelium inhibits platelet aggregation. In septic shock there is overproduction of NO resulting in hypotension and capillary leakage.
- Respiratory – endogenous NO provides an important basal vasodilator tone in pulmonary and bronchial vessels, which may be reversed in hypoxia. When inhaled in concentrations of up to 40 ppm it may reduce V/Q mismatching in acute respiratory distress syndrome (ARDS) and reduce pulmonary hypertension in neonates. Inhaled NO has no effect on the systemic circulation due to its rapid inactivation within red blood cells. Its affinity for haemoglobin is 1500 times that of carbon monoxide. It has no bronchodilator properties.
- Immune – NO synthesized in macrophages and neutrophils can be toxic to certain pathogens and may be an important host defence mechanism.
- Haematological – NO inhibits platelet aggregation.
- Neuronal – nerves containing NO are widely distributed throughout the central nervous system. Proposed roles include modulation of the state of arousal, pain perception, programmed cell death and long-term neuronal depression and excitation whereby neurones may 'remember' previous signals. Peripheral neurones containing NO control regional blood flow in the corpus cavernosum.

N-monomethyl-L-arginine (L-NMMA) is a guanidino substituted analogue of L-arginine, which inhibits NOS. While L-NMMA has been used to antagonize NOS, resulting in an increased blood pressure in septic shock, it does not alter the course of the underlying pathology and has not been shown to alter survival.

Sodium nitroprusside and the organic nitrates (e.g. glyceryl trinitrate) exert their effect by the spontaneous release of nitric oxide or metabolism to nitric oxide in smooth muscle cells.

UK guidelines for the use of inhaled NO in adult intensive care units

An expert group of physicians and representatives from the department of health and industry issued the following guidelines in 1997:

Indications: severe ARDS (optimally ventilated, $PaO_2 < 12$ kPa with $F_IO_2 = 1$), or right-sided cardiac failure.

Dose: maximum = 40 ppm, but use minimum effective dose.

Equipment: a synchronized inspiratory injection system is considered optimal. If a continuous delivery system is used it must be through a calibrated flowmeter. Stainless steel pressure regulators and connectors should be used.

Monitoring: chemiluminescence or electrochemical analyzers should be used and are accurate to 1 ppm. Methaemoglobinaemia is only very rarely significant and is more likely in paediatric patients or those with methaemoglobin reductase deficiency but levels should be checked before and after starting NO, and daily thereafter.

Exposure: Environmental NO levels should not exceed 25 ppm for 8 hours (time-weighted average). Scavenging is not required in a well ventilated unit.

Contraindications: Methaemoglobinaemia (bleeding diathesis, intracranial haemorrhage, severe left ventricular failure).

Helium

Helium (He) is an inert gas presented as either Heliox (79% He, 21% O_2) in brown cylinders with white shoulders or as 100% helium in brown cylinders at 137 bar. It does not support combustion.

Its key physical characteristic is its lower density (and hence specific gravity) than both air and oxygen.

	Helium	Heliox	Oxygen	Air
Specific gravity	0.178	0.337	1.091	1

Therefore, during turbulent flow the velocity will be higher when Heliox is used. This will reduce the work of breathing and improve oxygenation in patients with an upper airway obstruction such as a tumour. Helium/oxygen mixtures are also used for deep water diving to avoid nitrogen narcosis. The lower density of helium/oxygen mixtures produces higher frequency vocal sounds, giving the typical squeaky voice.

Carbon dioxide

Carbon dioxide (CO_2) is a colourless gas with a pungent odour at high concentrations. It is stored as a liquid at 51 bar at 20°C in grey cylinders (C = 450 litres up to E = 1800 litres).

Physiochemical properties
- Boiling point −78.5°C
- Critical temperature 31°C
- Critical pressure 73.8 bar

Uses
It is used as the insufflating gas during laparoscopic procedures and occasionally to stimulate respiration following general anaesthesia. It is also used in cryotherapy.

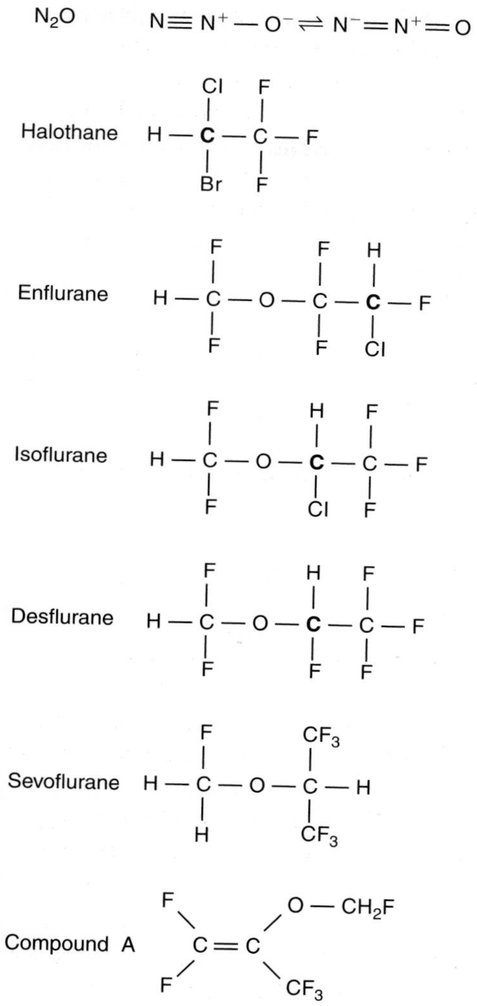

N_2O $N\equiv N^+ - O^- \rightleftharpoons N^- = N^+ = O$

Halothane

$$H - \overset{\overset{\displaystyle Cl}{|}}{\underset{\underset{\displaystyle Br}{|}}{C}} - \overset{\overset{\displaystyle F}{|}}{\underset{\underset{\displaystyle F}{|}}{C}} - F$$

Enflurane

$$H - \overset{\overset{\displaystyle F}{|}}{\underset{\underset{\displaystyle F}{|}}{C}} - O - \overset{\overset{\displaystyle F}{|}}{\underset{\underset{\displaystyle F}{|}}{C}} - \overset{\overset{\displaystyle H}{|}}{\underset{\underset{\displaystyle Cl}{|}}{C}} - F$$

Isoflurane

$$H - \overset{\overset{\displaystyle F}{|}}{\underset{\underset{\displaystyle F}{|}}{C}} - O - \overset{\overset{\displaystyle H}{|}}{\underset{\underset{\displaystyle Cl}{|}}{C}} - \overset{\overset{\displaystyle F}{|}}{\underset{\underset{\displaystyle F}{|}}{C}} - F$$

Desflurane

$$H - \overset{\overset{\displaystyle F}{|}}{\underset{\underset{\displaystyle F}{|}}{C}} - O - \overset{\overset{\displaystyle H}{|}}{\underset{\underset{\displaystyle F}{|}}{C}} - \overset{\overset{\displaystyle F}{|}}{\underset{\underset{\displaystyle F}{|}}{C}} - F$$

Sevoflurane

$$H - \overset{\overset{\displaystyle F}{|}}{\underset{\underset{\displaystyle H}{|}}{C}} - O - \overset{\overset{\displaystyle CF_3}{|}}{\underset{\underset{\displaystyle CF_3}{|}}{C}} - H$$

Compound A

$$\underset{F}{\overset{F}{>}}C = C\underset{CF_3}{\overset{O - CH_2F}{<}}$$

Figure 8.10. Structure of some inhaled anaesthetics and Compound A. **C** represents a chiral centre.

Effects

- Cardiovascular – by sympathetic stimulation it increases heart rate, blood pressure, cardiac output and dilates the coronary arteries. Arrhythmias are more likely in the presence of a raised $PaCO_2$.
- Respiratory – the respiratory centre and peripheral chemoreceptors respond to a raised $PaCO_2$ resulting in an increased minute volume and bronchodilation. However, a $PaCO_2$ above 10 kPa may result in respiratory depression.

- Central nervous system – as $PaCO_2$ rises so does cerebral blood flow and intracranial pressure. Beyond 10 kPa narcosis may ensue.

Carbon dioxide absorbents

Absorbents consume CO_2 to prevent rebreathing in a circle system. In the UK they are mainly sodium hydroxide (sodalime) based while in the US they are potassium hydroxide based (baralyme). There are three steps in the chemical reaction:

$$H_2O + CO_2 \rightarrow H_2CO_3$$
$$H_2CO_3 + 2NaOH \rightarrow Na_2CO_3 + 2H_2O$$
$$Na_2CO_3 + Ca(OH)_2 \rightarrow CaCO_3 + 2NaOH.$$

Analgesics

Pain is defined as an unpleasant sensory and emotional experience associated with actual or potential tissue damage. Since pain is so highly subjective, it may also be described as being what the patient says it is.

Pain may be classified according to its presumed aetiology. Nociceptive pain is the result of the stimulation of nociceptors by noxious stimuli, whilst neuropathic pain is the result of dysfunction of the nervous system. These may exist together as mixed pain. There is also visceral pain, the clearest example being that associated with gallstones.

An alternative classification is based on chronicity. The point at which acute pain becomes chronic has been suggested at about 12 weeks or when the pain is no longer thought to be due to the initial insult.

Physiology

Nociceptive impulses are triggered by the stimulation of nociceptors that respond to chemical, mechanical or thermal damage. The chemical mediators that initiate (H^+, K^+, acetylcholine, histamine, serotonin (5-HT), bradykinin), and sensitize (prostaglandins, leukotrienes, substance P, neurokinin A, calcitonin gene-related peptide) the nociceptors are legion. Two types of primary afferent fibres exist:
- small myelinated Aδ fibres (diameter 2–5 μm) that conduct sharp pain rapidly (40 m.s^{-1})
- unmyelinated C fibres (diameter < 2 μm) that conduct dull pain slowly (2 m.s^{-1})

These fibres enter the dorsal horn of the spinal cord and synapse at different sites (Aδ at Rexed laminae II and V; C at Rexed laminae II). The substantia gelatinosa (lamina II) integrates these inputs, from where second-order neurones form the ascending spinothalamic and spinoreticular pathways on the contralateral side. Descending pathways and the larger Aβ fibres conducting 'touch' stimulate inhibitory interneurones within the substantia gelatinosa and inhibit C fibre nociceptive inputs. This forms the basis of the 'gate theory' of pain (Figure 9.1).

Pain may be modified by altering the neural pathway from its origin at the nociceptor to its interpretation within the central nervous system. The commonly used agents are discussed below under the following headings:
- **Opioids and related drugs**
- **Non-steroidal anti-inflammatory drugs (NSAIDs)**

Table 9.1. Classification of opioid receptors.

Receptor	Effects
MOP, μ, mu	analgesia, meiosis, euphoria, respiratory depression, bradycardia, inhibition of gut motility
KOP, κ, kappa	analgesia, sedation, meiosis
DOP, δ, delta	analgesia, respiratory depression
NOP	

Other important agents such as local anaesthetics, antidepressants, anti-epileptics, guanethidine, ketamine and clonidine are often used to treat pain and are discussed elsewhere.

Opioids and related drugs

The term 'opiate' refers to all naturally occurring substances with morphine like properties, while 'opioid' is a more general term that includes synthetic substances that have an affinity for opioid receptors. Opioids are basic amines.

Receptor Classification

Classical receptor classification, that is, kappa and delta, was based on either the name of the agonist that acted at that receptor, *mu* (μ)– *morphine*, *kapppa* (κ) – *ketcyclazocine* or the location of the receptor, *delta* (δ) – vas *deferens*. The latest reclassification is listed in Table 9.1. and includes an additional non-classical receptor, NOP, which was discovered at the time of receptor cloning. It is known as the nociceptin/orphanin FQ peptide receptor.

Both receptor types are serpentine (i.e. span the membrane seven times) and are linked to inhibitory G-proteins so that when stimulated by an appropriate opioid

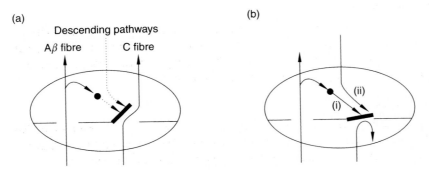

Figure 9.1. Principle of the gate theory of pain within the dorsal horn of the spinal cord. (a) Pain mediated via C fibres passes through the gate centrally; (b) the gate is shut as Aβ fibres stimulate inhibitory interneurones (i) and by descending pathways, preventing the central passage of pain (ii).

Table 9.2. Opioid receptor subtypes and their ligands.

Ligand	Receptor			
	μ	κ	δ	NOP
Endorphins	+++	+++	+++	
Enkephalins	+		+++	
Dynorphins	+	+++		
N/OFQ				+++
Morphine	+++	+	+	
Fentanyl	+++	+		
Naloxone	+++	++	++	

Note: + represents receptor affinity, blank represents no receptor affinity.

agonist (e.g. morphine to μ) the following sequence occurs: voltage sensitive Ca^{2+} channels are closed, hyperpolarization by K^+ efflux and adenylase cyclase inhibition leading to reduced cAMP. These processes result in inhibition of transmitter release between nerve cells.

MOP or μ-receptor

The μ-receptor is located thoughout the CNS including the cerebral cortex, the basal ganglia, the spinal cord (presynaptically on primary afferent neurons within the dorsal horn) and the periaqueductal grey (as the origin of the descending inhibitory control pathway). Apart from analgesia μ-receptor stimulation produces wide-ranging effects including respiratory depression (by reducing chemoreceptor sensitivity to carbon dioxide), constipation (reduced secretions and peristalsis) and cardiovascular depression.

KOP or κ-receptor

The original κ-receptor agonist was ketocyclazacine, which demonstrated a different set of effects when compared with μ-receptor stimulation. The main advantage of κ-receptor stimulation relates to a lack of respiratory depression, although κ-agonists do seem to have μ-antagonist effects thus limiting their use.

DOP or δ-receptor

The δ-receptor was the first to be cloned and is less widely spread throughout the central nervous system. Like μ-receptors, when stimulated they inhibit neurotransmitter release. It may also be involved in regulating mood and movement.

NOP-receptor

When stimulated by nociceptin/orphanin FQ the NOP-receptor produces effects similar to μ-receptor stimulation. It acts at both spinal and supraspinal levels to

Table 9.3. Various pharmacological properties of some opioids.

	Elimination half-life (min)	Clearance (ml.min^{-1}.kg^{-1})	Volume of distribution (l.kg^{-1})	Plasma protein bound (%)	pK$_a$	Percentage unionized (at pH 7.4)	Relative lipid solubility (from octanol:water coefficient)
Morphine	170	16	3.5	35	8.0	23	1
Pethidine	210	12	4.0	60	8.7	5	30
Fentanyl	190	13	4.0	83	8.4	9	600
Alfentanil	100	6	0.6	90	6.5	89	90
Remifentanil	10	40	0.3	70	7.1	68	20

Table 9.4. Summary of actions of some partial agonists at various opioid receptors.

	Agonist action at:	Antagonist action at:
Nalorphine	κ	μ
Pentazocine	κ (partial)	μ
	δ (partial)	
Buprenorphine	μ (partial)	
	NOP (partial)	
Nalbuphine	κ (partial)	μ (partial)

produce hyperalgesia at low doses but analgesia at high doses. NOP-receptor antagonists produce long-lasting analgesia and prevent morphine tolerance, and may be useful in the future.

Morphine

Morphine is a naturally occurring phenanthrene derivative. It has a complex structure (Figure 9.2) and is the reference opioid with which all others are compared. It is a μ-receptor agonist.

Presentation and uses

Morphine is formulated as tablets, suspensions and suppositories, and as slow-release capsules and granules in a wide range of strengths. The oral dose of morphine is 5–20 mg 4 hourly. The parenteral preparation contains 10–30 mg.ml^{-1} and may be given intravenously or intramuscularly. The intramuscular dose is 0.1–0.2 mg.kg^{-1} 4 hourly. Intravenous morphine should be titrated to effect, but the total dose is similar. It should be noted that these doses are only guidelines and the frequency of administration and/or the dose may have to be increased. The subcutaneous route is usually avoided due to its relatively low lipid solubility and therefore slow absorption. Delayed respiratory depression following intrathecal or epidural administration may occur and is again due to its relatively low lipid solubility.

Effects

- Analgesia – particularly effective for visceral pain while less effective for sharp or superficial pain. Occasionally increased doses may be required but this is usually due to a change in pathophysiology rather than dependence.
- Respiratory depression – the sensitivity of the brain stem to carbon dioxide is reduced following morphine while its response to hypoxia is less affected. However if the hypoxic stimulus is removed by supplementary oxygen then respiratory. depression may be potentiated. The respiratory rate falls more than the tidal

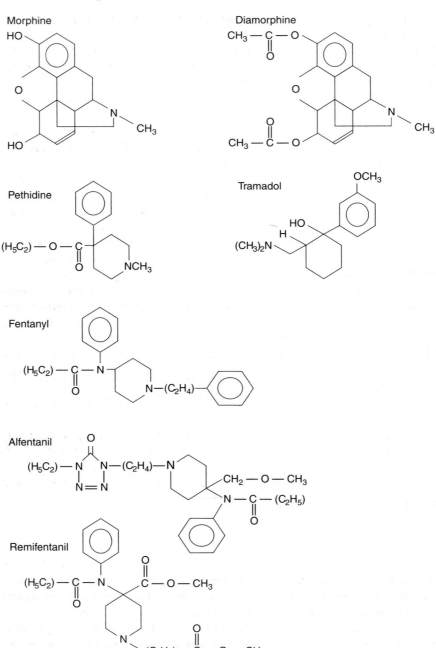

Figure 9.2. Structure of some opioids.

volume Morphine is anti-tussive. It may precipitate histamine release and bronchospasm.

- Nausea and vomiting – the chemoreceptor trigger zone is stimulated via 5-HT$_3$ and dopamine receptors. The cells within the vomiting centre are depressed by morphine and do not stimulate vomiting.
- Central nervous system – sedation, euphoria and dysphoria occur with increasing doses.
- Circulatory – morphine may induce a mild bradycardia and hypotension secondary to histamine release and a reduction in sympathetic tone. It has no direct myocardial depressant effects.
- Gut – morphine constricts the sphincters of the gut. Constipation results from a state of spastic immobility of the bowel. Whilst the sphincter of Oddi is contracted by morphine thereby raising the pressure within the biliary tree the clinical significance of this is unknown.
- Histamine release – reducing the rate of administration will help to limit histamine-induced bronchospasm and hypotension. Histamine release may result in a rash and pruritus but this may be reversed by naloxone.
- Pruritus – most marked following intrathecal or epidural use. However, this does not appear to be due to histamine release and is generally not associated with a rash. Paradoxically, antihistamines may be effective treatment for pruritus, possibly as a result of their sedative effects.
- Muscle rigidity – occasionally, morphine (and other opioids) can precipitate chest wall rigidity, which is thought to be due to opioid receptor interaction with dopaminergic and GABA pathways in the substantia nigra and striatum.
- Meiosis – due to stimulation of the Edinger–Westphal nucleus, which can be reversed by atropine.
- Endocrine – morphine inhibits the release of adrenocorticotrophic hormone (ACTH), prolactin and gonadotrophic hormones. Antidiuretic hormone (ADH) secretion is increased and may cause impaired water excretion and hyponatraemia.
- Urinary – the tone of the bladder detrusor and vesical sphincter is increased and may precipitate urinary retention. Ureteric tone is also increased.

Kinetics

When given orally morphine is ionized in the acidic gastric environment (because it is a weak base, pK$_a$ = 8.0) so that absorption is delayed until it reaches the relatively alkaline environment of the small bowel where it becomes unionized. Its oral bioavailability of 30% is due to hepatic first pass metabolism. Its peak effects following intravenous or intramuscular injection are reached after 10 and 30 minutes, respectively, and it has a duration of action of 3–4 hours. It has been given by the epidural (2–4 mg) and intrathecal (0.2–1.0 mg) routes but this has been associated with delayed respiratory depression.

Morphine concentration in the brain falls slowly due to its low lipid solubility, and consequently plasma concentrations do not correlate with its effects.

Morphine metabolism occurs mainly in the liver but also in the kidneys. Up to 70% is metabolized to morphine 3-glucuronide which appears to have effects on arousal and is possibly a μ-receptor antagonist. The other major metabolite is morphine 6-glucuronide, which is 13 times more potent than morphine and has a similar duration of action. They are both excreted in urine and accumulate in renal failure. Morphine is also N-demethylated. Neonates are more sensitive than adults to morphine due to reduced hepatic conjugating capacity, and in the elderly peak plasma levels are higher due to a reduced volume of distribution.

Diamorphine

Diamorphine is a diacetylated morphine derivative with no affinity for opioid receptors. It is a prodrug whose active metabolites are responsible for its effects. It is said to be approximately two times as potent as morphine.

Presentation and uses

Diamorphine is available as 10 mg tablets and as a white powder for injection containing 5, 10, 30, 100 or 500 mg diamorphine hydrochloride, which is readily dissolved before administration. It is used parenterally for the relief of severe pain and dyspnoea associated with pulmonary oedema at 2.5–10 mg. It is used intrathecally (0.1–0.4 mg) and via the epidural route (1–3 mg) for analgesia where, due to a higher lipid solubility, it is theoretically less likely to cause delayed respiratory depression when compared with morphine.

Kinetics

Owing to its high lipid solubility it is well absorbed from the gut but has a low oral bioavailability due to an extensive first-pass metabolism. Its high lipid solubility enables it to be administered effectively by the subcutaneous route. Once in the plasma it is 40% protein bound. It has a $pK_a = 7.6$ so that 37% is in the unionized form at pH 7.4. Metabolism occurs rapidly in the liver, plasma and central nervous system by ester hydrolysis to 6-monoacetylmorphine and morphine, which confer its analgesic and other effects. The plasma half-life of diamorphine itself is aproximately five minutes.

It produces the greatest degree of euphoria of the opioids and subsequently has become a drug of abuse.

Papaveretum

Papaveretum is a semi-synthetic mixture of the anhydrous hydrochlorides of the alkaloids of opium. It contains morphine, codeine and papaverine. Noscapine was removed from its formulation after it had been shown to be teratogenic in animal studies resulting in a standard dose of 15.4 mg, which is approximately equivalent to 10 mg morphine. It is not given via the intrathecal or epidural route due to preservatives. Its effects are essentially the same as morphine and are antagonized by naloxone.

Methadone

The notable features of methadone are its relatively low first-pass metabolism resulting in a relatively high oral bioavailability of 75% and a long plasma half-life. Thus it may be used orally, and as such it is used to treat those addicted to intravenous opioids, that is, diamorphine, by means of slow weaning programs. It is less sedative than morphine.

Methadone may also act as an antagonist at the NMDA receptor and this is thought to be especially beneficial in the treatment of certain neuropathic pain that would be otherwise resistant to typical opioids.

Kinetics

Methadone is 90% plasma protein bound and metabolism occurs in the liver to a number of inactive metabolites. Its plasma half-life is 18–36 hours. Up to 40% is excreted as unchanged drug in the urine, which is enhanced in acidic conditions.

Codeine

Codeine (methylmorphine) is 10 times less potent than morphine and not suitable for severe pain. The oral and intramuscular adult dose is 30–60 mg, the paediatric dose is 0.5–1 mg.kg^{-1} The intravenous route tends to cause hypotension probably via histamine release and is therefore avoided. It has been suggested codeine acts as no more than a prodrug for morphine.

Kinetics

The presence of a methyl group reduces hepatic conjugation resulting in an oral bioavailability of 50%. Post-operative oral bioavailability is much more variable and ranges from 20% to 80%.

A small proportion (5–15%) of codeine is eliminated unchanged in the urine while the remainder is eliminated via one of three metabolic pathways in the liver. The predominant metabolic pathway is 6-hydroxy glucuronidation, although 10–20% undergoes N-demethylation to norcodeine, and 5–15% undergoes O-demethylation to morphine. A number of other metabolites, such as normorphine and hydrocodone, have also been identified. Of these metabolites only morphine has significant activity at μ-receptors. O-demethylation is dependent on the non-inducible cytochrome P450 (CYP2D6), which exhibits genetic polymorphism so that poor metabolizers experience little pain relief. The frequency of poor metabolizers varies and is estimated at 9% of the UK population but 30% in the Hong Kong Chinese population.

Dihydrocodeine

Dihydrocodeine is a synthetic opioid, which is structurally similar to codeine but is approximately twice as potent. Like codeine its metabolism is subject to genetic polymorphism by virtue of the cytochrome P450 (CYP2D6).

Pethidine

Pethidine is a synthetic phenylpiperidine derivative originally designed as an anticholinergic agent but was subsequently shown to have analgesic properties.

Presentation

Pethidine is available as tablets and as a solution for injection containing 10–50 mg.ml^{-1}. The intravenous and intramuscular dose is 0.5–1.0 mg.kg^{-1} and may be repeated 2–3 hourly. In common with all opioids the dose should be titrated to effect.

Uses

Pethidine is often used during labour. Its high lipid solubility enables significant amounts to cross the placenta and reach the foetus. Following its metabolism, the less lipid-soluble norpethidine accumulates in the foetus, levels peaking about 4 hours after the initial maternal intramuscular dose. Owing to reduced foetal clearance, the half-lives of both pethidine and norpethidine are prolonged by a factor of three.

Effects

Pethidine shares the common opioid effects with morphine. However, differences are seen:

- Anticholinergic effects – it produces less marked meiosis and possibly a degree of mydriasis, a dry mouth and sometimes tachycardia.
- Gut – it is said to produce less biliary tract spasm than morphine but the clinical significance of this is unclear.
- Interactions – pethidine may produce a serious interaction if administered with monoamine oxidase inhibitors (MAOI). This is probably due to central serotoninenergic hyperactivity caused by pethidine inhibition of serotonin re-uptake in combination with an MAOI induced reduction in amine breakdown. Effects include coma, labile circulation, convulsions and hyperpyrexia. Other opioids are safe.

Kinetics

Pethidine is more lipid-soluble than morphine resulting in a faster onset of action. It has an oral bioavailability of 50%. It is metabolized in the liver by ester hydrolysis to the inactive pethidinic acid and by N-demethylation to norpethidine, which has half the analgesic activity of pethidine. Norpethidine has a longer elimination half-life

(14–21 hours) than pethidine and accumulates in renal failure. It has been associated with hallucinations and grand mal seizures following its accumulation. Its effects are not reversed by naloxone. Norpethidine and pethidinic acid are excreted in the urine along with small amounts of unchanged pethidine. The duration of action of pethidine is 120–150 minutes.

Fentanyl

Fentanyl is a synthetic phenylpiperidine derivative with a rapid onset of action. It is a μ-receptor agonist and as such shares morphine's effects. However, it is less likely to precipitate histamine release. High doses (50–150 μg.kg^{-1}) significantly reduce or even eliminate the metabolic stress response to surgery but are associated with bradycardia and chest wall rigidity.

Presentation

Fentanyl is prepared as a colourless solution for injection containing 50 μg.ml^{-1}, as transdermal patches that release between 25 and 100 μg per hour for 72 hours and as lozenges releasing 200 μg – 1.6 mg over 15 minutes.

Uses

Doses vary enormously depending on the duration of analgesia and sedation required. For pain associated with minor surgery, 1–2 μg.kg^{-1} is used intravenously and has a duration of about 30 minutes. Higher doses are generally required to obtund the stimulation of laryngoscopy. High doses (50–100 μg.kg^{-1}) are used for an opioid-based anaesthetic (although a hypnotic is also required), and here its duration of action is extended to about 6 hours. Following prolonged administration by continuous infusion only its elimination half-life is apparent, leading to a more prolonged duration of action.

Fentanyl has also been used to augment the effects of local anaesthetics in spinal and epidural anaesthesia at 10–25 μg and 25–100 μg, respectively. Its high lipid solubility ensures that a typical intrathecal dose does not cause delayed respiratory depression as it diffuses rapidly from cerebrospinal fluid (CSF) into the spinal cord. This contrasts with morphine, which enters the spinal cord slowly leaving some to be transported in the CSF by bulk flow up to the midbrain. However, respiratory depression is observed when epidural fentanyl is administered by continuous infusion or as repeated boluses.

Kinetics

Its onset of action is rapid following intravenous administration due to its high lipid solubility (nearly 600 times more lipid-soluble than morphine). However, following the application of a transdermal patch, plasma levels take 12 hours to reach equilibrium. At low doses (<3 μg.kg^{-1} intravenous) its short duration of action is due solely to distribution. However, following prolonged administration or with high doses, its duration of action is significantly prolonged as tissues become saturated. Its clearance is similar to and its elimination half-life is longer than that of morphine, reflecting its higher lipid solubility and volume of distribution. Fentanyl may become trapped in the acidic environment of the stomach where more than 99.9% is ionized. As it passes into the alkaline environment of the small bowel it becomes unionized and, therefore, available for systemic absorption. However, this is unlikely to raise systemic levels significantly due to a rapid hepatic first-pass metabolism, where it is N-demethylated to norfentanyl, which along with fentanyl is further hydroxylated. These inactive metabolites are excreted in the urine.

Alfentanil

Alfentanil is a synthetic phenylpiperidine derivative. It is a μ-receptor agonist but with some significant differences from fentanyl.

Presentation and uses

Alfentanil is presented as a colourless solution containing 500 μg or 5 mg.ml^{-1}. For short-term analgesia it is used in boluses of 5–25 μg.kg^{-1}. It is also used by infusion for sedation where its duration of action is significantly prolonged.

Kinetics

Alfentanil has a pK_a = 6.5; at a pH of 7.4, 89% is present in the unionized form and is, therefore, available to cross lipid membranes. Fentanyl has a pK_a = 8.4, so only 9% is unionized at a pH of 7.4. So despite a significantly lower lipid solubility than fentanyl, it has a faster onset of action (when given in equipotent doses). Alfentanil has a much smaller initial volume of distribution so that despite a smaller clearance its elimination half-life is also shorter.

Metabolism occurs in the liver by N-demethylation to noralfentanil. This and other metabolites are conjugated and excreted in the urine. Midazolam is metabolized by the same hepatic enzymes (CYP3A3/4) so when administered concurrently both elimination half-lives are significantly increased. Erythromycin may prolong alfentanil's activity by inhibiting hepatic CYP450.

Remifentanil

The pure μ-receptor agonist remifentanil is a synthetic phenylpiperidine derivative of fentanyl with a similar potency. While it shares many of the effects associated with the opioids its metabolism makes it unique in this class of drug. It is not a controlled drug.

Presentation

Remifentanil is presented as a crystalline white powder in glass vials containing 1, 2 or 5 mg remifentanil hydrochloride. The preparation also contains glycine and is not licensed for spinal or epidural administration.

Uses

Remifentanil is administered intravenously by infusion. It should be diluted before use with 5% dextrose, 0.9 or 0.45% saline, in which it is stable for 24 hours. It is not recommended for use as a sole induction agent and is given as an initial bolus of $1 \mu g.kg^{-1}$ over not less than 30 seconds, followed by an infusion that will vary according to the choice of supplemental anaesthesia. The usual dose range is 0.05–2.00 $\mu g.kg^{-1}.min^{-1}$.

While it is capable of producing intense analgesia during administration, it should be remembered that additional post-operative analgesia is required following painful procedures due to its short duration of action.

Effects

Remifentanil shares many of morphine's effects including respiratory depression and chest wall rigidity. However, due to its ultra-short duration of action nausea and vomiting seem to be less common. It characteristically causes a fall in heart rate and blood pressure, which may be reversed by glycopyrrolate. Its analgesic effects are reversed by naloxone.

Kinetics

Remifentanil is rapidly broken down by non-specific plasma and tissue esterases resulting in an elimination half-life of 3–10 minutes. Its duration of action is, therefore, determined by metabolism and not distribution (cf. alfentanil and fentanyl). Owing to the abundance of these esterases the duration of administration does not effect the duration of action, that is, the context-sensitive half-time (c.f. p77) does not change. This is in contrast to the other opioids whose half-time is context-sensitive, being dependent on the duration of infusion. It is a poor substrate for plasma cholinesterases and as such is unaffected by cholinesterase deficiency. Anti-cholinesterase drugs do not alter its metabolism. An essentially inactive carboxylic acid metabolite (1/4600th as potent) is excreted in the urine. The half-life of this metabolite in the healthy adult is 2 hours. Impaired hepatic and renal function do not prolong its effects.

Tramadol

Tramadol is a cyclohexanol derivative. It is a racemic mixture, each enantiomer producing specific actions.

Presentation

Tramadol is available as tablets, capsules or sachets in a variety of strengths (50–400 mg modified release) and as a solution for intravenous or intramuscular injection containing 100 mg in 2 ml. Its analgesic potency is one-fifth to one-tenth that of morphine.

Mechanism of action

Tramadol has agonist properties at all opioid receptors but particularly at μ-receptors but has not been classified as a controlled drug. It also inhibits the re-uptake of noradrenaline and 5-HT, and stimulates presynaptic 5-HT release, which provides an alternative pathway for analgesia involving the descending inhibitory pathways within the spinal cord.

Effects

In equi-analgesic doses to morphine, tramadol produces less respiratory depression and constipation. In other respects it has similar actions to morphine. Respiratory depression and analgesia are reversed by naloxone.

Interactions

Tramadol has the potential to interact with drugs that inhibit central 5-HT or noradrenaline re-uptake, that is, the tricyclic antidepressants and selective serotonin re-uptake inhibitors, resulting in seizures. It should not be used in patients with epilepsy.

Kinetics

Tramadol is well absorbed from the gut with an oral bioavailability of 70% which increases to more than 90% after repeated doses. It is metabolized in the liver by demethylation and subsequent glucuronidation to a number of metabolites, only one of which (O-desmethyltramadol) has been shown to have analgesic activity. These products are excreted in the urine. Its volume of distribution is $4 \, \text{l.kg}^{-1}$ and its elimination half-life is 5–6 hours.

Naloxone

Naloxone is a pure opioid antagonist and will reverse opioid effects at μ-, κ- and δ-receptors, although its affinity is highest for μ-receptors. Other occasional effects include hypertension, pulmonary oedema and cardiac arrhythmias and antanalgesia in opioid naive subjects.

At 1–$4 \, \mu\text{g.kg}^{-1}$ intravenously it is the drug of choice in opioid overdose. However, its duration of action at 30–40 minutes is shorter than morphine and high-dose fentanyl so that supplementary doses or an infusion of naloxone may be required.

Opioid partial agonists

This group of drugs has been used to control pain and to reverse opioid-induced respiratory depression with variable success. They are not widely used.

Nalorphine was the first partial agonist to be introduced as a morphine antagonist but was subsequently found to have analgesic effects of its own. It produced a high incidence of psychomimetic effects at analgesic doses and is no longer available in the UK.

Pentazocine produces analgesia with little respiratory depression. However, side effects including nausea, vomiting, hallucinations and dysphoria have meant that it is rarely used.

Buprenorphine is structurally similar to and more potent than morphine with a duration of up to 10 hours due to receptor binding. Due to its receptor-binding profile it produces analgesia at low concentrations (μ-receptor) but with increasing doses the NOP effects take over to produce anti-analgesic effects. Nausea and vomiting are severe and prolonged.

Nalbuphine is equipotent to morphine but appears to have a ceiling effect with respect to its respiratory depression. Unfortunately it also appears to have a ceiling effect with respect to its analgesic actions. Its actions may be reversed with naloxone.

Non-steroidal anti-inflammatory drugs (NSAIDs)

Non-steroidal anti-inflammatory drugs are used widely to treat mild to moderate pain and also to reduce opioid consumption in the peri-operative period.

The route of administration is usually oral or rectal although some agents may be administered intravenously (tenoxicam, ketorolac, parecoxib). Absorption is rapid through the small bowel. NSAIDs are highly protein bound in the plasma and have low volumes of distribution. The effects of other highly protein bound drugs (e.g. warfarin) may be potentiated as they become displaced. Characteristically these drugs are metabolized in the liver and excreted in an inactive form in the urine and bile.

Mechanism of action

Non-steroidal anti-inflammatory drugs inhibit the enzyme cyclo-oxy-genase thereby preventing the production of both prostaglandins (including prostacyclin) and thromboxanes from membrane phospholipids (Figure 9.3). Thromboxane is produced by platelets when activated by exposure to adenosine, collagen or adrenaline, and promotes haemostasis by vasoconstriction and platelet aggregation. Conversely, endothelial prostacyclin promotes vasodilatation and inhibits platelet aggregation.

Low-dose aspirin prevents arterial thromboembolism by selectively inhibiting platelet thromboxane production. Platelets have no nuclei and are therefore not able to regenerate new cyclo-oxygenase so that aspirin's effects last for the life span

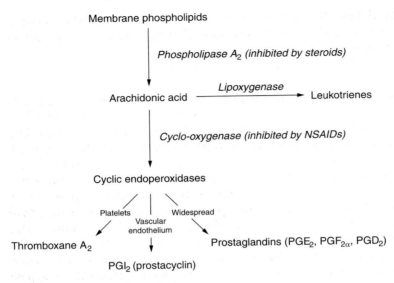

Figure 9.3. Prostaglandin synthesis.

of the platelet. The production of prostacyclin in vascular endothelium is not affected in this way, so the overall effect is selective inhibition of thromboxane.

The other NSAIDs produce reversible enzyme inhibition, the activity of cyclo-oxygenase resuming when plasma levels fall. Decreased PGE_2 and $PGF_{2\alpha}$ synthesis account for their anti-inflammatory effect, while reduced thromboxane synthesis leads to reduced platelet aggregation and adhesiveness. Their antipyretic actions are due to inhibition of centrally produced prostaglandins that stimulate pyrexia. Reduced prostaglandin synthesis in gastric mucosal cells may lead to mucosal ulceration. Lipoxygenase is not inhibited by NSAIDs and the production of leukotrienes is unaltered.

Cyclo-oxygenase (COX) exists as two isoenzymes, COX-1 and COX-2. The main molecular difference between COX-1 and COX-2 lies in the substitution of isoleucine for valine, which allows access to a hydrophobic side pocket that acts as an alternative specific binding site for drugs.

COX-1 (the constitutive form) is responsible for the production of prostaglandins that control renal blood flow and form the protective gastric mucosal barrier. In addition COX-1 mediates synthesis of thromboxane. (A variant of COX-1, which has been called COX-3 and exists centrally, is possibly the mechanism by which paracetamol reduces pain and pyrexia.)

COX-2 (the inducible form) is produced in response to tissue damage and facilitates the inflammatory response. COX-2 also mediates production of prostacyclin

(PGI$_2$) in vascular endothelium. As a result, COX-2 inhibitors may alter the delicate thromboxane/prostacyclin balance in favour of platelet aggregation, vasoconstriction and thromboembolism.

Other effects

- Gastric irritation – intestinal erosions not limited to the stomach are commonly encountered during prolonged administration of NSAIDs. These lesions result in a spectrum of adverse effects from mild pain to iron deficiency anaemia and fatal haemorrhage. Many elements (mucous layer, bicarbonate secretion, rapid cell turnover and an abundant blood supply) are involved in the protection of the intestinal mucosa against acid and enzyme attack. Prostaglandins are involved in many of these elements so that when their synthesis is inhibited, protection is reduced. During aspirin therapy acetylsalicylate and salicylate ions are trapped in the alkaline environment of the mucosal cells thereby increasing their potential for side-effects. The potential for haemorrhage is increased due to its effect on platelet function. Meloxicam is more selective towards COX-2 and has been associated with reduced gastric ulceration although a similar renal toxicity profile when compared with other NSAIDs. Diclofenac blocks both forms equally while indomethacin and aspirin have a much higher affinity for COX-1.
- NSAID sensitive asthma – acute severe asthma may be precipitated in up to 20% of asthmatics when given NSAIDs and is associated with chronic rhinitis or nasal polyps. Those affected are usually middle-aged – children are relatively spared. By inhibiting cyclo-oxygenase, more arachidonic acid is converted to leukotrienes which are known to cause bronchospasm. Aspirin also causes an abnormal reaction to the platelets of susceptible patients causing the release of cytotoxic mediators.
- Renal function – renally produced prostaglandins (PGE$_2$ and PGI$_2$) are essential in maintaining adequate renal perfusion when the level of circulating vasoconstrictors (renin, angiotensin, noradrenaline) is high. Aspirin and other NSAIDs may alter this delicate balance by inhibiting their production, reducing renal perfusion and potentially leading to acute renal failure. At low doses of aspirin (<2 g.day^{-1}), urate is retained as its tubular secretion is inhibited. At higher doses (>5 g.day^{-1}), aspirin becomes uricosuric as re-absorption of urates is inhibited to a greater degree. It is rarely used for this purpose as the side effects at higher doses are unacceptable. Analgesic nephropathy may develop after prolonged use of aspirin. The features are papillary necrosis and interstitial fibrosis. NSAIDs may precipitate fluid retention and this may become significant in those with heart failure. COX-2 inhibitors appear to lead to a greater degree of fluid retention and hypertension.
- Platelet function – while altered platelet function may be advantageous in certain circumstances (acute myocardial infarction and prevention of stroke), during the peri-operative period it may cause increased blood loss. The reduced production

Table 9.5. Classification of NSAIDs.

Group	Class	Drug
Non-specific COX inhibitors	salicylates	aspirin
	acetic acid derivatives	diclofenac, ketorolac, indomethacin
	anthralinic acids	mefanamic acid
	pyrazolones	phenylbutazone,
	proprionic acids	ibuprofen, naproxen
	para-aminophenols	paracetamol
	oxicams	tenoxicam, piroxicam
Preferential COX-2 inhibitors	oxicams	meloxicam
Specific COX-2 inhibitors	pyrazole	parecoxib, celecoxib, rofecoxib
	methylsulphone	etoricoxib
	phenylacetic acid derivative	lumaricoxib

of cyclic endoperoxidases and thromboxane A_2 prevents platelet aggregation and vasoconstriction and, therefore, inhibits the haemostatic process. The effects of aspirin on platelets last for the life span of the platelet for two reasons: platelets are unable to generate new cyclo-oxygenase and the enzyme inhibition is irreversible. Up to 14 days are required to generate new platelets. COX-2 inhibition has no effect on platelet function even at high doses.

- Drug interactions – caution should be exercised when NSAIDs are administered with anticoagulants such as heparin or warfarin, especially as the latter may be displaced from its plasma protein-binding sites, increasing its effects. Serum lithium may be increased when administered with NSAIDs and its levels should, therefore, be monitored.
- Hepatotoxicity – this is normally observed following prolonged or excessive use of NSAIDs. Up to 15% of patients may experience a rise in serum transaminase levels, even following short courses.

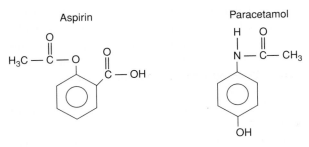

Figure 9.4. Structures of aspirin and paracetamol.

Non-specific COX inhibitors

Salicylates

Aspirin

Uses

Aspirin (acetylsalicylic acid) is widely used for its analgesic and anti-inflammatory effects. It is also used for its effects on platelet function in acute myocardial infarction and the prevention of stroke.

Mechanism of action

At low dose, aspirin selectively inhibits platelet cyclo-oxygenase while preserving vessel wall cyclo-oxygenase. This has the effect of reducing TXA_2-induced vaso-constriction and platelet aggregation while leaving vessel wall synthesis of prostag-landins unaltered and, therefore, dilated.

Other effects

- Metabolic – aspirin also has effects on the metabolic state, which are usually of little significance, but in overdose these become significant. It uncouples oxida-tive phosphorylation, thereby increasing oxygen consumption and carbon dioxide production. Initially minute ventilation is increased to keep $PaCO_2$ static. However, when aspirin levels are increased significantly the respiratory centre is stimulated directly causing a respiratory alkalosis. The picture is complicated in the premor-bid state by a metabolic acidosis. However, in children the respiratory centre is depressed by rising aspirin levels, and a metabolic acidosis occurs earlier so that a mixed respiratory and metabolic acidosis is more common.

Features of aspirin overdose

Common

- Usually conscious – only unconscious in massive overdose
- Sweaty
- Tinnitus
- Blurred vision
- Tachycardia
- Pyrexia
  - Hyperventilation
  - Respiratory alkalosis (subsequently complicated by metabolic acidosis)

Rare

- Nausea and vomiting, epigastric pain
- Oliguria
- Gastrointestinal bleed

- Pulmonary oedema (due to increased capillary permeability)
- Coagulopathy
- Hypokalaemia
- Hypo- or hyperglycaemia
- Encephalopathic, unconscious

Treatment

- Activated charcoal
- Forced alkaline diuresis
- Haemofiltration/haemodialysis

Reye's syndrome is uncommon and affects mainly children. Its aetiology has been linked to aspirin. It causes widespread mitochondrial damage, fatty changes in the liver progressing to hepatic failure, encephalopathy with cerebral oedema and has a mortality rate of up to 40%. Therefore, aspirin is only recommended for children below 12 years of age when specifically indicated, for example, for juvenile arthritis (Still's disease).

Kinetics

Aspirin is a weak acid with a $pK_a = 3$ and is present essentially in the unionized form in the stomach allowing gastric absorption, but due to the relatively alkaline nature of the mucosal cells salicylate ions may become trapped and unable to reach the systemic circulation. However, due to total surface area the small bowel absorbs more drug. Once in the systemic circulation, 85% is protein bound, mainly by albumin. It is rapidly hydrolyzed by intestinal and hepatic esterases to salicylate, which undergoes further hepatic metabolism to salicyluric acid and glucuronide derivatives. Salicylate and its metabolites are excreted in the urine (enhanced under alkaline conditions). The elimination half-life varies because glycine conjugation (converting salicylate to salicyluric acid) may become saturated in overdose resulting in zero-order kinetics.

Para-aminophenols

Paracetamol

While paracetamol has essentially no effect on cyclo-oxygenase in vitro it has been classified as a NSAID because of its moderate analgesic and antipyretic properties. It has been proposed that its antipyretic actions are due to inhibition of prostaglandin synthesis within the central nervous system, by inhibition of COX-3, a COX-1 variant.

Presentation and uses

Paracetamol is presented as 500 mg tablets alone and in combination with weak opioids. Suppositories contain 125 mg and 1 g and the paediatric elixir contains

120 mg in 5 ml. A preparation containing 100 mg methionine and 500 mg paracetamol is available but at increased cost. A solution of 1 g in 100 mls is available for intravenous use. The adult dose is 4 g.day^{-1} in divided doses. The initial paediatric dose is 15–30 mg.kg^{-1} which is then reduced to 10–15 mg.kg^{-1} every 4 hours with a maximum dose of 90 mg.kg^{-1}.day^{-1}.

Kinetics

Paracetamol is well absorbed from the small bowel and has an oral bioavailability of 80%. Unlike the other NSAIDs it does not cause gastric irritation, is less protein bound (10%) and has a larger volume of distribution. Paracetamol is metabolized by the liver mainly to glucuronide conjugates but also to sulphate and cysteine conjugates. These are actively excreted in the urine, only a small fraction being excreted unchanged. N-acetyl-p-amino-benzoquinoneimine is a highly toxic metabolite of paracetamol that is produced in small amounts following therapeutic doses. It is rapidly conjugated with hepatic glutathione to render it harmless.

Toxicity

Following a toxic dose, the normal hepatic conjugation pathways become saturated so that more N-acetyl-p-amino-benzoquinoneimine is produced which rapidly exhausts hepatic glutathione. It is then free to form covalent bonds with sulphydryl groups on hepatocytes resulting in cell death and centrilobular hepatic necrosis. Treatment with oral methionine and oral or intravenous acetylcysteine is directed at replenishing hepatic glutathione. Methionine enhances glutathione synthesis while acetylcysteine is hydrolyzed to cysteine, which is a glutathione precursor. Intravenous acetylcysteine is preferred as vomiting is common in paracetamol overdose.

Features of paracetamol overdose

- Normally remain conscious
- Nausea and vomiting
- Epigastric pain
- Sweating
- Erythema, urticaria, mucosal lesions
- Acute haemolytic anaemia
- Peripheral vasodilatation and shock following massive overdose
- Delayed hyperglycaemia
- Hepatic failure after 48 hours
  - LFT and clotting (INR) worst at 3–5 days
  - Cholestasis
  - Fulminant hepatic failure at 3–7 days

Treatment
- Activated charcoal
- Intravenous glucose
- Acetylcysteine or methionine
- Early referral to specialist centre

Acetic acid derivatives

Diclofenac

Diclofenac is a phenylacetic acid derivative.

Presentation

Diclofenac is available in a parenteral as well as an oral and rectal formulation. The intravenous preparation should be diluted and administered over a minimum of 30 minutes. It is also available in combination with misoprostil, which provides prophylaxis against gastric and duodenal ulceration. The maximum adult dose is 150 mg.day^{-1} in divided doses. The paediatric dose is 1 mg.kg^{-1} tds for pain associated with minor surgery (tonsillectomy, inguinal herniotomy).

Uses

Diclofenac may be used alone to treat mild to moderate post-operative pain or to reduce opioid consumption when treating severe pain. It is particularly useful in treating renal colic. Owing to its effects on cyclo-oxygenase it may also precipitate gastric irritation, acute renal impairment and reduced platelet function, which often prevents it from being used in major surgery.

Other effects

- Gut – diclofenac produces less gastric irritation than both indomethacin and aspirin.
- Pain – the parenteral formulation is highly irritant and intramuscular injection may be very painful and is associated with muscle damage. Intravenous injection causes local thrombosis.
- Interactions – plasma concentrations of lithium and digoxin may be increased. In general it does not effect either oral anticoagulants or oral hypoglycaemic agents, but isolated reports would suggest that close monitoring is used.

Kinetics

In keeping with other drugs in its class diclofenac is well absorbed from the gut, highly plasma protein bound (99%) and has a small volume of distribution (0.15 l.kg^{-1}). It undergoes hepatic hydroxylation and conjugation to inactive metabolites that are excreted in the urine (60%) and bile (40%).

Table 9.6. Clinical and kinetic data for some NSAIDs.

Drug	Maximum daily dose	Elimination half-life (h)	Plasma protein-binding (%)	Analgesic and antipyretic activity	Anti-inflammatory activity
Aspirin	4 g	variable[*]	85	+++	++
Paracetamol	4 g	2	10	+++	++
Diclofenac	150 mg	1–2	99	+	+++
Ketorolac	40 mg	5	99	++	+
Indomethacin	200 mg	6	95	+	+++
Phenylbutazone	300 mg	50–100	98	+	++++
Tenoxicam	20 mg	72	99	+	++
Meloxicam	15 mg	20	99	+	++
Ibuprofen	1.8 g	2–3	99	+	+

[*] When obeying first-order kinetics the $t_{1/2}$ elimination of aspirin is short (15–30 min). However, this is significantly prolonged when enzyme systems become saturated and its kinetics become zero-order.

Ketorolac

Ketorolac is an acetic acid derivative with potent analgesic activity but limited anti-inflammatory activity. It is also a potent antipyretic. It may be given orally or parenterally and has a duration of action of up to 6 hours. It shares the side-effect profile common to all NSAIDs.

Indomethacin

Indomethacin is a potent anti-inflammatory agent but is a less effective analgesic. Rectal use has been associated not only with a reduced peri-operative opioid requirement, but also with reduced platelet function resulting in wound haematoma and increased blood loss. It is used to promote closure of the ductus arteriosus in the premature infant by inhibiting prostaglandin synthesis. It shares the other effects common to NSAIDs but has been particularly linked with headache. It may also impair hepatic function and antagonize the effects of diuretics and angiotensin-converting enzyme inhibitors.

Kinetics

Indomethacin is well absorbed from the gut with an oral bioavailability of 80%. It is more than 99% bound by plasma proteins and is metabolized to inactive metabolites that are excreted in the urine and bile. Five percent is excreted unchanged.

Pyrazolones

Phenylbutazone

Phenylbutazone is a potent anti-inflammatory agent. Its use has been limited to hospital patients with ankylosing spondylitis due to serious haematological side effects including agranulocytosis and aplastic anaemia. It is significantly bound by plasma proteins and will interact with other highly bound drugs. It may also impair hepatic function, produce a rash, and cause sodium and water retention.

Proprionic acids

Ibuprofen

Ibuprofen is prepared as 200–600 mg tablets and as a paediatric elixir containing 20 mg.ml^{-1}. It is not recommended for children below 1 year of age. The paediatric dose is 20 mg.kg^{-1}.day^{-1} in divided doses. It has mild anti-inflammatory and analgesic effects but has the lowest incidence of side effects of the most commonly used NSAIDs.

Oxicams

Tenoxicam

Tenoxicam exhibits many of the features common with other NSAIDs. Two specific features make it particularly useful in the peri-operative period:
- It may be given intravenously resulting in a rapid onset of action.
- It has a long elimination half-life (72 hours) resulting in a long duration of action and allowing once-daily dosage.

However, these advantages may become disadvantages if side effects become significant.

Kinetics

Tenoxicam is well absorbed from the gut and has a high oral bioavailability. It is highly plasma protein bound (99%). Clearance from the body is due to metabolism to an inactive metabolite that is excreted in the urine (66%) and in bile (33%). The dose is 20 mg.day^{-1}.

Preferential COX–2 inhibitors

Meloxicam

Meloxicam is available as tablets and suppositories and the initial dose is 7.5 mg.day^{-1}, which may be doubled.

Meloxicam has limited preferential selectivity for COX-2 and is quoted as being between 3 to 50 times as potent against COX-2. At a dose of 7.5 mg.day^{-1} it has a reduced gastrointestinal side-effect profile when compared with diclofenac, although its renal side-effect profile appears to be equivalent to other NSAIDs.

Kinetics

Meloxicam is slowly but almost completely absorbed from the gut with an oral bioavailability of 90%. It is 99% protein bound, essentially to albumin. Metabolism occurs in the liver to inactive metabolites that are excreted in the urine (50%) and bile

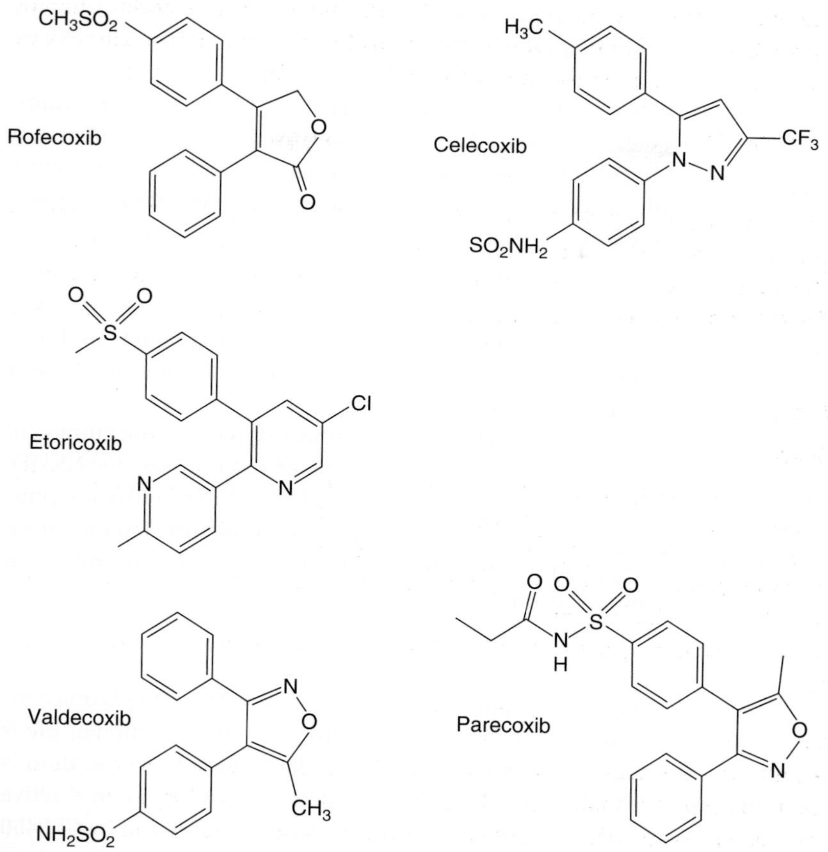

Figure 9.5. Structures of some COX-2 inhibitors.

(50%). Three percent is excreted unchanged in the urine. The elimination half-life is 20 hours.

Specific COX-2 inhibitors

It is possible that by the time this edition goes to print further COX-2 inhibitors will have been withdrawn from the market due to concerns about myocardial infarction (MI) and stroke. It is currently unclear if these concerns revolve around individual drugs or the entire class of COX-2 inhibitors.

Initially, large studies suggested that there was a significantly reduced incidence of gastrointestinal side effects associated with COX-2 inhibitors compared with standard NSAIDs. However, the Food and Drug Administration (FDA) later presented further data that exposed the increased MI and stroke rates but also a gastrointestinal side-effect rate equal to standard NSAIDs after 12 months therapy as well as a number of other side-effects – hypertension, heart failure, hepatotoxicity and oedema.

The Committee on Safety of Medicines have advised that COX-2 use is contraindicated in patients with ischaemic heart disease, cerebrovascular disease, mild heart failure and peripheral vascular disease. Careful consideration should be given before their use in patients with risk factors for cardiovascular events (hypertension, hyperlipidaemia, diabetes, smoking).

Rofecoxib

Rofecoxib (withdrawn September 2004) is presented as 12.5 mg tablets and as a suspension containing 12.5 mg per 5 mls. The daily dose is 12.5–25 mg. It has a COX-1:COX-2 inhibitory ratio of 1:276.

The VIGOR study demonstrated that rofecoxib significantly reduces the number of clinically important gastric complications when compared to a non-specific NSAID. However, more comprehensive analysis of further data beyond 12 months, not published with the original article, revealed a much less favourable picture. The incidence of MI was 1.7% in those taking rofecoxib compared with 0.7% in the control group which prompted its withdrawl from the market.

Kinetics

Rofecoxib is well absorbed from the gut (oral bioavailability >90%) with plasma concentration peaking at 3 hours. It is 85% protein bound and the plasma half-life is around 17 hours allowing once-daily administration. Its volume of distribution is 1.2 l.kg. It is metabolized in the liver by cytosolic reduction (not CYP450) to inactive products that are excreted in the urine. As rofecoxib is not metabolized by CYP450 it has fewer potential interactions than celecoxib. Rofecoxib appears to be safe in subjects with previous adverse cutaneous reactions (erythema, urticaria angioedema) to non-specific NSAIDs.

Celecoxib

Celecoxib is presented as 100 mg tablets and used to a maximum dose of 200 mg bd for osteoarthritis and rheumatoid arthritis. It has a COX-1:COX-2 inhibitory ratio of 1:30.

The CLASS trial demonstrated the incidence of ulcer complications in patients treated with celecoxib was similar to those treated with non-specific NSAIDs, although this may have been confused by concurrent aspirin therapy. Also the incidence of stroke and MI was not increased by celecoxib. Other studies designed to assess the ability of celecoxib to prevent colon cancer have confused the picture regarding stroke and MI because on this point they did not agree.

Kinetics

Celecoxib reaches peak plasma concentration after 2–3 hours and has an elimination half-life of 8–12 hours. It is 97% protein bound and has a volume of distribution of 5.7 l.kg. It is metabolized by hepatic CYP2C9 to inactive metabolites so that only a small amount appears unchanged in the urine. Drugs that inhibit (omeprazole) or induce (carbamazepine) CYP2C9 will increase or decrease plasma concentrations.

It has a sulphonamide group and therefore should not be used in patients with a sulphonamide allergy.

Valdecoxib and parecoxib

Parecoxib is a prodrug, which is converted to the active moiety valdecoxib. Its half-life is 45 minutes and has no actions of its own. Valdecoxib has been withdrawn (April 2005) due to serious dermatological side effects (see below). At the time of writing paracoxib remains in use and has not been associated with similar dermatological side effects probably due to its short-term use. It has a COX-1:COX-2 inhibitory ratio of 1:61.

Parecoxib is a parenteral COX-2 antagonist and should be reconstituted with 0.9% saline prior to administration. The initial dose is 40 mg (i.m. or i.v.) followed by 20–40 mg 6–12 hourly up to a maximum dose of 80 mg per day.

Kinetics

Parecoxib is converted to valdecoxib by enzymatic hydrolysis in the liver. Valdecoxib undergoes hepatic metabolism by CYP2C9, CYP3A4 and glucuronidation to many metabolites, one of which antagonizes COX-2. Due to its hepatic elimination, renal impairment does not influence its kinetics, but it is not recommended in severe hepatic impairment.

The dose should be reduced when coadministered with fluconazole due to inhibition of CYP2C9, although no adjustment is necessary when coadministered with ketoconazole or midazolam which is metabolized by CYP3A4. Valdecoxib appears to inhibit other cytochrome P450 enzymes and may increase the plasma concentration of flecanide and metoprolol (CYP2D6 inhibition), and omeprazole, phenytoin and diazepam (CYP2C19 inhibition).

Parecoxib has a plasma half-life of 20 minutes while valdecoxib has an elimination half-life of 8 hours.

Hypersensitivity reactions including exfoliative dermatitis, Stevens–Johnson syndrome, toxic dermal necrosis and angiodema have been reported following valdecoxib in those who also have sulphonamide sensitivity. The overall reporting rate is in the order of 8 per million patients. It is, therefore, contraindicated in this group. However, parecoxib has a non-aromatic sulphonamide group similar to frusemide and tolbutamide, neither of which is contraindicated in sulphonamide sensitivity.

Etoricoxib

Etoricoxib is a highly selective COX-2 inhibitor that has a UK license but is awaiting FDA approval. It is a methylsulphone.

It has been shown to be efficacious in providing effective pain control when compared to COX-1 inhibitors. It has a COX-1:COX-2 inhibitory ratio of 1:344.

Kinetics

Etoricoxib is absorbed efficiently producing an oral bioavailability of > 95%. It has a volume of distribution of 1.5 l.kg^{-1} and is 90% plasma protein bound. Its elimination half-life is 22 hours. It is metabolized in the liver through cytochrome P450 oxidation, CYP3A4 being the predominant isoenzyme. However, other isoenzymes are involved and may become more involved with specific CYP3A4 inhibition. It is a weak inhibitor of CYP-2D6, -3A, and -2C9. Its elimination half-life increases in hepatic failure, but in isolated renal failure no change is seen.

Its side effects (or lack of them) are predictable. Its rate of gastric irritation is similar to placebo and significantly lower than COX-1 inhibitors, although this effect decreases beyond 9–12 months therapy. There is currently insufficient data to confirm that etoricoxib will be free from the cardiovascular effects that caused rofecoxib to be withdrawn from the market.

Lumaricoxib

Lumaricoxib is a phenylacetic acid derivative and as such is structurally different from the other COX-2 inhibitors, bearing a closer resemblance to diclofenac. It has a COX-1:COX-2 inhibitory ratio of 1:700. Due to its structure it has a lower volume of distribution compared with the other COX-2 inhibitors.

Following reports of serious hepatoxicity including cases resulting in death or liver transplantation, lumaricoxib is now contraindicated in patients with any current liver disease or a history of drug induced elevation of transaminases. In addition liver function tests are required during treatment.

Kinetics

It has the shortest elimination half-life of 5 hours.

Local anaesthetics

Physiology

Individual nerve fibres are made up of a central core (axoplasm) and a phospholipid membrane containing integral proteins, some of which function as ion channels.

The resting membrane potential

The neuronal membrane contains the enzyme Na^+/K^+ ATPase that actively maintains a thirty fold K^+ concentration gradient (greater concentration inside) and a ten fold Na^+ concentration gradient (greater concentration outside). K^+ tends to flow down its concentration gradient out of the cell due to the selective permeability of the membrane. However, intracellular anionic proteins tend to oppose this ionic flux, and the balance of these processes results in the resting membrane potential of -80 mV (negative inside). It can, therefore, be seen that the ratio of intracellular to extracellular K^+ alters the resting membrane potential. Hypokalaemia increases (makes more negative) the resting membrane potential while the Na^+ concentration has little effect, as the membrane is essentially impermeable to Na^+ when in the resting state.

The action potential

The action potential is generated by altered Na^+ permeability across the phospholipid membrane and lasts only 1–2 milliseconds. Electrical or chemical triggers initially cause a slow rise in membrane potential until the threshold potential (about -50 mV) is reached. Voltage sensitive Na^+ channels then open, increasing Na^+ permeability dramatically and the membrane potential briefly reaches $+30$ mV (approaching the Na^+ equilibrium potential of $+67$ mV) at which point the Na^+ channels close. The membrane potential returns to its resting value with an increased efflux of K^+. The Na^+/K^+ ATPase restores the concentration gradients although the total number of ions moving across the membrane is small. Conduction along unmyelinated fibres is relatively slow compared with myelinated fibres where current jumps from one node of Ranvier to another (saltatory conduction) and reaches 120 m.s^{-1}. Retrograde conduction is not possible under normal circumstances due to inactive Na^+ channels following the action potential.

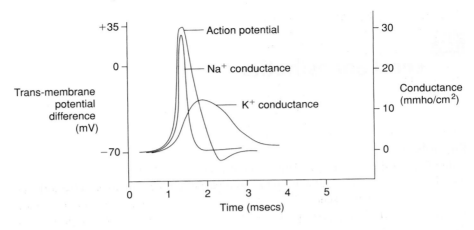

Figure 10.1. Changes in Na^+ and K^+ conductance during the action potential.

Local anaesthetics

Preparations

Local anaesthetics are formulated as the hydrochloride salt to render them water-soluble. They often contain the preservative sodium metabisulphite and a fungicide. Multi-dose bottles contain 1 mg.ml^{-1} of the preservative methyl parahydroxybenzoate. Only the single-dose ampoules without additives (apart from glucose at 80 mg.ml^{-1} used in 'heavy' bupivacaine) are suitable for subarachnoid administration as the preservatives carry the risk of producing arachnoiditis. Adrenaline or felypressin (a synthetic derivative of vasopressin with no antidiuretic effect) are added to some local anaesthetic solutions in an attempt to slow down absorption from the site of injection and to prolong the duration of action. Lidocaine is available in a large range of concentrations varying from 0.5% to 10%. The high concentrations are used as a spray to anaesthetize mucous membranes (note 1% $= 10$ mg.ml^{-1}).

Mechanism of action

Local anaesthetic action is dependent on blockade of the Na^+ channel. Unionized lipid-soluble drug passes through the phospholipid membrane where in the axoplasm it is protonated. In this ionized form it binds to the internal surface of a Na^+ channel, preventing it from leaving the inactive state. The degree of blockade in vitro is proportional to the rate of stimulation due to the attraction of local anaesthetic to 'open' Na^+ channels (Figure 10.2).

Alternatively, 'membrane expansion' may offer an additional mechanism of action. Unionized drug dissolves into the phospholipid membrane and may cause swelling of the Na^+ channel/lipoprotein matrix resulting in its inactivation.

Table 10.1. Classification of local anaesthetics.

Esters −CO.O−	Amides −NH.CO−
Procaine	Lidocaine
Amethocaine	Prilocaine
Cocaine	Bupivacaine
	Ropivacaine
	Dibucaine

Physiochemical characteristics

Local anaesthetics are weak bases and exist predominantly in the ionized form at neutral pH as their pK_a exceeds 7.4. They fall into one of two chemical groupings, ester or amide, which describes the linkage between the aromatic lipophilic group and the hydrophilic group that each group possesses. Esters are comparatively unstable in solution, unlike amides that have a shelf-life of up to 2 years (Table 10.1, Figure 10.3).

The individual structures confer different physiochemical and clinical character-istics.

- **Potency** is closely correlated to **lipid solubility** in vitro, but less so in vivo. Other fac-tors such as vasodilator properties and tissue distribution determine the amount of local anaesthetic that is available at the nerve.
- The **duration of action** is closely associated with the extent of **protein binding**. Local anaesthetics with limited protein binding have a short duration of action, and conversely those with more extensive protein binding have a longer duration of action.
- The **onset of action** is closely related to pK_a. Local anaesthetics are weak bases and exist mainly in the ionized form at normal pH. Those with a high pK_a have a greater fraction present in the ionized form, which is unable to penetrate the phospholipid membrane, resulting in a slow onset of action. Conversely, a low

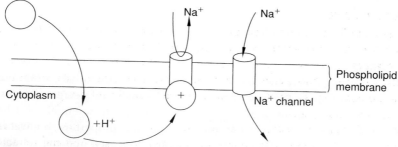

Figure 10.2. Mechanism of action of local anaesthetics.

pK_a reflects a higher fraction present in the unionized form and, therefore, a faster onset of action as more is available to cross the phospholipid membrane.

- The intrinsic **vasodilator activity** varies between drugs and influences **potency** and **duration of action**. In general, local anaesthetics cause vasodilatation in low concentrations (prilocaine > lidocaine > bupivacaine > ropivacaine) and vasoconstriction at higher concentrations. However, cocaine has solely vasoconstrictor actions by inhibiting neuronal uptake of catecholamines (uptake 1) and inhibiting MAO.

However, total dose and concentration of administered local anaesthetic will also have a significant effect on a given clinical situation.

Local anaesthetics are generally ineffective when used to anaesthetize infected tissue. The acidic environment further reduces the unionized fraction of drug available to diffuse into and block the nerve. There may also be increased local vascularity, which increases removal of drug from the site.

Lidocaine: $pK_a = 7.9$

At pH 7.4

$$pH = pKa + \log\left\{\frac{[B]}{[BH^+]}\right\}$$

$$7.4 = 7.9 + \log\left\{\frac{[B]}{[BH^+]}\right\}$$

$$-0.5 = \log\left\{\frac{[B]}{[BH^+]}\right\}$$

$$0.3 = \left\{\frac{[B]}{[BH^+]}\right\}$$

so 75% ionized and 25% unionized.

At pH of 7.1

$$7.1 = 7.9 + \log\left\{\frac{[B]}{[BH^+]}\right\}$$

$$0.16 = \left\{\frac{[B]}{[BH^+]}\right\}$$

so 86% ionized and 14% unionized (i.e. less available to penetrate nerves).

Other effects

- Cardiac – lidocaine may be used to treat ventricular arrhythmias, while bupivacaine is not. Both drugs block cardiac Na^+ channels and decrease the maximum rate of increase of phase 0 of the cardiac action potential (cf. Chapter 14). They also have direct myocardial depressant properties (bupivacaine > lidocaine). The PR and QRS intervals are also increased and the refractory period prolonged. However, bupivacaine is ten times slower at dissociating from the Na^+ channels, resulting in persistent depression. This may lead to re-entrant arrhythmias and ventricular fibrillation. In addition, tachycardia may enhance frequency-dependent blockade by bupivacaine, which adds to its cardiac toxicity. Life-threatening arrhythmias may also reflect disruption of Ca^{2+} and K^+ channels. Ropivacaine differs from bupivacaine both in the substitution of a propyl for a butyl group and in its preparation as a single, S, enantiomer. It dissociates more rapidly from cardiac Na^+ channels and produces less direct myocardial depression than bupivacaine, and is, therefore, less toxic. However, it has a slightly shorter duration of action and is slightly less potent than bupivacaine resulting in a slightly larger dose requirement for an equivalent block.

- Central nervous system – local anaesthetics penetrate the brain rapidly and have a bi-phasic effect. Initially inhibitory interneurones are blocked resulting in excitatory phenomenon – circumoral tingling, visual disturbance, tremors, and dizziness. This is followed by convulsions. Finally, all central neurones are depressed leading to coma and apnoea.

Kinetics

Absorption

The absorption of local anaesthetics into the systemic circulation varies depending on the characteristics of the agent used, the presence of added vasoconstrictor and the site of injection.

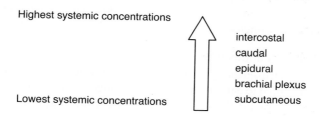

Highest systemic concentrations

intercostal
caudal
epidural
brachial plexus
Lowest systemic concentrations
subcutaneous

Clearly, if local anaesthetic is inadvertently injected into a vein or artery, very high systemic levels will result and possibly cause central nervous system or cardiovascular toxicity. Less than 10 mg lidocaine inadvertently injected into the carotid or vertebral artery will result in a rapid rise in central nervous system concentrations and will cause coma and possibly apnoea and cardiac arrest.

Distribution

Ester local anaesthetics are minimally bound while amides are more extensively bound (bupivacaine > ropivacaine > lidocaine > prilocaine) in the plasma. α_1-Acid glycoprotein binds local anaesthetic with high affinity although albumin binds a greater quantity due to its relative abundance. When protein binding is increased (pregnancy, myocardial infarction, renal failure, post-operatively and in infancy) the free fraction of drug is reduced.

The degree of protein binding will affect the degree of placental transfer. Bupivacaine is more highly bound than lidocaine, so less crosses the placenta. If the foetus becomes acidotic there will be an increase in the ionized fraction and local anaesthetic will accumulate in the foetus (ion trapping). Ester local anaesthetics do not cross the placenta in significant amounts due to their rapid metabolism.

Metabolism and elimination

Esters are hydrolyzed rapidly by plasma cholinesterases and other esterases to inactive compounds. Para-aminobenzoate is one of the main metabolites and has been associated with hypersensitivity reactions especially in the atopic patient. This rapid hydrolysis results in a short elimination half-life. Cocaine is the exception, undergoing hepatic hydrolysis to water-soluble metabolites that are excreted in the urine.

Amides undergo hepatic metabolism by amidases. Amidase metabolism is much slower than plasma hydrolysis and so amides are more prone to accumulation when administered by continuous infusion. Reduced hepatic blood flow or hepatic dysfunction can decrease amide metabolism.

Toxic doses

Raised systemic blood levels of local anaesthetic lead initially to the central nervous system and then to cardiovascular toxicity. However, the absorption of local anaesthetic varies widely depending on the site of administration and presence of vasoconstrictors. Therefore, the concept of a toxic dose without regard to the site of administration is meaningless. The toxic plasma levels are given in Table 10.2.

Intravenous regional anaesthesia

Bupivacaine has been used for intravenous regional techniques, but following a number of deaths attributed to cardiac toxicity it is no longer used in this way. Prilocaine (0.5%) is commonly used in this setting although lidocaine may also be used.

Lidocaine

Lidocaine is an amide local anaesthetic that is also used to control ventricular tachyarrhythmias. It has class Ib anti-arrhythmic actions (see Chapter 14).

Preparations

Lidocaine is formulated as the hydrochloride and is presented as a colourless solution (0.5–2%) with or without adrenaline (1 in 80–200 000); a 2% gel; a 5% ointment; a spray delivering 10 mg.dose^{-1} and a 4% solution for topical use on mucous membranes.

Kinetics

Lidocaine is 70% protein bound to α_1-acid glycoprotein. It is extensively metabolized in the liver by dealkylation to monoethylglycine-xylidide and acetaldehyde.

Table 10.2. Some pharmacological properties of various local anaesthetics.

	Relative potency	Onset	Duration of action	Toxic plasma concentration ($\mu g.ml^{-1}$)	pK_a	Percentage unionized (at pH 7.4)	Plasma protein bound (%)	Relative lipid solubility	Elimination half-life (min)
Amethocaine	8	slow	long		8.5	7	75	200	80
Cocaine	2	moderate	short	0.5	8.6	5	95		100
Lidocaine	2	fast	moderate	>5	7.9	25	70	150	100
Prilocaine	2	fast	moderate	>5	7.7	33	55	50	100
Bupivacaine	8	moderate	long	>1.5	8.1	15	95	1000	160
Ropivacaine	8	moderate	long	>4	8.1	15	94	300	120
Mepivacaine	2	slow	moderate	>5	7.6	40	77	50	115

The former is further hydrolyzed while the latter is hydroxylated to 4-hydroxy–2, 6-xylidine forming the main metabolite, which is excreted in the urine. Some of the metabolic products of lidocaine have anti-arrhythmic properties while others may potentiate lidocaine-induced seizures.

Clearance is reduced in the presence of hepatic or cardiac failure.

Eutectic mixture of local anaesthetic (EMLA)

When two compounds are mixed to produce a substance that behaves with a single set of physical characteristics, it is said to be eutectic. Eutectic mixture of local anaesthetic (5%) contains a mixture of crystalline bases of 2.5% lidocaine and 2.5% prilocaine in a white oil:water emulsion. The mixture has a lower melting point, being an oil at room temperature, while the individual components would be crystalline solids.

Presentation and uses

Eutectic mixture of local anaesthetic is presented as an emulsion in tubes containing 5 g or 30 g. It is used to anaesthetize skin before vascular cannulation or harvesting for skin grafts. It should be applied to intact skin under an occlusive dressing for at least 60 minutes to ensure adequate anaesthesia.

Cautions

EMLA cream should be avoided in patients with congenital or idiopathic methaemoglobinaemia, or in infants less than 12 months of age who are receiving treatment with methaemoglobin-inducing drugs. Patients taking drugs associated with methaemoglobinaemia (e.g. sulphonamides or phenytoin) are at greater risk of developing methaemoglobinaemia if concurrently treated with EMLA cream. Methaemoglobinaemia is caused by o-toluidine, a metabolite of prilocaine.

EMLA should not be used on mucous membranes due to rapid systemic absorption. EMLA should be used with caution in patients receiving class I anti-arrhythmic drugs (e.g. tocainide, mexiletine) because the toxic effects are additive and potentially synergistic.

Bupivacaine

Presentation and uses

Bupivacaine is prepared as a 0.25% and 0.5% (with or without 1:200 000 adrenaline) solution. A 0.5% preparation containing 80 mg.ml^{-1} glucose (specific gravity 1.026) is available for subarachnoid block.

It remains the mainstay of epidural infusions in labour and post-operatively despite concerns regarding its potential cardiac toxicity and the availability of newer drugs (ropivacaine and levobupivacaine). The maximum dose is said to be 2 mg.kg^{-1}.

Kinetics

The onset of action is intermediate or slow and significantly slower than that of lidocaine. It is the most highly protein bound amide local anaesthetic and is metabolized in the liver by dealkylation to pipecolic acid and pipecolylxylidine.

Levobupivacaine

Levobupivacaine is the S-enantiomer of bupivacaine, which is the racemic mixture of the S- and R-enantiomer.

Presentation and uses

Levobupivacaine is prepared as a 2.5, 5 and 7.5 mg.ml^{-1} solution. It is used in a manner similar to that of bupivacaine. A maximum single dose of 150 mg is recommended with a maximum dose over 24 hours of 400 mg.

Toxicity profile

The single advantage of levobupivacaine over bupivacaine and other local anaesthetics is its potential for reduced toxicity. While extrapolation of research from animal models to humans may be confusing, combined with limited human volunteer work it appears that levobupivacaine has two potentially useful properties. First, the dose required to produce myocardial depression (by blocking cardiac K$^+$ channels) is higher for levobupivacaine compared with bupivacaine, and second, excitatory central nervous system effects or convulsions occur at lower doses with bupivacaine than levobupivacaine.

Ropivacaine

Presentation and uses

The amide local anaesthetic ropivacaine is prepared in three concentrations (2, 7.5 and 10 mg.ml^{-1}), in two volumes (10 and 100 ml) and as the pure S-enantiomer. It is not prepared in combination with a vasoconstrictor as this does not alter its duration of action or uptake from tissues. The R-enantiomer is less potent and more toxic. It has a propyl group on its piperidine nitrogen in contrast to the butyl group present in bupivacaine and the methyl group present in mepivacaine (Figure 10.3).

The main differences from bupivacaine lie in its pure enantiomeric formulation, improved toxic profile and lower lipid solubility. Its lower lipid solubility may result in reduced penetration of the large myelinated Aβ motor fibres, so that initially these fibres are relatively spared from local anaesthetic. However, during continuous infusion they too will become blocked by local anaesthetic resulting in similar degrees of block between Aβ fibres and the smaller unmyelinated C fibres. Therefore, the motor block produced by ropivacaine is slower in onset, less dense and of shorter duration when compared with an equivalent dose of bupivacaine. Theoretically it

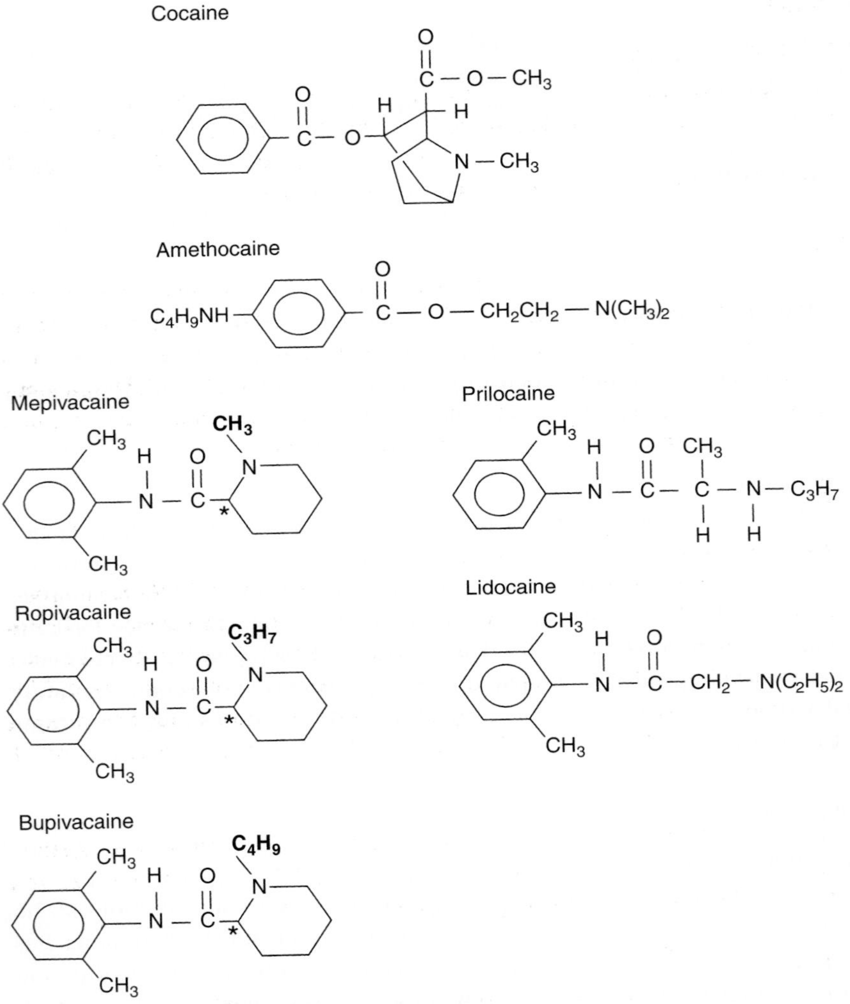

Figure 10.3. Structure of some local anaesthetics. Asterisk marks chiral centre.

would appear more appropriate than bupivacaine for epidural infusion due to its sensory/motor discrimination and greater clearance.

Kinetics

Ropivacaine is metabolized in the liver by aromatic hydroxylation, mainly to 3-hydroxy-ropivacaine, but also to 4-hydroxy-ropivacaine, both of which have some local anaesthetic activity.

Prilocaine

Presentation and uses

Prilocaine is presented as a 0.5–2.0% solution. It is also available as a 3% solution with felypressin (0.03 unit.ml^{-1}) for dental use. It has similar indications to lidocaine but is most frequently used for intravenous regional anaesthesia. The maximum dose is 6 mg.kg^{-1} or 8 mg.kg^{-1} when administered with felypressin.

Kinetics

Prilocaine is the most rapidly metabolized amide local anaesthetic, metabolism occurring not only in the liver, but also the kidney and lung. When given in large doses one of its metabolites, o-toluidine, may precipitate methaemoglobinaemia. This may require treatment with ascorbic acid or methylene blue, which act as reducing agents. The neonate is at special risk as its red blood cells are deficient in methaemoglobin reductase. EMLA cream may precipitate the same reaction.

Cocaine

Presentation and uses

Cocaine is an ester local anaesthetic derived from the leaves of *Erythroxylon coca*, a plant indigenous to Bolivia and Peru. It is used for topical anaesthesia and local vasoconstriction. Moffatt's solution (2 ml 8% cocaine, 2 ml 1% sodium bicarbonate, 1 ml 1:1000 adrenaline) has been used in the nasal cavities, although its potential for side effects has rendered it less popular. Cocaine is also formulated as a paste ranging from 1% to 4%. A maximum dose of 1.5 mg.kg^{-1} or 100 mg is currently recommended.

Mechanism of action

Cocaine blocks uptake 1 and MAO while also stimulating the central nervous system. These combined effects increase the likelihood of precipitating hypertension and arrhythmias. Its use also provokes hyperthermia.

Side effects

When taken or administered in high doses it can cause confusion, hallucinations, seizures, arrhythmias and cardiac rupture.

Kinetics

Cocaine is absorbed well from mucous membranes and is highly protein bound (about 95%). Unlike other esters it undergoes significant hepatic hydrolysis to inactive products, which are excreted in the urine.

Amethocaine

Amethocaine is an ester local anaesthetic used for topical anaesthesia. It is presented as 0.5% and 1% drops for topical use before local anaesthetic block or as a sole agent for lens surgery. It may produce a burning sensation on initial instillation. It is also available as a 4% cream for topical anaesthesia to the skin and is used in a similar fashion to EMLA cream. However, it has a faster onset of action, producing good topical anaesthesia by 30 minutes, following which it may be removed. Its effects last for 4–6 hours. It produces some local vasodilatation and erythema, which may assist venous cannulation.

Muscle relaxants and anticholinesterases

Physiology

The neuromuscular junction (NMJ) forms a chemical bridge between the motor neurone and skeletal muscle. The final short section of the motor nerve is unmyelinated and comes to lie in a gutter on the surface of the muscle fibre at its mid-point – each being innervated by a single axonal terminal from a fast Aα neurone (*en plaque* appearance). However, for the intra-occular, intrinsic laryngeal and some facial muscles the pattern of innervation is different with multiple terminals from slower Aγ neurones scattered over the muscle surface (*en grappe* appearance). Here, muscle contraction depends on a wave of impulses throughout the terminals.

The post-synaptic membrane has many folds; the shoulders contain ACh receptors while the clefts contain the enzyme acetylcholinesterase (AChE), which is responsible for the hydrolysis of ACh (Figure 11.1).

Acetylcholine

Synthesis

The synthesis of ACh (Figure 11.2) is dependent on acetyl-coenzyme A and choline, which is derived from the diet and recycled from the breakdown of ACh. Once synthesized in the axoplasm it is transferred into small synaptic vesicles where it is stored prior to release.

Release

When an action potential arrives at a nerve terminal it triggers Ca^{2+} influx, which then combines with various proteins to trigger the release of vesicular ACh. About 200 such vesicles (each containing about 10 000 ACh molecules) are released in response to each action potential.

Acetylcholine receptor

Nicotinic ACh receptors are in groups on the edges of the junctional folds on the post-synaptic membrane. They are integral membrane proteins with a molecular weight of 250 000 Da and consist of five subunits (two α, and a single β, ϵ and δ in adults). They are configured with a central ion channel that opens when the α subunits (each of 40 000 Da) bind ACh. Binding the initial molecule of ACh increases the affinity of the second α subunit for ACh. These receptors are also present on

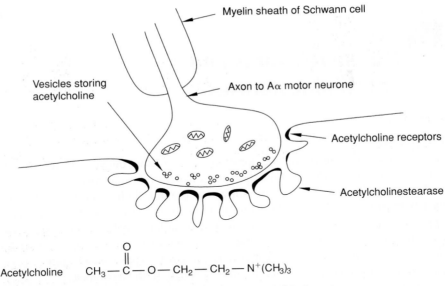

Acetylcholine

$$CH_3 - \overset{\overset{\displaystyle O}{\|}}{C} - O - CH_2 - CH_2 - N^+(CH_3)_3$$

Figure 11.1. Neuromuscular junction and structure of acetylcholine.

the prejunctional membrane and provide positive feedback to maintain transmitter release during periods of high activity. When blocked by non-depolarizing muscle relaxants they may be responsible for 'fade' (Figure 11.3).

The ACh receptor ion channel is non-specific, allowing Na^+, K^+ and Ca^{2+} across the membrane, generating a miniature end-plate potential. These summate until the threshold potential is reached at which point voltage-gated Na^+ channels are opened, causing a rapid depolarization, leading to the propagation of an action potential across the muscle surface. On reaching the T tubular system, Ca^{2+} is released from the sarcoplasmic reticulum which initiates muscle contraction.

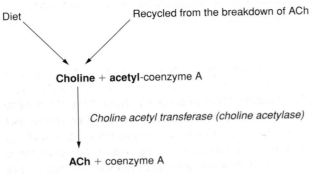

Figure 11.2. Synthesis of acetylcholine (ACh).

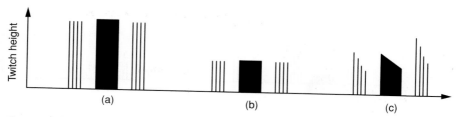

Figure 11.3. Types of neuromuscular block in response to a train-of-four, tetanic stimulus, repeat train-of-four. (a) Control, no muscle relaxant present; (b) partial depolarizing block, reduced but equal twitch height, no post-tetanic facilitation; (c) partial non-depolarizing block, reducing twitch height, fade on tetanic stimulation, post-tetanic facilitation.

Metabolism

ACh is metabolized by AChE, which is located on the junctional clefts of the post-synaptic membrane. AChE has an anionic and an esteratic binding site. The anionic site binds with the positively charged quaternary ammonium moiety while the esteratic site binds the ester group of ACh. At the point of ACh breakdown choline is released and AChE becomes acetylated. The acetylated enzyme is rapidly hydrolyzed and acetic acid is produced.

Monitoring neuromuscular block

Muscle relaxants are monitored by examining the effect they have on muscle contraction following stimulation of the relevant nerve. Nerve stimulators must generate a supramaximal stimulus (60–80 mA) to ensure that all the composite nerve fibres are depolarized. The duration of the stimulus is 0.1 msec. The negative electrode should be directly over the nerve while the positive electrode should be placed where it cannot affect the muscle in question.

There are five main patterns of stimulation that are used and the characteristic responses observed in the relevant muscle reveal information about the block.

Single twitch stimulation

This is the simplest form of neurostimulation and requires a baseline twitch height for it to reveal useful information. It should be remembered that no reduction in twitch height will be observed until 75% of NMJ receptors have been occupied by muscle relaxant (Figure 11.4). This margin of safety exists because only a small number of receptors are required to generate a summated mini end-plate potential, which triggers an action potential within the muscle. Partial NMJ block with depolarizing muscle relaxants (DMRs) and non-depolarizing muscle relaxants (NDMRs) reduce the height of single twitch stimulation.

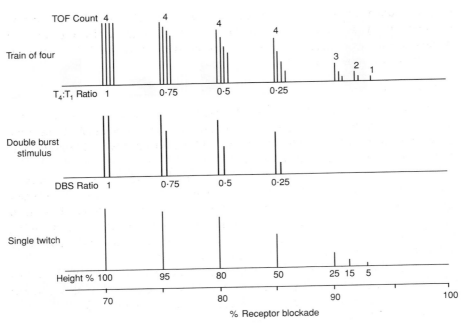

Figure 11.4. Patterns of non-depolarizing muscle-relaxant block against increasing NMJ, receptor blockade.

Tetanic stimulation

When individual stimuli are applied at a frequency >30 Hz the twitches observed in the muscle become fused into a sustained muscle contraction – tetany. The response may be larger in magnitude than a single stimulus as the elastic forces of the muscle do not need to be overcome for each twitch. Most stimulators deliver stimuli of 0.1 msec duration at a frequency of 50 Hz, which provides maximum sensitivity. In the presence of a partial NDMR the tetanic stimulation fades with time. This is due to blockade by the NDMR of presynaptic ACh receptors, thereby preventing the positive feedback (see above) used to mobilize ACh at times of peak activity. Partial DMR block reduces but does not exhibit fade in response to tetanic stimulation.

Post-tetanic potentiation and count

Following tetanic stimulation, subsequent twitches are seen to be larger. This may be due to increased synthesis and mobilization of ACh and or increased Ca^{2+} in the synaptic terminal. Post-tetanic potentiation forms the basis of the post-tetanic count where stimuli at 1 Hz are started 3 seconds after a tetanic stimulation. The number of twitches is inversely related to the depth of block. It is best used when the degree of receptor blockade is >95%, that is, when single twitch or train-of-four are unable to evoke muscle twitches. It should be remembered that the effects of tetanic stimulation may last for up to 6 minutes and may therefore give a false impression of inadequate block to single twitch or train-of-four analysis. Partial DMR block does not exhibit post tetanic potentiation.

Train-of-four

The train-of-four (TOF) is four 0.1 msec stimuli delivered at 2 Hz. The ratio of the fourth twitch height to the first twitch height (T_4:T_1), or the number of twitches may be recorded leading to the TOF ratio or the TOF count respectively (Figure 11.4). It does not require a baseline twitch height.

In a manner similar to that seen with tetanic stimulation the rapid stimuli lead to a reducing twitch height in the presence of partial non-depolarizing muscle relaxant blockade, that is, $T_4 < T_1$. As receptor occupancy rises above 70% T_4 will start to decrease in size. When T_4 has decreased by 25% T_1 starts to decrease, corresponding to 75–80% receptor occupancy. T_4 disappears when T_1 is approximately 25% of its original height. TOF ratio is difficult to assess in practise.

The TOF count records the number of twitches in response to a TOF. As receptor ocupancy exceeds 90% T_4 disappears and only T_1 is present at 95% receptor ocupancy. So the TOF count assesses the degree of deep NDMR block.

TOF ratio in the presence of partial DMR block is 1.

Double burst stimulation

Double burst stimulation (DBS) describes the delivery of two bursts of stimulation separated by 0.75 sec. Each burst consists of three 0.2 msec stimuli separated by 20 msec (i.e. at a 50 Hz). Double burst stimulation was developed to allow easy manual detection of small amounts of residual NMJ blockade so that when the magnitude of the two stmuli are equal clinically significant residual NMJ blockade does not exist. However, when assessed mechanically DBS is no more sensitive than TOF (Figure 11.4).

Depolarizing muscle relaxants

Suxamethonium

$$CH_2 - \overset{\overset{\displaystyle O}{\|}}{C} - O - CH_2 - CH_2 - N^+(CH_3)_3$$
$$CH_2 - \underset{\underset{\displaystyle O}{\|}}{C} - O - CH_2 - CH_2 - N^+(CH_3)_3$$

Suxamethonium was first introduced in 1952 and provided a significant advantage over tubocurarine as profound muscle relaxation of short duration was achieved

Table 11.1. Characteristics of partial neuromuscular blockade.

	Partial depolarizing or Phase I block	Partial non-depolarizing or Phase II block
Single twitch	reduced	reduced
Train-of-four ratio (T_4:T_1)	>0.7	<0.7
1 Hz stimulus	sustained	fade
Post-tetanic potentiation	no	yes
Effect of anticholinesterases	block augmented	block antagonized

rapidly. It can be thought of as two molecules of ACh joined back to back through their acetyl groups.

Presentation and uses

Suxamethonium is formulated as a colourless solution containing 50 mg.ml^{-1} and should be stored at 4°C. It is used to achieve rapid muscle relaxation required during rapid sequence induction and has also been used by infusion to facilitate short surgical procedures.

Mechanism of action

Suxamethonium mimics the action of ACh by attaching to the nicotinic ACh receptor and causing membrane depolarization. However, because its hydrolyzing enzyme (plasma or pseudo-cholinesterase) is not present at the NMJ its duration of action is longer than that of ACh. The persistent depolarization produced initiates local current circuits that render the voltage-sensitive Na$^+$ channels within 1–2 mm inactive. This area of electrical inexcitability prevents the transmission of further action potentials resulting in muscle relaxation.

Initially this depolarizing block is described as a Phase I block; however, if further doses of suxamethonium are given it may become a Phase II block. The characteristics of a Phase II block are similar to those of a non-depolarizing block, but the mechanism is thought to be different (probably a pre-synaptic effect) (Table 11.1, Figure 11.3).

Kinetics

Suxamethonium is rapidly hydrolyzed by plasma or pseudo-cholinesterase (an enzyme of the liver and plasma – none being present at the NMJ), to such an extent that only 20% of the initial intravenous dose reaches the NMJ, so that the rate of hydrolysis becomes a critical factor in determining the duration of the neuromuscular block. Suxamethonium is hydrolyzed to choline and succinylmonocholine, which is weakly active. Succinylmonocholine is metabolized further by plasma cholinesterase to succinic acid and choline. Because metabolism is rapid, less than 10% is excreted in the urine (Figure 11.5).

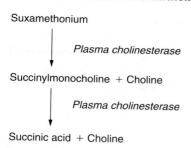

Suxamethonium

Plasma cholinesterase

Succinylmonocholine + Choline

Plasma cholinesterase

Succinic acid + Choline

Figure 11.5. Metabolism of suxamethonium.

Other effects

Apart from its useful effects at the NMJ, suxamethonium has many other effects all of which are detrimental:

- Arrhythmias – sinus or nodal bradycardia, and ventricular arrhythmias can occur following suxamethonium, via stimulation of the muscarinic receptors in the sinus node. The bradycardia is often more severe after a second dose but may be prevented by atropine. This phenomenon is often more pronounced in children.

- Hyperkalaemia – a small rise in serum K^+ is expected following suxamethonium in the normal subject as depolarization involves K^+ efflux into extracellular fluid. Patients with burns (of >10%) and neuromuscular disorders are susceptible to a sudden release of K^+, which may be large enough to provoke cardiac arrest. Burn patients are at risk from about 24 hours after injury and for up to 18 months. Extrajunctional ACh receptors (which contain a fetal γ subunit in place of an adult ϵ subunit) proliferate over the surface of the muscle, and when activated release K^+ into the circulation. Patients with paraplegia, progressive muscle disease or trauma-induced immobility are at risk via a similar mechanism. The period of particular risk in those with paraplegia is during the first 6 months but it continues in those with progressive muscle disease, becoming more severe as more muscle is involved.

   Those with renal failure are not at increased risk of a sudden hyperkalaemic response to suxamethonium per se. However, serum K^+ may be grossly deranged in acute renal failure leading to an increased risk of arrhythmias.

- Myalgia – muscle pains are commonest in young females mobilizing rapidly in the post-operative period. Pre-treatment with a small dose of non-depolarizing muscle relaxant (e.g. gallamine), diazepam or dantrolene have all been used with limited success in an attempt to reduce this unpleasant side effect.

- Intra-occular pressure (IOP) – is raised by about 10 mmHg for a matter of minutes following suxamethonium (normal range 10–15 mmHg) and is significant in the presence of a globe perforation. However, concurrently administered thiopental will offset this rise so that IOP remains static or may even fall. The mechanism by which suxamethonium increases IOP has not been clearly defined, but it is known to involve contraction of tonic myofibrils and transient dilation of choroidal blood vessels.

- Intragastric pressure – rises by about 10 cmH_2O, but as the lower oesophageal sphincter tone increases simultaneously there is no increased risk of reflux.
- Anaphylaxis – suxamethonium makes up a significant proportion of the cases of anaphylaxis caused by muscle relaxants.
- Malignant hyperthermia (see below).
- Prolonged neuromuscular block (see below).

Malignant hyperthermia (MH)
MH is a rare (1 in 200 000 in the UK), autosomal-dominant condition.

Mechanism

The exact mechanism has not been fully elucidated but the ryanodine receptor located on the membrane of the sarcoplasmic reticulum and encoded on chromosome 19 is intimately involved. There are three isoforms of the ryanodine receptor encoded by three distinct genes. Isoform 1 (RYR1) is located primarily in skeletal muscle, isoform 2 (RYR2) is located primarily in heart muscle and isoform 3 (RYR3) is located primarily is the brain. The RYR1 receptor functions as the main Ca^{2+} channel allowing stored Ca^{2+} from the sarcoplasmic reticulum into the cytoplasm, which in turn activates the contractile mechanisms within muscle. Abnormal RYR1 receptors allow excessive amounts of Ca^{2+} to pass, resulting in generalized muscle rigidity. ATP consumption is high as it is used in the process to return Ca^{2+} to the sarcolplasmic reticulum and as a result there is increased CO_2, heat and lactate production. Cells eventually break down resulting in myoglobinaemia and hyperkalaemia.

Treatment

This requires intravenous dantrolene (increments of 1 $mg.kg^{-1}$ up to 10 $mg.kg^{-1}$), aggressive cooling (using ice-cold saline to lavage bladder and peritoneum – if open), and correction of abnormal biochemical and haematological parameters. Treatment should continue on ITU and should only stop when symptoms have completely resolved, otherwise it may recur. Before the introduction of dantrolene in 1979 the mortality rate was as high as 70% but is now less than 5%.

Diagnosis

The diagnosis of MH is based on the response of biopsied muscle to 2% halothane and caffeine (2 $mmol.l^{-1}$). Patients are labelled either 'susceptible' (MHS) – when positive to both halothane and caffeine, 'equivocal' (MHE) – when positive to either halothane or caffeine, or 'non-susceptible' (MHN) – when negative to halothane and caffeine.

Safe drugs

These include opioids, thiopental, propofol, etomidate, ketamine, benzodiazepines, atropine, local anaesthetics and N_2O.

Patients suspected of having MH should be referred to the UK MH investigation unit in Leeds.

Dantrolene is used in the treatment (and prophylaxis) of MH, neuroleptic malignant syndrome, chronic spasticity of voluntary muscle and ecstacy intoxication. It is available as capsules and in vials as an orange powder containing dantrolene 20 mg, mannitol 3 g and sodium hydroxide. Each vial should be reconstituted with 60 ml water producing a solution of pH 9.5. It is highly irritant when extravasated and a diuresis follows intravenous administration reflecting its formulation with mannitol. Chronic use is associated with hepatitis and pleural effusion.

Mechanism of action

Dantrolene uncouples the excitation contraction process by binding to the ryanodine receptor thereby preventing the release of Ca^{2+} from the sarcoplasmic reticulum in striated muscle. As vascular smooth muscle and cardiac muscle are not primarily dependent on Ca^{2+} release for contraction, they are not usually affected. It has no effect on the muscle action potential and usually has little effect on the clinical duration of the non-depolarizing muscle relaxants. It may, however, produce respiratory failure secondary to skeletal muscle weakness.

Kinetics

Oral bioavailability is variable and it is approximately 85% bound in the plasma to albumin. It is metabolized in the liver and excreted in the urine.

Prolonged block (suxamethonium apnoea)

Plasma cholinesterase activity may be reduced due to genetic variability or acquired conditions, leading to prolonged neuromuscular block. Single amino acid substitutions are responsible for genetically altered enzymatic activity. Four alleles – usual (normal), atypical (dibucaine-resistant), silent (absent) and fluoride-resistant – have been identified at a single locus of chromosome 3 and make up the 10 genotypes.

Ninety-six percent of the population is homozygous for the normal Eu gene and metabolize suxamethonium rapidly. Up to 4% may be heterozygotes resulting in a mildly prolonged block of up to 10 minutes while a very small fraction may have a genotype that confers a block of a few hours. This prolonged block may be reversed by administration of fresh frozen plasma, which provides a source of plasma cholinesterase. Alternatively the patient may be sedated and ventilated while the block wears off naturally.

Table 11.2. Some genetic variants of plasma cholinesterase.

Genotype	Incidence	Duration of block	Dibucaine number
Eu:Eu	96%	normal	80
Eu:Ea	1:25	+	60
Eu:Es	1:90	+	80
Eu:Ef	1:200	+	75
Ea:Ea	1:2800	++++	20
Ea:Ef	1:20 000	++	50
Es:Ea	1:29 000	++++	20
Es:Es	1:100 000	++++	–
Ef:Es	1:150 000	++	60
Ef:Ef	1:154 000	++	70

Dibucaine (cinchocaine) is an amide local anaesthetic that inhibits normal plasma cholinesterase. However, it inhibits the variant forms of plasma cholinesterase less effectively. At a concentration of 10^{-5} mol.l^{-1}, using benzylcholine as a substrate, dibucaine inhibits the Eu:Eu form by 80% but the Ea:Ea form by only 20%. Other combinations are inhibited by 20–80% depending on the type involved. The percentage inhibition is known as the 'Dibucaine number' and indicates the genetic makeup for an individual but makes no assessment of the quantity of enzyme in the plasma (Table 11.2).

Acquired factors associated with reduced plasma cholinesterase activity include:
- Pregnancy
- Liver disease
- Renal failure
- Cardiac failure
- Thyrotoxicosis
- Cancer
- Drugs – either directly or by acting as substrate or inhibitor to AChE. Metoclopramide, ketamine, the oral contraceptive pill, lithium, lidocaine, ester local anaesthetics, cytotoxic agents, edrophonium, neostigmine and trimetaphan

Non-depolarizing muscle relaxants

Non-depolarizing muscle relaxants inhibit the actions of ACh at the NMJ by binding competitively to the α subunit of the nicotinic ACh receptor on the post-junctional membrane.

There is a wide safety margin at the NMJ to ensure muscle contraction, so that more than 70% of receptors need to be occupied by muscle relaxant before neuromuscular blockade can be detected by a peripheral nerve stimulator. The non-depolarizing block has essentially the same characteristics as the Phase II block (Table 11.1).

Non-depolarizing muscle relaxants fall into one of two chemical groupings:
- Aminosteroidal compounds – vecuronium, rocuronium, pancuronium
- Benzylisoquinolinium compounds – atracurium, mivacurium, tubocurarine

Across the two chemical groups the drugs can be divided according to their duration of action:
- Short – mivacurium
- Intermediate – atracurium
- Long – pancuronium

Owing to their relatively polar nature, non-depolarizing drugs are unable to cross lipid membranes resulting in a small volume of distribution. Some are hydrolyzed in the plasma (atracurium, mivacurium) while others undergo a degree of hepatic metabolism (pancuronium, vecuronium). The unmetabolized fraction is excreted in the urine or bile.

Muscle relaxants are never given in isolation and so their potential for drug interaction should be considered (Table 11.3).

Vecuronium

Vecuronium is a 'clean' drug, so called because it does not affect the cardiovascular system or precipitate the release of histamine. Its chemical structure differs from pancuronium by a single methyl group making it the monoquaternary analogue.

Presentation and uses

Vecuronium is potentially unstable in solution and so is presented as 10 mg freeze-dried powder containing mannitol and sodium hydroxide and is dissolved in 5 ml water before administration. At 0.1 mg.kg^{-1} satisfactory intubating conditions are reached in about 90–120 seconds. It has a medium duration of action.

Other effects

- Cardiovascular – vecuronium has no cardiac effects but, unlike pancuronium or tubocurarine, it may leave unchecked the bradycardias associated with fentanyl and propofol.
- Critical illness myopathy – this is seen most frequently in critically ill patients in association with corticosteroids and/or muscle relaxants and may involve a prolonged recovery.

Kinetics

Like pancuronium, vecuronium is metabolized in the liver by de-acetylation to 3- and 17-hydroxy and 3,17-dihydroxy-vecuronium. Again the 3-hydroxy metabolite carries significant muscle-relaxant properties, but unlike 3-hydroxypancuronium it has a very short half-life and is of little clinical significance with normal renal

Table 11.3. Pharmacological and physiological interactions of muscle relaxants.

	Effect on blockade	Mechanism
Pharmacological		
Volatile anaesthetics	prolonged	depression of somatic reflexes in CNS (reducing transmitter release at the NMJ)
Aminoglycosides (large intraperitoneal doses), polymyxins and tetracycline	prolonged	decreased ACh release possibly by competition with Ca^{2+} (which unpredictably reverses the block)
Local anaesthetics	variable	low doses of local anaesthetic may enhance blockade by causing a degree of Na^+ channel blockade
Lithium	prolonged	Na^+ channel blockade
Diuretics	variable	variable effect on cAMP. May have effects via serum K^+
Ca^{2+} channel antagonists	prolonged	reduced Ca^{2+} influx leading to reduced ACh release
Physiological		
Hypothermia	prolonged	reduced metabolism of muscle relaxant
Acidosis	variable	prolonged in most, but reduced for gallamine. The tertiary amine group of dTC becomes protonated increasing its affinity for the ACh receptor
Hypokalaemia	variable	acute hypokalaemia increases (i.e. makes more negative) the resting membrane potential. Non-depolarizing relaxants are potentiated while depolarizing relaxants are antagonized. The reverse is true in hyperkalaemia
Hypermagnesaemia	prolonged	decreased ACh release by competition with Ca^{2+}, and stabilization of the post-junctional membrane. When used at supranormal levels (e.g. pre-eclampsia) Mg^{2+} can cause apnoea via a similar mechanism

function. With only a single charged quaternary ammonium group, it is more lipid-soluble than pancuronium and despite the metabolism of a similar proportion in the liver, a far greater proportion is excreted in the bile. It may accumulate during administration by infusion.

Rocuronium

This aminosteroidal drug was developed from vecuronium and is structurally different at only four positions. Its main advantage is its rapid onset (intubating conditions within 60–90 seconds), which in turn is due to its low potency.

A muscle relaxant with a low potency must be given at a higher dose to achieve a clinically significant effect. A higher number of molecules result in a greater concentration gradient from the plasma to the NMJ so that diffusion is faster and onset time is reduced.

Presentation and uses

Rocuronium is prepared as a colourless solution containing 50 mg in 5 ml. At 0.6 mg.kg^{-1} intubating conditions are reached within 100–120 seconds, although this may be reduced to 60 seconds with higher doses (0.9–1.2 mg.kg^{-1}). Its duration of action is similar to that of vecuronium.

Other effects

- Cardiovascular – like vecuronium it has minimal cardiovascular effects, although at high doses when used to facilitate a more rapid tracheal intubation, it may cause an increase in heart rate.

Kinetics

Rocuronium is mainly excreted unchanged in the bile and to a lesser extent in the urine, although some de-acetylated metabolites may be produced. Its duration of action may be prolonged in hepatic and renal failure.

Pancuronium

Pancuronium is a bisquaternary aminosteroidal compound.

Presentation and uses

Pancuronium is presented as a colourless solution containing 4 mg in 2 ml and should be stored at 4°C. At 0.1 mg.kg^{-1} intubating conditions are reached within 90–150 seconds. Its duration of action is about 45 minutes.

Other effects

- Cardiovascular – pancuronium causes a tachycardia by blocking cardiac muscarinic receptors. It may also have indirect sympathomimetic actions by preventing the uptake of noradrenaline at post-ganglionic nerve endings.

Kinetics

Between 10% and 40% is plasma protein bound, and in keeping with other drugs in its class pancuronium has a low volume of distribution. About 35% is metabolized in

Table 11.4. Properties of some non-depolarizing muscle relaxants.

	Intubating dose $(mg.kg^{-1})$	Speed of onset	Duration	Cardiovascular effects	Histamine release
Vecuronium	0.1	medium	medium	none/bradycardia	rare
Rocuronium	0.6	rapid	medium	none	rare
Pancuronium	0.1	medium	long	tachycardia	rare
Atracurium	0.5	medium	medium	none	slight
Cis-atracurium	0.2	medium	medium	none	rare
Mivacurium	0.2	medium	short	none	slight
Gallamine	2.0	fast	medium	tachycardia	rare
Tubocurarine	0.5	slow	long	hypotension	common

the liver by de-acetylation to 3- and 17-hydroxy and 3,17-dihydroxy-pancuronium, the former of which is half as potent as pancuronium. Unchanged drug is eliminated mainly in the urine while its metabolites are excreted in bile.

Tubocurarine (dTC)

Curare is a generic term used to describe various alkaloids from the plant species *Chondrodendron*. It was used in South America to poison the tips of hunting arrows.

Tubocurarine, which was first used as an aid to anaesthesia in 1942, is a mono-quaternary alkaloid with a tertiary amine group, which is largely protonated at body pH.

Presentation and uses

Tubocurarine is presented as a colourless solution containing 10 mg.ml^{-1}. At 0.5 mg.kg^{-1} intubating conditions are reached within 3 minutes. Its duration of action is about 40 minutes, but this is variable.

Other effects

- Cardiovascular – dTC causes the greatest degree of autonomic ganglion blockade and histamine release of all the non-depolarizing muscle relaxants, which results in a fall in blood pressure. Reflex tachycardia is uncommon due to the ganglion blockade. It appears to protect against arrhythmias.
- Gut – it increases salivation.
- Toxicity – anaphylaxis is associated with its use.

Kinetics

dTC is 30–50% protein bound. Under acidic conditions the tertiary amine group (pK$_a$ 8.0) becomes increasingly protonated, resulting in increased potency. However, as pH varies, [K$^+$] also varies, which alters the membrane potential and may offset altered potency. Elimination is independent of metabolism with 70% excreted in the urine and 30% in bile as unchanged drug. It accumulates in patients with renal failure in whom a greater proportion is excreted in the bile.

Atracurium

Atracurium is a benzylisoquinolinium compound that is formulated as a mixture of 10 stereoisomers, resulting from the presence of 4 chiral centres.

Presentation and uses

Atracurium is presented as a colourless solution containing $10 \, mg.ml^{-1}$ in 2.5, 5 and 25 ml vials and should be stored at $4°C$. At $0.5 \, mg.kg^{-1}$ intubating conditions are reached within 90–120 seconds.

Other effects

- Cardiorespiratory – following rapid administration it may precipitate the release of histamine, which may be localized to the site of injection but may be generalized resulting in bronchospasm and hypotension. Slow intravenous injection minimizes these effects.
- Myopathy – in a manner similar to that of vecuronium, atracurium is associated with critical illness myopathy.

Kinetics

Atracurium has a unique metabolic pathway, undergoing ester hydrolysis and Hofmann elimination.

- Ester hydrolysis – non-specific esterases unrelated to plasma cholinesterase are responsible for hydrolysis and account for 60% of atracurium's metabolism. The breakdown products are a quaternary alcohol, a quaternary acid and laudanosine. Unlike Hofmann elimination, acidic conditions accelerate this metabolic pathway. However, pH changes in the clinical range probably do not alter the rate of ester hydrolysis of atracurium.
- Hofmann elimination – while atracurium is stable at pH 4 and at $4°C$, Hofmann elimination describes its spontaneous breakdown to laudanosine and a quaternary monoacrylate when placed at normal body temperature and pH. Acidosis and hypothermia will slow the process. Both breakdown products have been shown to have potentially serious side effects (i.e. seizures), but at concentrations in excess of those encountered clinically. Laudanosine, while being a glycine antagonist, has no neuromuscular-blocking properties and is cleared by the kidneys.

These metabolic pathways result in a drug whose elimination is independent of hepatic or renal function, which in certain clinical situations is advantageous.

Cis-atracurium

Cis-atracurium is one of the ten stereoisomers present in atracurium.

Table 11.5. Kinetics some non-depolarizing muscle relaxants.

	Protein bound (%)	Volume of distribution (l.kg^{-1})	Metabolized (%)	Elimination (%)	
				Bile	Urine
Pancuronium	20–60	0.27	30	20	80
Vecuronium	10	0.23	20	70	30
Rocuronium	10	0.20	<5	60	40
Atracurium	15	0.15	90	0	10
Cis-atracurium	15	0.15	95	0	5
Mivacurium	10	*0.21–0.32	90	0	5
Tubocurarine	30–50	0.30	0	30	70
Gallamine	10	0.23	0	0	100

*Isomer specific

Presentation and uses

Cis-atracurium is presented as a colourless solution containing 2 or 5 mg.ml^{-1} and should be stored at 4°C. It is about three to four times more potent than atracurium and, therefore, has a slower onset time. However, the onset time can be improved by increasing the dose as its potential for histamine release is extremely low.

Kinetics

Cis-atracurium has a similar kinetic profile to atracurium. However, it does not undergo direct hydrolysis by plasma esterases and the predominant pathway for its elimination is Hofmann elimination to laudanosine and a monoquaternary acrylate. This is then hydrolyzed by non-specific plasma esterases to a monoquaternary alcohol and acrylic acid. All of its metabolites are void of neuromuscular-blocking properties.

It has been used safely in children from 2 years of age and in elderly patients with minimal alteration of its kinetics. There is no change in its kinetic profile in patients with end-stage renal or hepatic impairment (Table 11.5).

Mivacurium

Mivacurium (a benzylisoquinolinium ester – similar to atracurium) is a chiral mixture of three stereospecific isomers in the following proportions:

- 36% cis-trans
- 58% trans-trans
- 6% cis-cis

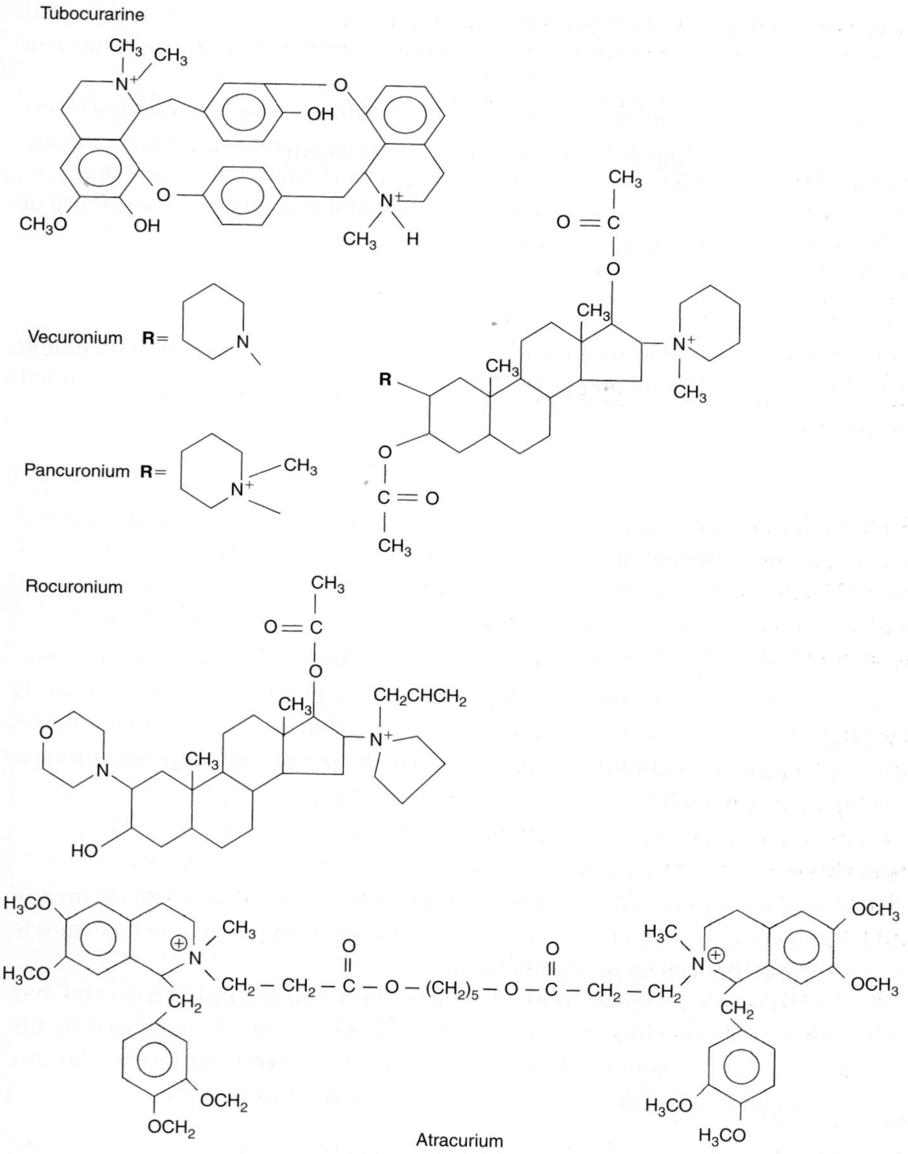

Figure 11.6. Structure of some non-depolarizing muscle relaxants.

The cis-cis isomer has about 10% of the potency of the other two isomers and is not metabolized enzymatically. Its half-life is ten times that of the other two isomers.

The main advantage of mivacurium is its short duration of action. Routine reversal of mivacurium with neostigmine may not be required due to its rapid enzymatic metabolism. In addition, neostigmine inhibits plasma cholinesterase and may prevent its metabolism. Edrophonium may be a more suitable agent for the reversal of neuromuscular block secondary to mivacurium.

Presentation and uses
Mivacurium is presented as an acidic (pH 3.5–5.0) aqueous solution containing 2 mg.ml^{-1} in 5 and 10 ml ampoules. It has a shelf-life of 18 months when stored below 25°C.

Effects
- Cardiorespiratory – high doses may release histamine, resulting in a fall in blood pressure and bronchospasm.

Kinetics
Plasma cholinesterase is responsible for the metabolism of the cis-trans and trans-trans isomers, so those patients with genetically low plasma cholinesterase levels (cf. suxamethonium apnoea) are subject to prolonged neuromuscular blockade. Its duration of action is significantly prolonged in patients with end-stage liver disease, mainly due to reduced plasma cholinesterase activity.

Gallamine
Gallamine was introduced into anaesthesia in 1947 as the first synthetic muscle relaxant. It currently has a limited role in anaesthesia, being used to reduce muscle fasciculations induced by suxamethonium.

It selectively blocks cardiac muscarinic receptors causing a tachycardia and may also activate the sympathetic nervous system. As it is excreted unchanged by the kidneys, renal failure significantly prolongs its half-life. Unlike other muscle relaxants an alkalosis prolongs its duration of action while an acidosis shortens it.

Anticholinesterases
The enzyme AChE hydrolyzes ACh, terminating its effects. Anticholinesterases antagonize AChE so that more ACh is available at the NMJ. However, the actions of anticholinesterases are not specific to the NMJ and autonomic cholinergic effects (bradycardia, salivation) are also seen. For this reason they are often given with an anticholinergic (atropine or glycopyrrolate).

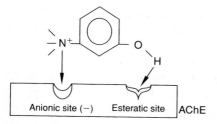

Anionic site (−)   Esteratic site   AChE

Figure 11.7. Edrophonium forms an easily reversible enzyme complex.

Three groups are defined based on their mechanism of action:
- Easily reversible inhibition
- Formation of a carbamylated enzyme complex
- Irreversible inactivation by organophosphorous compounds

Easily reversible inhibition

Edrophonium

Edrophonium is the only drug in this group. It is a phenolic quaternary amine.

Uses

At an intravenous dose of 2–10 mg it rapidly distinguishes between a myasthenic crisis (where muscle power is improved) and a cholinergic crisis (where the clinical picture is worsened).

Mechanism of action

The quaternary amine group of edrophonium is attracted to the anionic site of AChE while its hydroxyl group forms a hydrogen bond at the esteratic site and stabilizes the complex (Figure 11.7). ACh is now unable to reach the active site of AChE. However, ACh competes with edrophonium for AChE because a true covalent bond is not formed between edrophonium and AChE. Edrophonium also causes increased ACh release.

Kinetics

Owing to its quaternary amine structure edrophonium has a low lipid solubility and is not absorbed following oral administration. For similar reasons, it does not cross the BBB or the placenta. It has a faster onset of action than neostigmine. Up to 65% is excreted unchanged in the urine, the rest undergoes glucuronidation in the liver and subsequent excretion in the bile. It has only slight muscarinic side-effects but may still cause a bradycardia and salivation.

Formation of a carbamylated enzyme complex

Neostigmine, pyridostigmine, physostigmine (Figure 11.8).

193

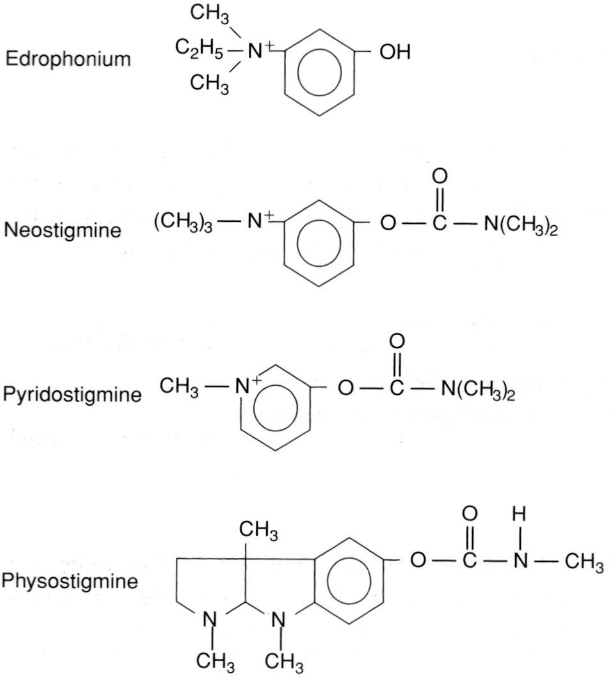

Edrophonium $C_2H_5 \overset{\displaystyle CH_3}{\underset{\displaystyle CH_3}{\diagup}} N^+ \langle \bigcirc \rangle OH$

Neostigmine $(CH_3)_3 - N^+ \langle \bigcirc \rangle O - \overset{\displaystyle O}{\overset{\|}{C}} - N(CH_3)_2$

Pyridostigmine $CH_3 - N^+ \langle \bigcirc \rangle O - \overset{\displaystyle O}{\overset{\|}{C}} - N(CH_3)_2$

Physostigmine

$\overset{CH_3}{} \qquad O - \overset{\displaystyle O}{\overset{\|}{C}} - \overset{\displaystyle H}{\overset{|}{N}} - CH_3$

N—CH₃ N—CH₃

Figure 11.8. Chemical structure of some anticholinesterases.

Mechanism of action

Both ACh and the carbamate esters are hydrolyzed when they react with AChE. However, ACh acetylates AChE while the carbamate esters produce a carbamylated enzyme (Figure 11.9). The later has a much slower rate of hydrolysis and so is unable to work for longer, hence, it stops AChE hydrolyzing ACh. The carbamate esters are also known as acid-transferring or time-dependent AChE inhibitors. Neostigmine also inhibits plasma cholinesterase and as such may prolong the actions of suxamethonium.

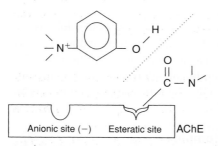

Figure 11.9. Neostigmine forms a carmabylated enzyme complex.

Neostigmine

Neostigmine is a quaternary amine.

Presentation and uses

Neostigmine is available as tablets and in solution for intravenous injection (and in combination with glycopyrrolate). It is used to reverse the effects of non-depolarizing muscle relaxants (0.05 mg.kg^{-1} intravenously), in the treatment of myasthenia gravis (15–30 mg orally where effects last up to 4 hours) and in urinary retention.

Effects

- Cardiovascular – if administered alone it will precipitate a bradycardia. It has a limited role in the treatment of supraventricular tachycardia.
- Respiratory – it may precipitate bronchospasm in asthmatics.
- Gut – it increases salivation and intestinal motility, which may result in abdominal cramps.

Kinetics

Neostigmine is poorly absorbed from the gut and has a low oral bioavailability. It is minimally protein bound, has a low volume of distribution and is partially metabolized in the liver. Approximately 55% is excreted unchanged in the urine.

Pyridostigmine

Pyridostigmine is also a quaternary amine used mainly in the treatment of myasthenia gravis, where it is preferred to neostigmine because it has a longer duration of action and has fewer autonomic effects.

Kinetics

Pyridostigmine has a slower onset of action than neostigmine and its duration of action is longer. It relies on renal elimination more than neostigmine (75% excreted unchanged).

Like neostigmine it does not cross the blood–brain barrier.

Physostigmine has a tertiary amine structure and it, therefore, has different properties. It is well absorbed from the gut and crosses the blood–brain barrier. In the past it has been used in the treatment of anticholinergic poisoning.

Organophosphorous compounds

Organophosphorous compounds are highly toxic and are mainly used as insecticides (e.g. tetraethylpyrophosphate (TEPP)), or nerve gases (sarin (GB)). However, ecothiopate iodide has been used to treat glaucoma by relaxing the ciliary muscle and thereby improving drainage channels of the trabecular meshwork.

These agents are highly lipid-soluble and are, therefore, rapidly absorbed across skin.

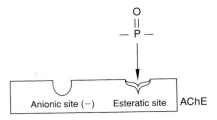

Figure 11.10. Organophosphorus compounds phosphorylate AChE, forming a very stable complex.

Mechanism of action

The esteratic site of AChE, is phosphorylated by organophosphorous compounds resulting in inhibition of the enzyme (Figure 11.10). The complex that is formed is very stable and, unlike the carbamate esters, is resistant to hydrolysis or reactivation. In practice recovery depends on synthesis of new enzyme. These drugs also inhibit plasma cholinesterase.

Toxic manifestations include nicotinic and muscarinic effects, autonomic instability and initially central excitation progressing to depression, coma and apnoea.

Pralidoxime and **obidoxine** are reactivators of phosphorylated AChE by promoting hydrolysis. Atropine, anticonvulsants and ventilation may also be necessary in organophosphorous poisoning.

Cyclodextrins

Cyclodextrins are inert doughnut-shaped molecules that have the ability to encapsulate other specific molecules. The gamma cyclodextrin Org25969 is currently undergoing Phase III trials for its efficacy in encapsulating rocuronium. Encapsulation effectively removes rocuronium from the plasma and as further drug diffuses away from the NMJ its effect there is reversed. It appears to be effective in reversing rocuronium, even from profound levels of NMJ blockade, and quickly. In addition it has no other effects unlike the anticholinesterases. The cyclodextrin/rocuronium complex is eliminated via the kidneys.

Org25969 offers a significant advance in the reversal of NDMR blockade.

SECTION III Cardiovascular drugs

12 Sympathomimetics

Physiology

Autonomic nervous system (ANS)

The ANS is a complex system of neurones that controls the body's internal milieu. It is not under voluntary control and is anatomically distinct from the somatic nervous system. Its efferent limb controls individual organs and smooth muscle, while its afferent limb relays information (occasionally in somatic nerves) concerning visceral sensation and may result in reflex arcs.

The hypothalamus is the central point of integration of the ANS, but is itself under the control of the neocortex. However, not all autonomic activity involves the hypothalamus: locally, the gut coordinates its secretions; some reflex activity is processed within the spinal cord; and the control of vital functions by baroreceptors is processed within the medulla. The ANS is divided into the parasympathetic and sympathetic nervous systems.

Parasympathetic nervous system (PNS)

The PNS is made up of pre- and post-ganglionic fibres. The pre-ganglionic fibres arise from two locations (Figure 12.1):
- Cranial nerves (III, VII, IX, X) – which supply the eye, salivary glands, heart, bronchi, upper gastrointestinal tract (to the splenic flexure) and ureters
- Sacral fibres (S2,3,4) – which supply distal bowel, bladder and genitals

All these fibres synapse within ganglia that are close to, or within, the effector organ. The post-ganglionic neurone releases acetylcholine, which acts via nicotinic receptors.

The PNS may be modulated by anticholinergics (see Chapter 18) and anticholinesterases (see Chapter 11).

Sympathetic nervous system (SNS)

The SNS is also made up of pre- and post-ganglionic fibres. The pre-ganglionic fibres arise within the lateral horns of the spinal cord at the thoracic and upper lumbar levels (T1–L2) and pass into the anterior primary rami, and via the white rami communicans into the sympathetic chain or ganglia where they may either synapse at that or an adjacent level, or pass anteriorly through a splanchnic nerve to synapse in a prevertebral ganglion (Figure 12.2). The unmyelinated post-ganglionic

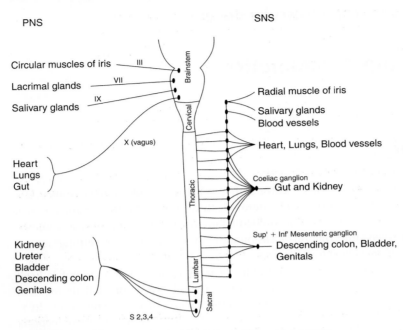

Figure 12.1. Simplified diagram of the autonomic nervous system.

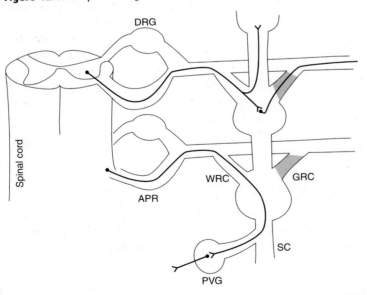

Figure 12.2. Various connections of the sympathetic nervous system. DRG, dorsal root ganglion; APR, anterior primary rami; WRC, white rami communicans; GRC, grey rami communicans; PVG, prevertebral ganglion; SC, sympathetic chain.

Table 12.1. Summary of transmitters within the autonomic nervous system.

	Pre-ganglionic	Post-ganglionic
PNS	acetylcholine	acetylcholine
SNS	acetylcholine	noradrenaline
Adrenal medulla	acetylcholine	—
Sweat glands	acetylcholine	acetylcholine

fibres then pass into the adjacent spinal nerve via the grey rami communicans. They release noradrenaline, which acts via adrenoceptors.

The adrenal medulla receives presynaptic fibres that synapse directly with its chromaffin cells using acetylcholine as the transmitter. It releases adrenaline into the circulation, which, therefore, acts as a hormone, not a transmitter.

Post-ganglionic sympathetic fibres release acetylcholine to innervate sweat glands.

All pre-ganglionic ANS fibres are myelinated and release acetylcholine, which acts via nicotinic receptors (Table 12.1).

Sympathomimetics

Sympathomimetics exert their effects via adrenoceptors or dopamine receptors either directly or indirectly. **Direct-acting** sympathomimetics attach to and act directly via these receptors, while **indirect-acting** sympathomimetics cause the release of noradrenaline to produce their effects via these receptors.

The structure of sympathomimetics is based on a benzene ring with various amine side chains attached at the C1 position. Where a hydroxyl group is present at the C3 and C4 positions the agent is known as a **catechol**amine (because 3,4-dihydroxybenzene is otherwise known as 'catechol').

Sympathomimetic and other inotropic agents will be discussed under the following headings:

- **Naturally occurring catecholamines**
- **Synthetic agents**
- **Other inotropic agents**

Naturally occurring catecholamines

Adrenaline, noradrenaline and dopamine are the naturally occurring catecholamines and their synthesis is interrelated (Figure 12.3). They act via adrenergic and dopaminergic receptors, which are summarized in Table 12.2.

Adrenaline

Presentation and uses

Adrenaline is presented as a clear solution containing 0.1–1 $mg.ml^{-1}$ for administration as a bolus in asystole or anaphylaxis or by infusion (dose range

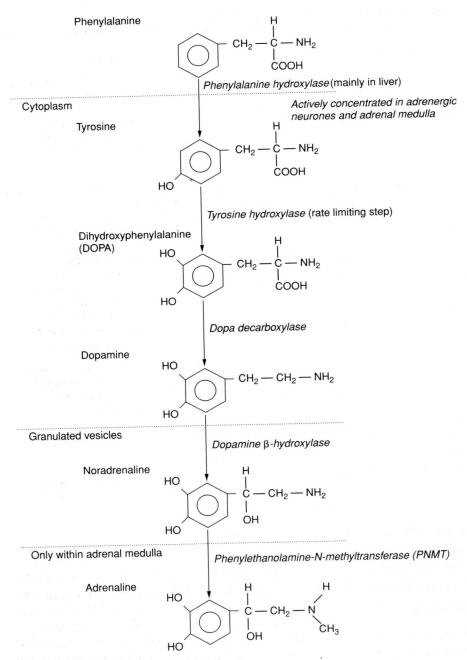

Figure 12.3. Catecholamine synthesis.

Table 12.2. Actions and mechanisms of adrenoceptors.

Receptor	Subtype	Location	Actions when stimulated	Mechanism
α	1	vascular smooth muscle	vasoconstriction	G_q-coupled phospholipase C activated → ↑ IP_3 → ↑ Ca^{2+}
	2	widespread throughout the nervous system	sedation, analgesia, attenuation of sympathetically mediated responses	G_i-coupled adenylate cyclase inhibited → ↑↓ cAMP
β	1	platelets heart	platelet aggregation +ve inotropic and chronotropic effect	G_s-coupled adenylate cyclase activated → ↑cAMP
	2	bronchi, vascular smooth muscle, uterus (and heart)	relaxation of smooth muscle	G_s-coupled adenylate cyclase activated → ↑cAMP → ↑ Na^+/K^+ ATPase activity and hyperpolarization
	3	adipose tissue	lipolysis	G_s-coupled adenylate cyclase activated → ↑cAMP
D	1	within the central nervous system	modulates extrapyramidal activity	G_s-coupled adenylate cyclase activated → ↑cAMP
		peripherally	vasodilatation of renal and mesenteric vasculature	
	2	within the central nervous system	reduced pituitary hormone output	G_i-coupled adenylate cyclase inhibited → ↑ cAMP
		peripherally	inhibit further noradrenaline release	

$0.01–0.5 \ \mu g.kg^{-1}.min^{-1}$) in the critically ill with circulatory failure. It may also be nebulized into the upper airway where its vasoconstrictor properties will temporarily reduce the swelling associated with acute upper airway obstruction. A 1% ophthalmic solution is used in open-angle glaucoma, and a metered dose inhaler delivering 280 μg for treatment of anaphylaxis associated with insect stings or drugs. In addition, it is presented in combination with local anaesthetic solutions at a strength of 1 in 80 000–200 000.

Mechanism of action

Adrenaline exerts its effects via α- and β-adrenoceptors. α_1-Adrenoceptor activation stimulates phospholipase C (via G_q), which hydrolyzes phosphatidylinositol bisphosphate (PIP_2). Inositol triphosphate (IP_3) is released, which leads to increased Ca^{2+} availability within the cell. α_2-Adrenoceptor activation is coupled to G_i-proteins that inhibit adenylate cyclase and reduce cAMP concentration. β-Adrenoceptors are coupled to G_s-proteins that activate adenylate cyclase, leading to an increase in cAMP and specific phosphorylation depending on the site of the adrenoceptor.

Effects

- Cardiovascular – the effects of adrenaline vary according to dose. When administered as a low-dose infusion, β effects predominate. This produces an increase in cardiac output, myocardial oxygen consumption, coronary artery dilatation and reduces the threshold for arrhythmias. Peripheral β effects may result in a fall in diastolic blood pressure and peripheral vascular resistance. At high doses by infusion or when given as a 1 mg bolus during cardiac arrest, α_1 effects predominate causing a rise in systemic vascular resistance. It is often used in combination with local anaesthetics to produce vasoconstriction before dissection during surgery. When used with halothane, the dose should be restricted to 100 μg per 10 minutes to avoid arrhythmias. It should not be infiltrated into areas supplied by end arteries lest their vascular supply become compromised. Extravasation can cause tissue necrosis.
- Respiratory – adrenaline produces a small increase in minute volume. It has potent bronchodilator effects although secretions may become more tenacious. Pulmonary vascular resistance is increased.
- Metabolic – adrenaline increases the basal metabolic rate. It raises plasma glucose by stimulating glycogenolysis (in liver and skeletal muscle), lipolysis and gluconeogenesis. Initially insulin secretion is increased (a β_2 effect) but is often overridden by an α effect, which inhibits its release and compounds the increased glucose production. Glucagon secretion and plasma lactate are also raised. Lipase activity is augmented resulting in increased free fatty acids, which leads to increased fatty acid oxidation in the liver and ketogenesis. These metabolic effects limit its use, especially in those with diabetes. Na^+ re-absorption is increased by direct stimulation of tubular Na^+ transport and by stimulating renin and, therefore, aldosterone production. β_2-Receptors are responsible for the increased transport of K^+ into cells, which follows an initial temporary rise as K^+ is released from the liver.
- Central nervous system – it increases MAC and increases the peripheral pain threshold.
- Renal – renal blood flow is moderately decreased and the increase in bladder sphincter tone may result in difficulty in micturition.

Kinetics

Adrenaline is not given orally due to inactivation. Subcutaneous absorption is less rapid than intramuscular. Tracheal absorption is erratic but may be used in emergencies where intravenous access is not available.

It is metabolized by mitochondrial MAO and catechol O-methyl transferase (COMT) within the liver, kidney and blood to the inactive 3-methoxy-4-hydroxymandelic acid (vanillylmandelic acid or VMA) and metadrenaline, which is conjugated with glucuronic acid or sulphates, both of which are excreted in the urine. It has a short half-life (about 2 minutes) due to rapid metabolism.

Noradrenaline

Presentation and uses

Noradrenaline is presented as a clear solution containing $0.2–2$ mg.ml^{-1} noradrenaline acid tartrate, which is equivalent to $0.1–1$ mg.ml^{-1} respectively of noradrenaline base, and contains the preservative sodium metabisulphite. It is used as an intravenous infusion (dose range $0.05–0.5$ μg.kg^{-1}.min^{-1}) to increase the systemic vascular resistance.

Mechanism of action

Its actions are mediated mainly via stimulation of α_1-adrenoceptors but also β-adrenoceptors.

Effects

- Cardiovascular – the effects of systemically infused noradrenaline are slightly different from those of endogenous noradrenaline. Systemically infused noradrenaline causes peripheral vasoconstriction, increases systolic and diastolic blood pressure and may cause a reflex bradycardia. Cardiac output may fall and myocardial oxygen consumption is increased. A vasodilated coronary circulation carries an increased coronary blood flow. Pulmonary vascular resistance may be increased and venous return is increased by venoconstriction. In excess it produces hypertension, bradycardia, headache and excessive peripheral vasoconstriction, occasionally leading to ischaemia and gangrene of extremities. Extravazation can cause tissue necrosis. Endogenously released noradrenaline causes tachycardia and a rise in cardiac output.
- Splanchnic – renal and hepatic blood flow falls due to vasoconstriction.
- Uterus – blood flow to the pregnant uterus is reduced and may result in foetal bradycardia. It may also exert a contractile effect and cause foetal asphyxia.
- Interactions – despite being a direct-acting sympathomimetic amine it should be used with caution in patients taking monoamine oxidase inhibitors (MAOI) as its effects may be exaggerated and prolonged.

Kinetics

For endogenously released noradrenaline, Uptake 1 describes its active uptake back into the nerve terminal where it is metabolized by MAO (COMT is not present in sympathetic nerves) or recycled. It forms the main mechanism by which noradrenaline is inactivated. Uptake 2 describes the diffusion away from the nerve and is less important. Noradrenaline reaches the circulation in this way and is metabolized by COMT to the inactive 3-methoxy–4-hydroxymandelic acid (vanillylmandelic acid or VMA) and normetadrenaline, which is conjugated with glucuronic acid or sulphates, both of which are excreted in the urine. It has a short half-life (about 2 minutes) due to rapid metabolism. Unlike adrenaline and dopamine, up to 25% is taken up as it passes through the lungs.

Dopamine

In certain cells within the brain and interneurones of the autonomic ganglia, dopamine is not converted to noradrenaline and is released as a neurotransmitter.

Presentation and uses

Dopamine is presented as a clear solution containing 200 or 800 mg in 5 ml water with sodium metabisulphite. It is used to improve haemodynamic parameters and urine output.

Mechanism of action

In addition to its effects on α and β adrenoceptors, dopamine also acts via dopamine (D_1 and D_2) receptors via G_s and G_i coupled adenylate cyclase leading to increased or decreased levels of cAMP.

Effects

- Cardiovascular – these depend on its rate of infusion and vary between patients. At lower rates (up to 10 μg.kg^{-1}.min^{-1}) β_1 effects predominate leading to increased contractility, heart rate, cardiac output and coronary blood flow. In addition to its direct effects, it also stimulates the release of endogenous noradrenaline. At higher rates (>10 μg.kg^{-1}.min^{-1}) α effects tend to predominate leading to increased systemic vascular resistance and venous return. In keeping with other inotropes an adequate preload is essential to help control tachycardia. It is less arrhythmogenic than adrenaline. Extravasation can cause tissue necrosis.
- Respiratory – infusions of dopamine attenuate the response of the carotid body to hypoxaemia. Pulmonary vascular resistance is increased.
- Splanchnic – dopamine has been shown to vasodilate mesenteric vessels via D_1 receptors. However, the improvement in urine output may be entirely due to

inhibition of proximal tubule Na^+ reabsorption and an improved cardiac output and blood pressure.

- Central nervous system – dopamine modulates extra-pyramidal movement and inhibits the secretion of prolactin from the pituitary gland. It cannot cross the blood–brain barrier, although its precursor L-dopa can.
- Miscellaneous – owing to stimulation of the chemoreceptor trigger zone it causes nausea and vomiting. Gastric transit time is also increased.
- Interactions – despite being a direct-acting sympathomimetic amine the effects of dopamine may be significantly exaggerated and prolonged during MAOI therapy.

Kinetics

Dopamine is only administered intravenously and preferably via a central vein. It acts within 5 minutes and has a duration of 10 minutes. Metabolism is via MAO and COMT in the liver, kidneys and plasma to inactive compounds (3,4-dihydroxyphenylacetic acid and homovanillic acid (HVA)) which are excreted in the urine as sulphate and glucuronide conjugates. About 25% of an administered dose is converted to noradrenaline in sympathetic nerve terminals. Its half-life is about 3 minutes.

Synthetic agents

Of the synthetic agents, only isoprenaline, dobutamine and dopexamine are classified as catecholamines as only they contain hydroxyl groups on the 3- and 4-positions of the benzene ring.

α_1-Agonists

Phenylephrine

Phenylephrine is a direct-acting sympathomimetic amine with potent α_1-agonist actions. It causes a rapid rise in systemic vascular resistance and blood pressure. It has no effect on β-adrenoceptors.

Presentation and uses

Phenylephrine is presented as a clear solution containing 10 mg in 1 ml. Phenylephrine is presented as a clear solution containing 10 mg in 1 ml. Bolus doses of 50–100 μg are used intravenously although 2–5 mg may be administered intramuscularly or subcutaneously for a more prolonged duration. It is used to increase a low systemic vascular resistance associated with spinal anaesthesia or systemically administered drugs. In certain patients, general anaesthesia may drop the systemic vascular resistance and reverse a left-to-right intracardiac shunt, this may be reversed by phenylephrine. It is also available for use as a nasal decongestant and mydriatic agent. It may have a limited use in the treatment of supraventricular tachycardia associated with hypotension.

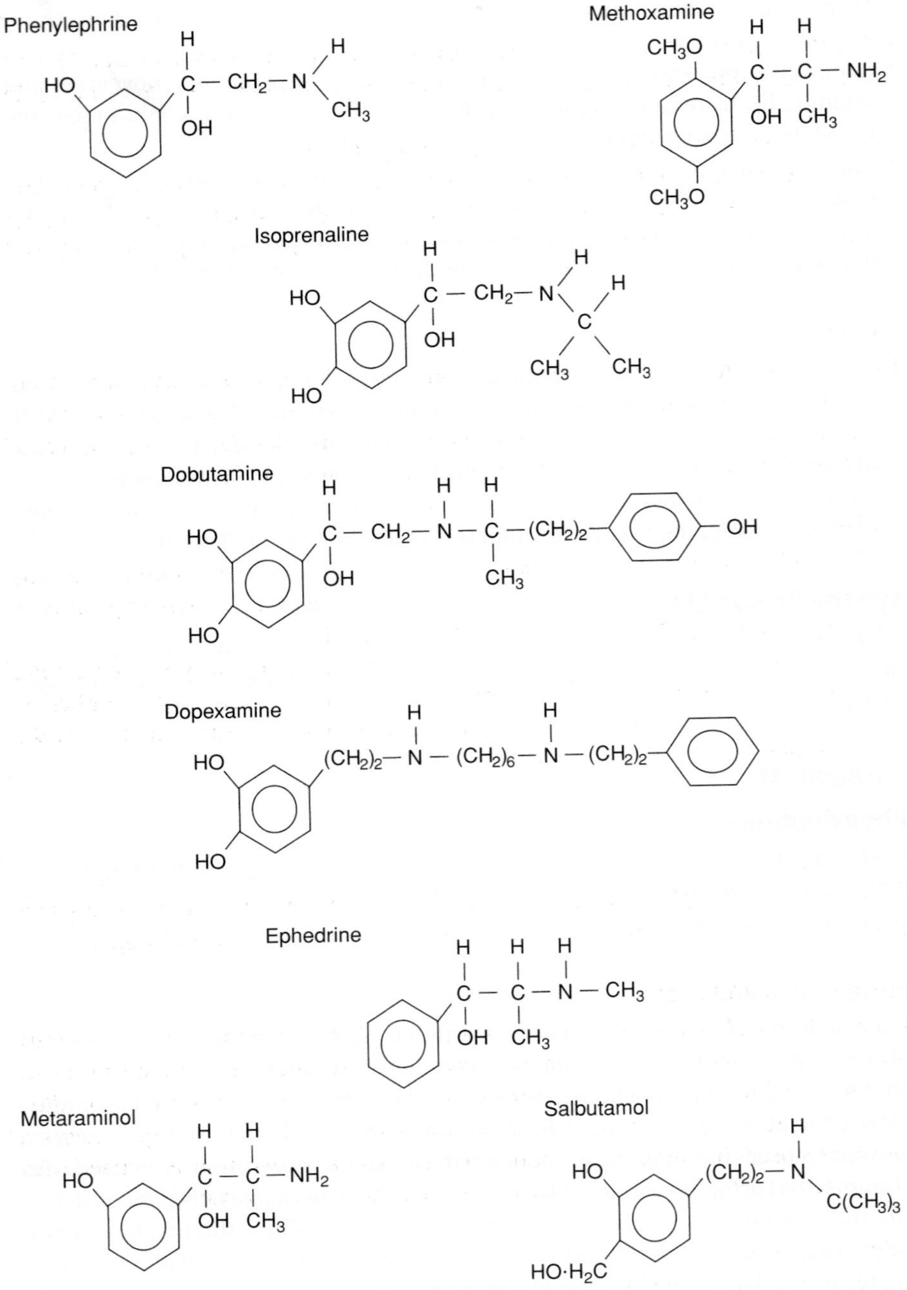

Section III **Cardiovascular drugs**

Figure 12.4. Structure of some synthetic sympathomimetic amines.

Effects

- Cardiovascular – phenylephrine raises the systemic vascular resistance and blood pressure and may result in a reflex bradycardia, all of which results in a drop in cardiac output. It is not arrhythmogenic.
- Central nervous system – it has no stimulatory effects.
- Renal – blood flow falls in a manner similar to that demonstrated by noradrenaline.
- Uterus – while its use in obstetrics results in a more favorable cord gas profile it has not yet gained widespread acceptance due to the possibility of accidental overdose.

Kinetics

Intravenous administration results in a rapid rise in blood pressure, which lasts 5–10 minutes, while intramuscular or subcutaneous injection takes 15 minutes to work but lasts up to 1 hour. It is metabolized in the liver by MAO. The products of metabolism and their route of elimination have not been identified.

Methoxamine

Methoxamine (no longer in production) is a direct-acting sympathomimetic amine with specific α_1-agonist actions. Consequently it has similar effects to phenylephrine. It is presented as a clear solution containing 20 mg.ml^{-1}.

An intravenous bolus of 1 mg usually produces a rapid rise in systemic vascular resistance and, therefore, blood pressure, often with an accompanying reflex bradycardia. It may also be given intramuscularly or subcutaneously at a higher dose for a more prolonged duration of action.

β-Agonists

Isoprenaline

Isoprenaline is a highly potent synthetic catecholamine with actions at β_1- and β_2-adrenoceptors. It has no α effects. It is not available in the UK any longer.

Presentation and uses

Isoprenaline is presented as a clear solution containing 1 mg.ml^{-1} for intravenous infusion and as a metered dose inhaler delivering 80 or 400 μg. It is no longer used to treat reversible airway obstruction as this was associated with an increased mortality. More specific β_2-agonists are now used (e.g. salbutamol). The 30 mg tablets are very rarely used. It is used intravenously to treat severe bradycardia associated with atrioventricular (AV) block or β-blockers (dose range 0.5–10 μg.min^{-1}).

Effects

- Cardiovascular – stimulation of β_1-adrenoceptors increases heart rate, myocardial contractility, automaticity and cardiac output. The effects on blood pressure are varied. The β_2 effects may drop the systemic vascular resistance so that the increase in cardiac output is insufficient to maintain blood pressure. Myocardial oxygen delivery may decrease significantly when tachycardia reduces diastolic coronary filling time and the reduced diastolic blood pressure reduces coronary perfusion. Some coronary vasodilatation occurs to attenuate this.

- Respiratory – it is a potent bronchodilator and inhibits histamine release in the lungs, improving mucous flow. Anatomical dead space and ventilation perfusion mismatching increases, which may lead to systemic hypoxaemia.
- Central nervous system – isoprenaline has stimulant effects on the CNS.
- Splanchnic – mesenteric and renal blood flow is increased.
- Metabolic – its β effects lead to a raised blood glucose and free fatty acids.

Kinetics

When administered orally it is well absorbed but extensive first-pass metabolism results in a low oral bioavailability, being rapidly metabolized by COMT within the liver. A significant fraction is excreted unchanged in the urine along with conjugated metabolites.

Dobutamine

Dobutamine is a direct-acting synthetic catecholamine derivative of isoprenaline. β_1 effects predominate but it retains a small effect at β_2-adrenoceptors.

Presentation and uses

Dobutamine is presented in 20 ml water containing 250 mg dobutamine and sodium metabisulphite or in 5 ml water containing 250 mg dobutamine and ascorbic acid. It is used to augment low cardiac output states associated with myocardial infarction, cardiac surgery and cardiogenic shock (dose range 0.5–20 μg.kg^{-1}.min^{-1}). It is also used in cardiac stress testing as an alternative to exercise.

Effects

- Cardiovascular – its main actions are direct stimulation of β_1-receptors resulting in increased contractility, heart rate and myocardial oxygen requirement. The blood pressure is usually increased despite a limited fall in systemic vascular resistance via β_2 stimulation. It may precipitate arrhythmias including an increased ventricular response rate in patients with atrial fibrillation or flutter, due to increased AV conduction. It should be avoided in patients with cardiac outflow obstruction (e.g. aortic stenosis, cardiac tamponade).
- Splanchnic – it has no effect on the splanchnic circulation although urine output may increase following a rise in cardiac output.

Kinetics

Dobutamine is only administered intravenously. It is rapidly metabolized by COMT to inactive metabolites that are conjugated and excreted in the urine. It has a half-life of 2 minutes.

Dopexamine

Dopexamine is a synthetic analogue of dopamine.

Presentation and uses

Dopexamine is presented as 50 mg in 5 ml (at pH 2.5) for intravenous use. It is used to improve cardiac output and improve mesenteric perfusion (dose range $0.5–6 \, \mu g.kg^{-1}.min^{-1}$).

Mechanism of action

Dopexamine stimulates β_2-adrenoceptors and dopamine (D_1) receptors and may also inhibit the re-uptake of noradrenaline. It has only minimal effect on D_2 and β_1-adrenoceptors, and no effect on α-adrenoceptors.

Effects

- Cardiovascular – while it has positive inotropic effects (due to cardiac β_2-receptors), improvements in cardiac output are aided by a reduced afterload due to peripheral β_2 stimulation, which may reduce the blood pressure. It produces a small increase in coronary blood flow and there is no change in myocardial oxygen extraction. The alterations in heart rate are varied and it only rarely precipitates arrhythmias.
- Mesenteric and renal – blood flow to the gut and kidneys increases due to an increased cardiac output and reduced regional vascular resistance. Urine output increases. It may cause nausea and vomiting.
- Respiratory – bronchodilation is mediated via β_2 stimulation.
- Miscellaneous – tremor and headache have been reported.

Kinetics

Dopexamine is cleared rapidly from the blood and has a half-life of 7 minutes.

Salbutamol

Salbutamol is a synthetic sympathomimetic amine with actions mainly at β_2-adreno-ceptors.

Presentation and uses

Salbutamol is presented as a clear solution containing $50–500 \, \mu g.ml^{-1}$ for intravenous infusion after dilution, a metered dose inhaler ($100 \, \mu g$) and a dry powder ($200–400 \, \mu g$) for inhalation, a solution containing $2.5–5 \, mg.ml^{-1}$ for nebulization, and oral preparations (syrup 0.4 mg.ml^{-1} and 2, 4 or 8 mg tablets). It is used in the treatment of reversible lower airway obstruction and occasionally in premature labour.

Effects

- Respiratory – its main effects are relaxation of bronchial smooth muscle. It reverses hypoxic pulmonary vasoconstriction, increasing shunt, and may lead to hypoxaemia. Adequate oxygen should, therefore, be administered with nebulized salbutamol.
- Cardiovascular – the administration of high doses, particularly intravenously, can cause stimulation of β_1-adrenoceptors resulting in tachycardia, which may limit the dose. Lower doses are sometimes associated with β_2-mediated vasodilatation, which may reduce the blood pressure. It may also precipitate arrhythmias, especially in the presence of hypokalaemia.
- Metabolic – Na$^+$/K$^+$ ATPase is stimulated and transports K$^+$ into cells resulting in hypokalaemia. Blood sugar rises especially in diabetic patients and is exacerbated by concurrently administered steroids.
- Uterus – it relaxes the gravid uterus. A small amount crosses the placenta to reach the foetus.
- Miscellaneous – a direct effect on skeletal muscle may produce tremor.

Kinetics

The absorption of salbutamol from the gut is incomplete and is subject to a significant hepatic first-pass metabolism. Following inhalation or intravenous administration, it has a rapid onset of action. It is 10% protein bound and has a half-life of 4–6 hours. It is metabolized in the liver to the inactive 4-O-sulphate, which is excreted along with salbutamol in the urine.

Salmeterol

Salmeterol is a long-acting β_2-agonist used in the treatment of nocturnal and exercise-induced asthma. It should not be used during acute attacks due to a relatively slow onset.

It has a long non-polar side chain, which binds to the β_2-adrenoceptor giving it a long duration of action (about 12 hours). It is 15 times more potent than salbutamol at the β_2-adrenoceptor, but four times less potent at the β_1-adrenoceptor. It prevents the release of histamine, leukotrienes and prostaglandin D$_2$ from mast cells, and also has additional anti-inflammatory effects that differ from those induced by steroids.

Its effects are similar to those of salbutamol.

Ritodrine

Ritodrine is a β_2-agonist that is used to treat premature labour. Tachycardia (β_1 effect) is often seen during treatment. It crosses the placenta and may result in foetal tachycardia.

Ritodrine has been associated with fatal maternal pulmonary oedema. It also causes hypokalaemia, hyperglycaemia and, at higher levels, vomiting, restlessness and seizures.

Terbutaline

Terbutaline is a β_2-agonist with some activity at β_1-adrenoceptors. It is used in the treatment of asthma and uncomplicated preterm labour. It has a similar side-effect profile to other drugs in its class.

Mixed (α and β)

Ephedrine

Ephedrine is found naturally in certain plants but is synthesized for medical use.

Presentation and uses

Ephedrine is formulated as tablets, an elixir, nasal drops and as a solution for injection containing 30 mg.ml^{-1}. It can exist as four isomers but only the L-isomer is active. It is used intravenously to treat hypotension associated with regional anaesthesia. In the obstetric setting this is now known to result in a poorer cord gas pH when compared to purer α agonists, but its widespread use persists due to the potential for the α agonists to cause a significant maternal hypertension. It is also used to treat bronchospasm, nocturnal enuresis and narcolepsy.

Mechanism of action

Ephedrine has both direct and indirect sympathomimetic actions. It also inhibits the actions of MAO on noradrenaline.

Owing to its indirect actions it is prone to tachyphylaxis as noradrenaline stores in sympathetic nerves become depleted.

Effects

- Cardiovascular – it increases the cardiac output, heart rate, blood pressure, coronary blood flow and myocardial oxygen consumption. Its use may precipitate arrhythmias.
- Respiratory – it is a respiratory stimulant and causes bronchodilation.
- Renal – renal blood flow is decreased and the glomerular filtration rate falls.
- Interactions – it should be used with extreme caution in those patients taking MAOI.

Kinetics

Ephedrine is well absorbed orally, intramuscularly and subcutaneously. Unlike adrenaline it is not metabolized by MAO or COMT and, therefore, has a longer duration of action and an elimination half-life of 4 hours. Some is metabolized in the liver but 65% is excreted unchanged in the urine.

Metaraminol

Metaraminol is a synthetic amine with both direct and indirect sympathomimetic actions. It acts mainly via α_1-adrenoceptors but also retains some β-adrenoceptor activity.

Presentation and uses

Metaraminol is presented as a clear solution containing 10 mg.ml^{-1}. It is used to correct hypotension associated with spinal or epidural anaesthesia. An intravenous bolus of 0.5–2 mg is usually sufficient.

Effects

- Cardiovascular – its main actions are to increase systemic vascular resistance, which leads to an increased blood pressure. Despite its activity at β-adrenoceptors the cardiac output often drops in the face of the raised systemic vascular resistance. Coronary artery flow increases by an indirect mechanism. Pulmonary vascular resistance is also increased leading to raised pulmonary artery pressure.

Other inotropic agents

Non-selective phosphodiesterase inhibitors

Aminophylline

Aminophylline is a methylxanthine derivative. It is a complex of 80% theophylline and 20% ethylenediamine (which has no therapeutic effect but improves solubility).

Presentation and uses

Aminophylline is available as tablets and as a solution for injection containing 25 mg.ml^{-1}. Oral preparations are often formulated as slow release due to its half-life of about 6 hours. It is used in the treatment of asthma where the dose ranges from 450 to 1250 mg daily. When given intravenously during acute severe asthma a loading dose of 6 mg.kg^{-1} over 20 minutes is given, followed by an infusion of 0.5 mg.kg^{-1}.h^{-1}. It may also be used to reduce the frequency of episodes of central apnoea in premature neonates. It is very occasionally used in the treatment of heart failure.

Theophylline

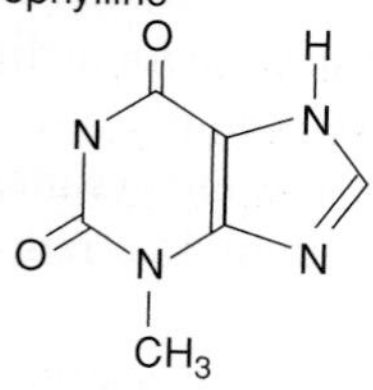

Enoximone

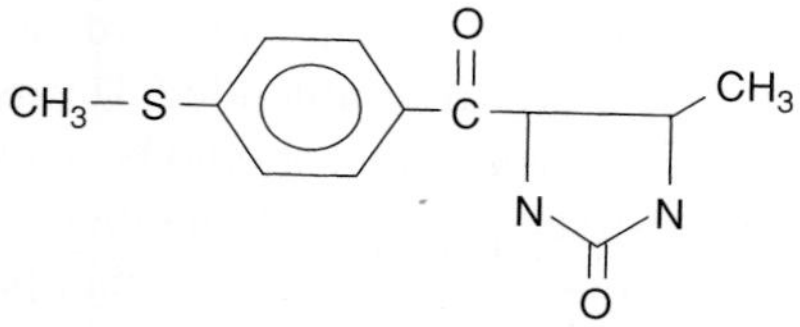

Milrinone

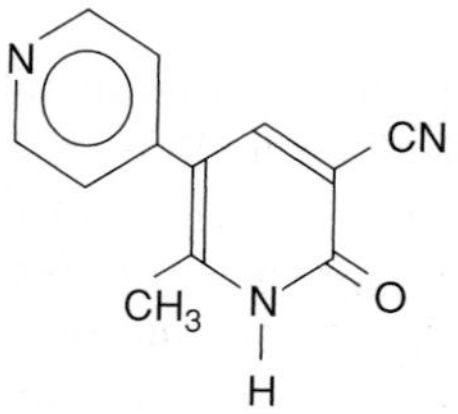

Figure 12.5. Structure of some phosphodiesterase inhibitors.

Mechanism of action

Aminophylline is a non-selective inhibitor of all five phosphodiesterase isoenzymes, which hydrolyze cAMP and possibly cGMP, thereby increasing their intracellular levels. It may also directly release noradrenaline from sympathetic neurones and demonstrate synergy with catecholamines, which act via adrenoceptors to increase intracellular cAMP. In addition it interferes with the translocation of Ca^{2+} into smooth muscle, inhibits the degranulation of mast cells by blocking their adenosine receptors and potentiates prostaglandin synthetase activity.

Effects

• Respiratory – aminophylline causes bronchodilation, improves the contractility of the diaphragm and increases the sensitivity of the respiratory centre to carbon dioxide. It works well in combination with β_2-agonists due to the different pathway used to increase cAMP.

- Cardiovascular – it has mild positive inotropic and chronotropic effects and causes some coronary and peripheral vasodilatation. It lowers the threshold for arrhythmias (particularly ventricular) especially in the presence of halothane.
- Central nervous system – the alkyl group at the 1-position (also present in caffeine) is responsible for its central nervous system stimulation, resulting in a reduced seizure threshold.
- Renal – the alkyl group at the 1-position is also responsible for its weak diuretic effects. Inhibition of tubular Na^+ reabsorption leads to a naturesis and may precipitate hypokalaemia.
- Interactions – co-administration of drugs that inhibit hepatic cytochrome P450 (cimetidine, erythromycin, ciprofloxacin and oral contraceptives) tend to delay the elimination of aminophylline and a reduction in dose is recommended. The use of certain selective serotonin re-uptake inhibitors (fluvoxamine) should be avoided with aminophylline as levels of the latter may rise sharply. Drugs that induce hepatic cytochrome P450 (phenytoin, carbamazepine, barbiturates and rifampicin) increase aminophylline clearance and the dose may need to be increased.

Kinetics

Aminophylline is well absorbed from the gut with a high oral bioavailability (>90%). About 50% is plasma protein bound. It is metabolized in the liver by cytochrome P450 to inactive metabolites and interacts with the metabolism of other drugs undergoing metabolism by a similar route. Owing to its low hepatic extraction ratio its metabolism is independent of liver blood flow. Approximately 10% is excreted unchanged in the urine. The effective therapeutic plasma concentration is 10–20 μg.ml^{-1}. Cigarette smoking increases the clearance of aminophylline.

Toxicity

Above 35 μg.ml^{-1}, hepatic enzymes become saturated and its kinetics change from first- to zero-order resulting in toxicity. Cardiac toxicity manifests itself as tachyarrhythmias including ventricular fibrillation. Central nervous system toxicity includes tremor, insomnia and seizures (especially following rapid intravenous administration). Nausea and vomiting are also a feature, as is rhabdomyolysis.

Selective phosphodiesterase inhibitors

Enoximone

The imidazolone derivative enoximone is a selective phosphodiesterase III inhibitor.

Presentation and uses

Enoximone is available as a yellow liquid (pH 12) for intravenous use containing 5 mg.ml^{-1}. It is supplied in propyl glycol and ethanol and should be stored between 5°C and 8°C. It is used to treat congestive heart failure and low cardiac output states associated with cardiac surgery. It should be diluted with an equal volume of water or 0.9% saline in plastic syringes (crystal formation is seen when mixed in glass syringes) and administered as an infusion of 5–20 μg.kg^{-1}.min^{-1}, which may be preceded by a loading dose of 0.5 mg.kg^{-1}, and can be repeated up to a maximum of 3 mg.kg^{-1}. Unlike catecholamines it may take up to 30 minutes to act.

Mechanism of action

Enoximone works by preventing the degradation of cAMP and possibly cGMP in cardiac and vascular smooth muscle. By effectively increasing cAMP within the myocardium, it increases the slow Ca^{2+} inward current during the cardiac action potential. This produces an increase in Ca^{2+} release from intracellular stores and an increase in the Ca^{2+} concentration in the vicinity of the contractile proteins, and hence to a positive inotropic effect. By interfering with Ca^{2+} flux into vascular smooth muscle it causes vasodilatation.

Effects

- Cardiovascular – enoximone has been termed an 'inodilator' due to its positive inotropic and vasodilator effects on the heart and vascular system. In patients with heart failure the cardiac output increases by about 30% while end diastolic filling pressures decrease by about 35%. The myocardial oxygen extraction ratio remains unchanged by virtue of a reduced ventricular wall tension and improved coronary artery perfusion. The blood pressure may remain unchanged or fall, the heart rate remains unchanged or rises slightly and arrhythmias occur only rarely. It shortens atrial, AV node and ventricular refractoriness. When used in patients with ischaemic heart disease, a reduction in coronary perfusion pressure and a rise in heart rate may outweigh the benefits of improved myocardial blood flow so that further ischaemia ensues.
- Miscellaneous – agranulocytosis has been reported.

Kinetics

While enoximone is well absorbed from the gut an extensive first-pass metabolism renders it useless when given orally. About 70% is plasma protein bound and metabolism occurs in the liver to a renally excreted active sulphoxide metabolite with 10% of the activity of enoximone and a terminal half-life of 7.5 hours. Only small amounts are excreted unchanged in the urine and by infusion enoximone has a terminal half-life of 4.5 hours. It has a wide therapeutic ratio and the risks of toxicity are low. The dose should be reduced in renal failure.

Milrinone

Milrinone is a bipyridine derivative and a selective phosphodiesterase III inhibitor with similar effects to enoximone. However, it has been associated with an increased mortality rate when administered orally to patients with severe heart failure.

Preparation and uses

Milrinone is formulated as a yellow solution containing 1 mg.ml^{-1} and may be stored at room temperature. It should be diluted before administration and should only be used intravenously for the short-term management of cardiac failure.

Kinetics

Approximately 70% is plasma protein bound. It has an elimination half-life of 1–2.5 hours and is 80% excreted in the urine unchanged. The dose should be reduced in renal failure.

Amrinone

Amrinone is not available in the UK. It has a similar pharmacological profile to the other selective phosphodiesterase inhibitors. Approximately 40% is excreted unchanged in the urine. One in 40 patients suffers a reversible dose-related thrombocytopenia.

Glucagon

Within the pancreas, α-cells secrete the polypeptide glucagon. The activation of glucagon receptors, via G-protein mediated mechanisms, stimulates adenylate cyclase and increases intracellular cAMP. It has only a limited role in cardiac failure, occasionally being used in the treatment of β-blocker overdose by an initial bolus of 10 mg followed by infusion of up to 5 mg.hr^{-1}. Hyperglycaemia and hyperkalaemia may complicate its use.

Ca^{2+}

While intravenously administered Ca^{2+} salts often improve blood pressure for a few minutes, their use should be restricted to circulatory collapse due to hyperkalaemia and Ca^{2+} channel antagonist overdose.

T_3

Thyroxine (T_4) and triiodothyronine (T_3) have positive inotropic and chronotropic effects via intracellular mechanisms. They are only used to treat hypothyroidism and are discussed in more detail in Chapter 25.

Adrenoceptor antagonists

- α-Adrenoceptor antagonists
- β-Adrenoceptor antagonists
- Combined α- and β-adrenoceptor antagonists

α-Adrenoceptor antagonists

α-Adrenoceptor antagonists (α-blockers) prevent the actions of sympathomimetic agents on α-adrenoceptors. Certain α-blockers (phentolamine, phenoxybenzamine) are non-specific and inhibit both α_1- and α_2-receptors, whereas others selectively inhibit α_1-receptors (prazosin) or α_2-receptors (yohimbine). The actions of specific α-adrenoceptor stimulation are shown in Table 13.1.

Non-selective α-blockade

Phentolamine

Phentolamine (an imidazolone) is a competitive non-selective α-blocker. Its affinity for α_1-adrenoceptors is three times that for α_2-adrenoceptors.

Presentation

It is presented as 10 mg phentolamine mesylate in 1 ml clear pale-yellow solution. The intravenous dose is 1–5 mg and should be titrated to effect. The onset of action is 1–2 minutes and its duration of action is 5–20 minutes.

Uses

Phentolamine is used in the treatment of hypertensive crises due to excessive sympathomimetics, MAOI reactions with tyramine and phaeochromocytoma, especially during tumour manipulation. It has a role in the assessment of sympathetically mediated chronic pain and has previously been used to treat pulmonary hypertension. Injection into the corpus cavernosum has been used to treat impotence due to erectile failure.

Effects

- Cardiovascular – α_1-blockade results in vasodilatation and hypotension while α_2-blockade facilitates noradrenaline release leading to tachycardia and a raised

217

Table 13.1. Actions of specific α-adrenoceptor stimulation.

Receptor type	Action
Post-synaptic	
α_1-Receptors	vasoconstriction
	mydriasis
	contraction of bladder sphincter
α_2-Receptors	platelet aggregation
	hyperpolarization of some CNS neurones
Presynaptic	
α_2-Receptors	inhibit noradrenaline release

cardiac output. Pulmonary artery pressure is also reduced. Vasodilatation of vessels in the nasal mucosa leads to marked nasal congestion.

- Respiratory – the presence of sulphites in phentolamine ampoules may lead to hypersensitivity reactions, which are manifest as acute bronchospasm in susceptible asthmatics.
- Gut – phentolamine increases secretions and motility of the gastrointestinal tract.
- Metabolic – it may precipitate hypoglycaemia secondary to increased insulin secretion.

Kinetics
The oral route is rarely used and has a bioavailability of 20%. It is 50% plasma protein bound and extensively metabolized, leaving about 10% to be excreted unchanged in the urine. Its elimination half-life is 20 minutes.

Phenoxybenzamine
Phenoxybenzamine is a long-acting non-selective α-blocker. It has a high affinity for α_1-adrenoceptors.

Presentation
It is presented as capsules containing 10 mg and as a clear, faintly straw-coloured solution for injection containing 100 mg/2 ml phenoxybenzamine hydrochloride with ethyl alcohol, hydrochloric acid and propylene glycol.

Uses
Phenoxybenzamine is used in the preoperative management of phaeochromocytoma (to allow expansion of the intravascular compartment), peri-operative management of some neonates undergoing cardiac surgery, hypertensive crises and occasionally as an adjunct to the treatment of severe shock. The oral dose starts at 10 mg and is increased daily until hypertension is controlled, the usual dose is 1–2 mg.kg^{-1}.day^{-1}. Intravenous administration should be via a central cannula and the

usual dose is 1 mg.kg^{-1}.day^{-1} given as a slow infusion in at least 200 ml 0.9% saline. β-blockade may be required to limit reflex tachycardia.

Mechanism of action

Its effects are mediated by a reactive intermediate that forms a covalent bond to the α-adrenoceptor resulting in irreversible blockade. In addition to receptor blockade, phenoxybenzamine inhibits neuronal and extra-neuronal uptake of catecholamines.

Effects

- Cardiovascular – hypotension, which may be orthostatic, and reflex tachycardia are characteristic. Overdose should be treated with noradrenaline. Adrenaline will lead to unopposed β effects thereby compounding the hypotension and tachycardia. There is an increase in cardiac output and blood flow to skin, viscera and nasal mucosa leading to nasal congestion.
- Central nervous system – it usually causes marked sedation although convulsions have been reported after rapid intravenous infusion. Meiosis is also seen.
- Miscellaneous – impotence, contact dermatitis.

Kinetics

Phenoxybenzamine is incompletely and variably absorbed from the gut (oral bioavailability about 25%). Its maximum effect is seen at 1 hour following an intravenous dose. The plasma half-life is about 24 hours and its effects may persist for 3 days while new α-adrenoceptors are synthesized. It is metabolized in the liver and excreted in urine and bile.

Selective α_1-blockade

Prazosin

Prazosin (a quinazoline derivative) is a highly selective α_1-adrenoceptor antagonist.

Presentation and uses

Prazosin is available as 0.5–2 mg tablets. It is used in the treatment of essential hypertension, congestive heart failure, Raynaud's syndrome and benign prostatic hypertrophy. The initial dose is 0.5 mg tds, which may be increased to 20 mg per day.

Effects

- Cardiovascular – prazosin produces vasodilatation of arteries and veins and a reduction of systemic vascular resistance with little or no reflex tachycardia. Diastolic pressures fall the most. Severe postural hypotension and syncope may follow the first dose. Cardiac output may increase in those with heart failure secondary to reduced filling pressures.

- Urinary – it relaxes the bladder trigone and sphincter muscle thereby improving urine flow in those with benign prostatic hypertrophy. Impotence and priapism have been reported.
- Central nervous system – fatigue, headache, vertigo and nausea all decrease with continued use.
- Miscellaneous – it may produce a false-positive when screening urine for metabolites of noradrenaline (VMA and MHPG seen in phaeochromocytoma).

Kinetics

Plasma levels peak about 90 minutes following an oral dose with a variable oral bioavailability of 50–80%. It is highly protein bound, mainly to albumin, and is extensively metabolized in the liver by demethylation and conjugation. Some of the metabolites are active. It has a plasma half-life of 3 hours. It may be used safely in patients with renal impairment as it is largely excreted in the bile.

Selective α_2-blockade

Yohimbine

The principal alkaloid of the bark of the yohimbe tree is formulated as the hydrochloride and has been used in the treatment of impotence. It has a variable effect on the cardiovascular system resulting in a raised heart rate and blood pressure but may precipitate orthostatic hypotension. In vitro it blocks the hypotensive responses of clonidine. It has an antidiuretic effect and can cause anxiety and manic reactions. It is contraindicated in renal or hepatic disease.

β-Adrenoceptor antagonists

β-Adrenoceptor antagonists (β-blockers) are widely used in the treatment of hypertension, angina and peri-myocardial infarction.

They are also used in patients with phaeochromocytoma (preventing the reflex tachycardia associated with α-blockade), hyperthyroidism (propranolol), hypertrophic obstructive cardiomyopathy (to control infundibular spasm), anxiety associated with high levels of catecholamines, topically in glaucoma, in the prophylaxis of migraine and to suppress the response to laryngoscopy and at extubation (esmolol).

They are all competitive antagonists with varying degrees of receptor selectivity. In addition some have intrinsic sympathomimetic activity (i.e. are partial agonists), whereas others demonstrate membrane stabilizing activity. These three features form the basis of their differing pharmacological profiles. Prolonged administration may result in an increase in the number of β-adrenoceptors.

Receptor selectivity

In suitable patients, the useful effects of β-blockers are mediated via antagonism of β_1-adrenoceptors, while antagonism of β_2-adrenoceptors results in unwanted

Table 13.2. Comparison between receptor selectivity, intrinsic sympathomimetic activity and membrane stabilizing activity of various β-blockers.

	β_1-receptor selectivity-cardioselectivity	Intrinsic sympathomimetic activity	Membrane stabilizing activity
Acebutolol	+	+	+
Atenolol	++	−	−
Esmolol	++	−	−
Metoprolol	++	−	+
Pindolol	−	++	+
Propranolol	−	−	++
Sotalol	−	−	−
Timolol	−	+	+
Labetalol	−	±	+

effects. Atenolol, esmolol and metoprolol demonstrate β_1-adrenoceptor selectivity (cardioselectivity) although when given in high dose β_2-antagonism may also be seen. All β-blockers should be used with extreme caution in patients with poor ventricular function as they may precipitate serious cardiac failure.

Intrinsic sympathomimetic activity – partial agonist activity

Partial agonists are drugs that are unable to elicit the same maximum response as a full agonist despite adequate receptor affinity. In theory, β-blockers with partial agonist activity will produce sympathomimetic effects when circulating levels of catecholamines are low, while producing antagonist effects when sympathetic tone is high. In patients with mild cardiac failure they should be less likely to induce bradycardia and heart failure. However, they should not be used in those with more severe heart failure as β-blockade will further reduce cardiac output.

Membrane stabilizing activity

These effects are probably of little clinical significance as the doses required to elicit them are higher than those seen in vivo.

Effects

- Cardiac – β-blockers have negative inotropic and chronotropic properties on cardiac muscle; sino-atrial (SA) node automaticity is decreased and atrioventricular (AV) node conduction time is prolonged leading to a bradycardia, while contractility is also reduced. The bradycardia lengthens the coronary artery perfusion time (during diastole) thereby increasing oxygen supply while reduced contractility diminishes oxygen demand. These effects are more important than those that tend to compromise the supply/demand equation, that is, prolonged systolic ejection

Table 13.3. Various pharmacological properties of some β-blockers.

Drug	Lipid solubility	Absorption (%)	Bioavailability (%)	Protein binding (%)	Elimination half-life (h)	Clearance	Active metabolites
Acebutolol	++	90	40	25	6	hepatic metabolism and renal excretion	yes
Atenolol	+	45	45	5	7	renal	no
Esmolol	+++	n/a	n/a	60	0.15	plasma hydrolysis	no
Metoprolol	+++	95	50	20	3–7*	hepatic metabolism	no
Oxprenolol	+++	80	40	80	2	hepatic metabolism	no
Pindolol	++	90	90	50	4	hepatic metabolism	no
Propranolol	+++	90	30	90	4	hepatic metabolism	yes
Sotalol	+	85	85	0	15	renal	no
Timolol	+++	90	50	10	4	hepatic metabolism and renal excretion	no
Labetalol	+++	70	25	50	5	hepatic metabolism	no

*Depends on genetic polymorphism – may be fast or slow hydroxylators.

time, dilation of the ventricles and increased coronary vascular resistance (due to antagonism of the vasodilatory β_2 coronary receptors). The improvement in the balance of oxygen supply/demand forms the basis for their use in angina and peri-myocardial infarction. However, in patients with poor left ventricular function β-blockade may lead to cardiac failure. β-blockers are class II anti-arrhythmic agents and are mainly used to treat arrhythmias associated with high levels of catecholamines (see Chapter 14).

- Circulatory – the mechanism by which β-blockers control blood pressure is not yet fully elucidated but probably includes a reduced heart rate and cardiac output, and inhibition of the renin-angiotensin system. Inhibition of β_1-receptors at the juxtaglomerular apparatus reduces renin release leading ultimately to a reduction in angiotensin II and its effects (vasoconstriction and augmenting aldosterone production). In addition, the baroreceptors may be set at a lower level, presynaptic β_2-receptors may inhibit noradrenaline release and some β-blockers may have central effects. However, due to antagonism of peripheral β_2-receptors there will be an element of vasoconstriction, which appears to have little hypertensive effect but may result in poor peripheral circulation and cold hands.

- Respiratory – all β-blockers given in sufficient dose will precipitate bronchospasm via β_2-antagonism. The relatively cardioselective drugs (atenolol, esmolol and metoprolol) are preferred but should still be used with extreme caution in patients with asthma.

- Metabolic – the control of blood sugar is complicated involving different tissue types (liver, pancreas, adipose), receptors (α-, β-adrenoceptors) and hormones (insulin, glucagon, catecholamines). Non-selective β-blockade may obtund the normal blood sugar response to exercise and hypoglycaemia although it may also increase the resting blood sugar levels in diabetics with hypertension. Therefore, non-selective β-blockers should not be used with hypoglycaemic agents. In addition, β-blockade may mask the normal symptoms of hypoglycaemia. Lipid metabolism may be altered resulting in increased triglycerides and reduced high density lipoproteins.

- Central nervous system – the more lipid-soluble β-blockers (metoprolol, propranolol) are more likely to produce CNS side effects. These include depression, hallucination, nightmares, paranoia and fatigue.

- Occular – intra-occular pressure is reduced, probably as a result of decreased production of aqueous humour.

- Gut – dry mouth and gastrointestinal disturbances.

Kinetics

Varying lipid solubility confers the main differences seen in the kinetics of β-blockers. Those with low lipid solubility (atenolol) are poorly absorbed from the gut, undergo little hepatic metabolism and are excreted largely unchanged in the urine. However, those with high lipid solubility are well absorbed from the gut and are extensively metabolized in the liver. They have a shorter half-life and consequently need more frequent administration. In addition, they cross the blood–brain barrier resulting in sedation and nightmares. Protein binding is variable.

Individual β-blockers

Acebutolol

Acebutolol is a relatively cardioselective β-blocker that is only available orally. It has limited intrinsic sympathomimetic activity and some membrane stabilizing properties. The adult dose is 400 mg bd but may be increased to 1.2 g.day^{-1} if required.

Kinetics

Acebutolol is well absorbed from the gut due to its moderately high lipid solubility, but due to a high first-pass metabolism its oral bioavailability is only 40%. Despite its lipid solubility it does not cross the BBB to any great extent. Hepatic metabolism produces the active metabolite diacetol, which has a longer half-life, and is less cardioselective than acebutolol. Both are excreted in bile and may undergo enterohepatic recycling. They are also excreted in urine and the dose should be reduced in the presence of renal impairment.

Atenolol

Atenolol is a relatively cardioselective β-blocker that is available as 25–100 mg tablets, a syrup containing 5 mg.ml^{-1} and as a colourless solution for intravenous use containing 5 mg in 10 ml. The oral dose is 50–100 mg.day^{-1} while the intravenous dose is 2.5 mg slowly, repeated up to a maximum of 10 mg, which may then be followed by an infusion.

Kinetics

Atenolol is incompletely absorbed from the gut. It is not significantly metabolized and has an oral bioavailability of 45%. Only 5% is protein bound. It is excreted unchanged in the urine and, therefore, the dose should be reduced in patients with renal impairment. It has an elimination half-life of 7 hours but its actions appear to persist for longer than this would suggest.

Esmolol

Esmolol is a highly lipophilic, cardioselective β-blocker with a rapid onset and offset. It is presented as a clear liquid with either 2.5 g or 100 mg in 10 ml. The former should be diluted before administration as an infusion (dose range 50–200 μg.kg^{-1}.min^{-1}), while the latter is titrated in 10 mg boluses to effect. It is used in the short-term management of tachycardia and hypertension in the peri-operative period, and for acute supraventricular tachycardia. It has no intrinsic sympathomimetic activity or membrane stabilizing properties.

Kinetics

Esmolol is only available intravenously and is 60% protein bound. Its volume of distribution is 3.5 l.kg^{-1}. It is rapidly metabolized by red blood cell esterases to an essentially inactive acid metabolite (with a long half-life) and methyl alcohol. Its rapid metabolism ensures a short half-life of 10 minutes. The esterases responsible for its hydrolysis are distinct from plasma cholinesterase so that it does not prolong the actions of suxamethonium.

Like other β-blockers it may also precipitate heart failure and bronchospasm, although its short duration of action limits these side effects.

It is irritant to veins and extravasation may lead to tissue necrosis.

Metoprolol

Metoprolol is a relatively cardioselective β-blocker with no intrinsic sympathomimetic activity. Early use of metoprolol in myocardial infarction reduces infarct size and the incidence of ventricular fibrillation. It is also used in hypertension, as an adjunct in thyrotoxicosis and for migraine prophylaxis. The dose is 50–200 mg daily. Up to 5 mg may be given intravenously for arrhythmias and in myocardial infarction.

Kinetics

Absorption is rapid and complete, but due to hepatic first-pass metabolism, its oral bioavailability is only 50%. However, this increases to 70% during continuous administration and is also increased when given with food. Hepatic metabolism may exhibit genetic polymorphism resulting in two different half-life profiles of 3 and 7 hours. Its high lipid solubility enables it to cross the blood–brain barrier and also into breast milk. Only 20% is plasma protein bound.

Propranolol

Propranolol is a non-selective β-blocker without intrinsic sympathomimetic activity. It exhibits the full range of effects described above at therapeutic concentrations. It is a racemic mixture, the S-isomer conferring most of its effects, although the R-isomer is responsible for preventing the peripheral conversion of T_4 to T_3.

Uses

Propranolol is used to treat hypertension, angina, essential tremor and in the prophylaxis of migraine. It is the β-blocker of choice in thyrotoxicosis as it not only inhibits the effects of the thyroid hormones, but also prevents the peripheral conversion of T_4 to T_3. Intravenous doses of 0.5 mg (up to 10 mg) are titrated to effect. The oral dose ranges from 160 mg to 320 mg daily, but due to increased clearance in thyrotoxicosis even higher doses may be required.

Kinetics

Owing to its high lipid solubility it is well absorbed from the gut but a high first-pass metabolism reduces its oral bioavailability to 30%. It is highly protein bound although this may be reduced by heparin. Hepatic metabolism of the R-isomer is more rapid than the S-isomer and one of their metabolites, 4-hydroxypropranolol, retains some activity. Its elimination is dependent on hepatic metabolism but is impaired in renal failure by an unknown mechanism. The duration of action is longer than its half-life of 4 hours would suggest.

Sotalol

Sotalol is a non-selective β-blocker with no intrinsic sympathomimetic properties. It also has class III anti-arrhythmic properties (see Chapter 14).

It is a racemic mixture, the D-isomer conferring the class III activity while the L-isomer has both class III and class II (β-blocking) actions.

Uses

Sotalol is used to treat ventricular tachyarrhythmias and for the prophylaxis of paroxysmal supraventricular tachycardias following direct current (DC) cardioversion. The ventricular rate is also well controlled if sinus rhythm degenerates back into atrial fibrillation. The CSM states that sotalol should not be used for angina, hypertension, thyrotoxicosis or peri-myocardial infarction. The oral dose is 80–160 mg bd and the intravenous dose is 50–100 mg over 20 minutes.

Other effects

The most serious side effect is precipitation of torsades de pointes, which is rare, occurring in less than 2% of those being treated for sustained ventricular tachycardia or fibrillation. It is more common with higher doses, a prolonged QT interval and electrolyte imbalance. It may precipitate heart failure.

Kinetics

Sotalol is completely absorbed from the gut and its oral bioavailability exceeds 90%. It is not protein bound or metabolized. Approximately 90% is excreted unchanged in urine while the remainder is excreted in bile. Renal impairment significantly reduces clearance.

Combined α- and β-adrenoceptor antagonists

Labetalol

Labetalol, as its name indicates, is an α- and β-adrenoceptor antagonist; α-blockade is specific to α_1-receptors while β-blockade is non-specific. It contains two asymmetric centres and exists as a mixture of four stereoisomers present in equal proportions. The (SR)-stereoisomer is probably responsible for the α_1 effects while the

(RR)-stereoisomer probably confers the β-blockade. The ratio of α_1:β-blocking effects is dependent on the route of administration: 1:3 for oral, 1:7 for intravenous.

Presentation and uses

Labetalol is available as 50–400 mg tablets and as a colourless solution containing 5 mg.ml^{-1}. It is used to treat hypertensive crises and to facilitate hypotension during anaesthesia. The intravenous dose is 5–20 mg titrated up to a maximum of 200 mg. The oral form is used to treat hypertension associated with angina and during pregnancy where the dose is 100–800 mg bd but may be increased to a maximum of 2.4 g daily.

Mechanism of action

Selective α_1-blockade produces peripheral vasodilatation while β-blockade prevents reflex tachycardia. Myocardial afterload and oxygen demand are decreased providing favourable conditions for those with angina.

Kinetics

Labetalol is well absorbed from the gut but due to an extensive hepatic first-pass metabolism its oral bioavailability is only 25%. However, this may increase markedly with increasing age and when administered with food. It is 50% protein bound. Metabolism occurs in the liver and produces several inactive conjugates.

Anti-arrhythmics

Physiology

Cardiac action potential

The heart is composed of pacemaker, conducting and contractile tissue. Each has a different action potential morphology allowing the heart to function as a coordinated unit.

The SA node is in the right atrium, and of all cardiac tissue it has the fastest rate of spontaneous depolarization so that it sets the heart rate. The slow spontaneous depolarization (pre-potential or pacemaker potential) of the membrane potential is due to increased Ca^{2+} conductance (directed inward). At −40 mV, slow voltage-gated Ca^{2+} channels (L channels) open resulting in membrane depolarization. Na^+ conductance changes very little. Repolarization is due to increased K^+ conductance while Ca^{2+} channels close (Figure 14.1a).

Contractile cardiac tissue has a more stable resting potential at −80 mV. Its action potential has been divided into five phases (Figure 14.1b):

- Phase 0 – describes the rapid depolarization (duration <1 ms) of the membrane, resulting from increased Na^+ (and possibly some Ca^{2+}) conductance through voltage-gated Na^+ channels.
- Phase 1 – represents closure of the Na^+ channels while Cl^- is expelled.
- Plateau phase 2 – due to Ca^{2+} influx via voltage-sensitive type-L Ca^{2+} channels and lasts up to 150 ms. This period is also known as the absolute refractory period in which the myocyte cannot be further depolarized. This prevents myocardial tetany.
- Phase 3 – commences when the Ca^{2+} channels are inactivated and there is an increase in K^+ conductance that returns the membrane potential to its resting value. This period is also known as the relative refractory period in which the myocyte requires a greater than normal stimulus to provoke a contraction.
- Phase 4 – during this the Na^+/K^+ ATPase maintains the ionic concentration gradient at about −80 mV, although there will be variable spontaneous 'diastolic' depolarization.

Arrhythmias

Tachyarrhythmias

- These may originate from **enhanced automaticity** where the resting potential of contractile tissue loses its stability and may reach its threshold for depolarization before that of the SA node. This is seen during ischaemia and hypokalaemia.
- Ischaemic myocardium may result in oscillations of the membrane potential. These **after-potentials** may reach the threshold potential and precipitate tachyarrhythmias.
- **Re-entry** or **circus** mechanisms describe how an ectopic focus may originate, leading to tachyarrhythmias (Figure 14.2).

Bradyarrhythmias

These are due to failure of conduction from the SA node to surrounding tissue. Second- and third-degree block becomes clinically significant. Atropine, β stimulation or pacing may be required.

Classification of anti-arrhythmics

Traditionally anti-arrhythmics have been classified according to the Vaughan–Williams classification. However, it does not include digoxin and more recently introduced drugs such as adenosine. In addition, individual agents do not fall neatly into one category, e.g. sotalol has class I, II and III activity.

Anti-arrhythmics may also be divided on the basis of their clinical use in the treatment of:

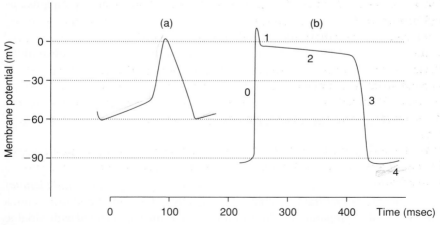

Figure 14.1. Action potentials of (a) pacemaker and (b) contractile tissue.

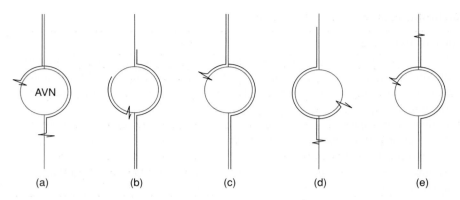

Figure 14.2. Atrioventricular nodal re-entrant tachycardia ($\curlywedge$ action potential followed by refractory period). In this situation, there are two anatomically and physiologically distinct conduction pathways within the atrioventricular node (AVN). The fast pathway has a long refractory period, whereas the slow pathway has a short refractory period. (a) A normal atrial action potential (AP) travels at different velocities through the two pathways. The AP in the slow pathway arrives at the refractory final common pathway and is therefore terminated (b). (b) also demonstrates how the slow pathway recovers from its refractory state more quickly than the fast pathway. If a premature atrial impulse arrives at the origins of the two pathways and finds the fast pathway still refractory it will only travel down the slow pathway (c). Because it travels slowly down the slow pathway it is not terminated by refractory tissue as in (b) and may travel on into the ventricles but also retrogradely up the fast pathway (d). Because of the short refractory period of the slow pathway the impulse may travel down the slow pathway (e) to continue the circus movement thereby generating the self-perpetuating tachycardia. The atrioventricular re-enterant tachcardia seen in WPW syndrome is generated in a similar manner except that the accessory pathway (bundle of Kent) is distinct from the AVN.

- **Supraventricular tachyarrhythmias** (**SVT**) (digoxin, adenosine, verapamil, β-blockers, quinidine)
- **Ventricular tachyarrhythmias** (**VT**) (lidocaine, mexiletine)
- **Both SVT and VT** (amiodarone, flecainide, procainamide, disopyramide, propafenone, sotalol)
- **Digoxin toxicity** (phenytoin)

Supraventricular tachyarrhythmias

Digoxin

Presentation

Digoxin is a glycoside that is extracted from the leaves of the foxglove (*Digitalis lanata*) and is available as oral (tablets of 62.5–250 μg, elixir 50 μg.ml^{-1}) and intravenous (100–250 μg.ml^{-1}) preparations. The intramuscular route is associated with variable absorption, pain and tissue necrosis.

14 Anti-arrhythmics

Table 14.1. Vaughan–Williams classification.

Class	Mechanism	Drugs
a	Na^+ channel blockade – prolongs the refractory period of cardiac muscle	quinidine, procainamide, disopyramide
Ib	Na^+ channel blockade – shortens the refractory period of cardiac muscle	lidocaine, mexiletine, phenytoin
Ic	Na^+ channel blockade – no effect on the refractory period of cardiac muscle	flecainide, propafenone
II	β-Adrenoceptor blockade	propranolol, atenolol, esmolol
III	K^+ channel blockade	amiodarone, bretylium, sotalol
IV	Ca^{2+} channel blockade	verapamil, diltiazem

Uses

Digoxin is widely used in the treatment of atrial fibrillation and atrial flutter. It has been used in heart failure but the initial effects on cardiac output may not be sustained and other agents may produce a better outcome. It has only minimal activity on the normal heart. It should be avoided in patients with ventricular extrasystoles or ventricular tachycardia (VT) as it may precipitate ventricular fibrillation (VF) due to increased cardiac excitability.

Treatment starts with the administration of a loading dose of between 1.0 and 1.5 mg in divided doses over 24 hours followed by a maintenance dose of 125–500 μg per day. The therapeutic range is 1–2 μg.l^{-1}.

Mechanism of action

Digoxin has direct and indirect actions on the heart.

- Direct – it binds to and inhibits cardiac Na^+/K^+ ATPase leading to increased intracellular Na^+ and decreased intracellular K^+ concentrations. The raised intracellular Na^+ concentration leads to an increased exchange with extracellular Ca^{2+} resulting in increased availability of intracellular Ca^{2+}, which has a positive inotropic effect, increasing excitability and force of contraction. The refractory period of the AV node and the bundle of His is increased and the conductivity reduced.
- Indirect – the release of acetylcholine at cardiac muscarinic receptors is enhanced. This slows conduction and further prolongs the refractory period in the AV node and the bundle of His.

In atrial fibrillation the atrial rate is too high to allow a 1:1 ventricular response. By slowing conduction through the AV node, the rate of ventricular response is reduced. This allows for a longer period of coronary blood flow and a greater degree of ventricular filling so that cardiac output is increased.

Side effects

Digoxin has a low therapeutic ratio and side effects are not uncommon:

- Cardiac – these include various arrhythmias and conduction disturbances – premature ventricular contractions, bigemini, all forms of AV block including third-degree block, junctional rhythm and atrial or ventricular tachycardia. Hypokalaemia, hypercalcaemia or altered pH may precipitate side effects. The ECG signs of prolonged PR interval, characteristic ST segment depression, T wave flattening and shortened QT interval are not signs of toxicity.

  DC cardioversion – severe ventricular arrhythmias may be precipitated in patients with toxic levels and it is recommended to withhold digoxin for 24 hours before elective cardioversion.

- Non-cardiac – anorexia, nausea and vomiting, diarrhoea and lethargy. Visual disturbances (including deranged red–green colour perception) and headache are common while gynaecomastia occurs during long-term administration. Skin rashes are rarely seen and may be accompanied by an eosinophilia.

- Interactions – plasma levels are increased by amiodarone, captopril, erythromycin and carbenoxolone. They are reduced by antacids, cholestyramine, phenytoin and metoclopramide. Ca^{2+} channel antagonists produce variable effects, verapamil will increase, while nifedipine and diltiazem may have no effect or produce a small rise in plasma levels.

Kinetics

The absorption of digoxin from the gut is variable depending on the specific formulation used, but the oral bioavailability is greater than 70%. It is about 25% plasma and has a volume of distribution of 5–10 $l.kg^{-1}$. Its volume of distribution is significantly increased in thyrotoxicosis and decreased in hypothyroidism. It undergoes only minimal hepatic metabolism, being excreted mainly in the unchanged form by filtration at the glomerulus and active tubular secretion. The elimination half-life is approximately 35 hours but is increased significantly in the presence of renal failure.

Toxicity

Plasma concentrations exceeding 2.5 $\mu g.l^{-1}$ are associated with toxicity although serious problems are unusual at levels below 10 $\mu g.l^{-1}$. Despite these figures the severity of toxicity does not correlate well with plasma levels. However, a dose of more than 30 mg is invariably associated with death unless digoxin-specific antibody fragments (Fab) are used.

Treatment of digoxin toxicity

Gastric lavage should be used with caution as any increase in vagal tone may precipitate further bradycardia or cardiac arrest. Owing to Na^+/K^+ ATPase inhibition, hyperkalaemia may be a feature and should be corrected. Hypokalaemia will exacerbate cardiac toxicity and should also be corrected. Where bradycardia is symptomatic atropine or pacing is preferred to infusions of catecholamines, which may precipitate further arrhythmias. Ventricular arrhythmias may be treated with lidocaine or phenytoin.

If plasma levels rise above 20 μg.l^{-1}, there are life-threatening arrhythmias or hyperkalaemia becomes uncontrolled, digoxin-specific Fab are indicated. These are IgG fragments. Digoxin is bound more avidly by Fab than by its receptor so that it is effectively removed from its site of action. The inactive digoxin–Fab complex is removed from the circulation by the kidneys. There is a danger of hypersensitivity or anaphylaxis on re-exposure to digoxin-specific Fab.

Adenosine

Adenosine is a naturally occurring purine nucleoside consisting of adenine (the purine base) and D-ribose (the pentose sugar), which is present in all cells.

Presentation

Adenosine is presented as a colourless solution in vials containing 3 mg.ml^{-1}. It should be stored at room temperature.

Uses

Adenosine is used to differentiate between SVT, where the rate is at least transiently slowed and VT, where the rate does not slow. Where SVT is due to re-entry circuits that involve the AV node, adenosine may covert the rhythm to sinus. Atrial fibrillation and flutter are not converted by adenosine to sinus rhythm as they are not generated by re-entry circuits involving the AV node, although its use in this setting will slow the ventricular response and aid ECG diagnosis.

Mechanism of action

Adenosine has specific actions on the SA and AV node mediated by adenosine A_1 receptors that are not found elsewhere within the heart. These adenosine-sensitive K^+ channels are opened, causing membrane hyperpolarization, and G_i-proteins cause a reduction in cAMP. This results in a dramatic negative chronotropic effect within the AV node.

Side effects

Because of its short half-life its side effects are also short lived but for the patient may be very distressing.

- Cardiac – it may induce atrial fibrillation or flutter as it decreases the atrial refractory period. It is contraindicated in those with second- or third-degree AV-block or with sick sinus syndrome.

- Non-cardiac – these include chest discomfort, shortness of breath and facial flushing. It should be used with caution in asthmatics as it may precipitate bronchospasm.
- Drug interactions – its effects may be enhanced by dipyridamole (by blocking its uptake) and antagonized by the methylxanthines especially aminophylline.

Kinetics

Adenosine is given in incremental doses from 3 to 12 mg as an intravenous bolus, preferably via a central cannula. It is rapidly de-aminated in the plasma and taken up by red blood cells so that its half-life is less than 10 seconds.

Verapamil

Verapamil is a competitive Ca^{2+} channel antagonist.

Presentation

It is presented as film-coated and modified-release tablets and as a solution for intravenous injection containing 2.5 mg.ml^{-1}.

Uses

Verapamil is used to treat SVT, atrial fibrillation or flutter, which it may slow or convert to a sinus rhythm. It is also used in the prophylaxis of angina and the treatment of hypertension.

Mechanism of action

Verapamil prevents the influx of Ca^{2+} through voltage-sensitive slow (L) channels in the SA and AV node, thereby reducing their automaticity. It has a much less marked effect on the contractile tissue of the heart, but does reduce Ca^{2+} influx during the plateau phase 2. Antagonism of these Ca^{2+} channels results in a reduced rate of conduction through the AV node and coronary artery dilatation.

Side effects

- Cardiac – if used to treat SVT complicating Wolff–Parkinson–White (WPW) syndrome, verapamil may precipitate VT due to increased conduction across the accessory pathway. In patients with poor left ventricular function it may precipitate cardiac failure. When administered concurrently with agents that also slow AV conduction (digoxin, β-blockers, halothane) it may precipitate serious bradycardia and AV block. It may increase the serum levels of digoxin. Grapefruit juice has been reported to increase serum levels and should be avoided during verapamil therapy.

  Although its effects are relatively specific to cardiac tissue it may also precipitate hypotension through vascular smooth muscle relaxation.

- Non-cardiac – cerebral artery vasodilatation occurs after the administration of verapamil.

Kinetics

Verapamil is used orally and intravenously. Although almost 90% is absorbed from the gut a high first-pass metabolism reduces its oral bioavailability to about 25%. Approximately 90% is bound to plasma proteins. It is metabolized in the liver to at least 12 inactive metabolites that are excreted in the urine. Its volume of distribution is 3–5 l.kg^{-1}. The elimination half-life of 3–7 hours is prolonged with higher doses as hepatic enzymes become saturated.

β-Blockers

The effects of catecholamines are antagonized by β-blockers. Therefore, they induce a bradycardia (by prolonging 'diastolic' depolarization – phase 4), depress myocardial contractility and prolong AV conduction. In addition, some β-blockers exhibit a degree of membrane stabilizing activity (class I) although this probably has little clinical significance. Sotalol also demonstrates class III activity by blocking K$^+$ channels and prolonging repolarization.

β-Blockers are used in the treatment of hypertension, angina, myocardial infarction, tachyarrhythmias, thyrotoxicosis, anxiety states, the prophylaxis of migraine and topically in glaucoma. Their use as an anti-arrhythmic is limited to treatment of paroxysmal SVT and sinus tachycardia due to increased levels of catecholamines. They have a role following acute myocardial infarction where they may reduce arrhythmias and prevent further infarction. Owing to their negative inotropic effects they should be avoided in those with poor ventricular function for fear of precipitating cardiac failure.

Esmolol

Esmolol is a relatively cardioselective β-blocker with a rapid onset and offset.

Presentation

It is presented as a clear liquid with either 2.5 g or 100 mg in 10 ml. The former should be diluted before administration as an infusion (dose range 50–200 μg.kg^{-1}.min^{-1}), while the latter is titrated in 10 mg boluses to effect.

Uses

Esmolol is used in the short-term management of tachycardia and hypertension in the peri-operative period, and for acute SVT. It has no intrinsic sympathomimetic activity or membrane-stabilizing properties.

Side effects
Although esmolol is relatively cardioselective it does demonstrate β_2-adrenoceptor antagonism at high doses and should therefore be used with caution in asthmatics. Like other β-blockers it may also precipitate heart failure. However, due to its short duration of action these side effects are also limited in time.

It is irritant to veins and extravasation may lead to tissue necrosis.

Kinetics
Esmolol is only available intravenously and is 60% plasma protein bound. Its volume of distribution is 3.5 l.kg^{-1}. It is rapidly metabolized by red blood cell esterases to an essentially inactive acid metabolite (with a long half-life) and methyl alcohol. Its rapid metabolism ensures a short half-life of 10 minutes. The esterases responsible for its hydrolysis are distinct from plasma cholinesterase so that it does not prolong the actions of suxamethonium.

Quinidine
The use of quinidine has declined as alternative treatments have become available with improved side-effect profiles. However, it may still be used to treat SVT, including atrial fibrillation and flutter, and ventricular ectopic beats.

Mechanism of action
Quinidine is a class Ia anti-arrhythmic and as such reduces the rate of rise of phase 0 of the action potential by blocking Na$^+$ channels. In addition, it raises the threshold potential and prolongs the refractory period without affecting the duration of the action potential. It also antagonizes vagal tone.

Side effects
These are common and become unacceptable in up to 30% of patients.
- Cardiac – quinidine may provoke other arrhythmias including heart block, sinus tachycardia (vagolytic action) and ventricular arrhythmias. The following ECG changes may be seen: prolonged PR interval, widened QRS and prolonged QT interval. When used to treat atrial fibrillation or flutter the patient should be pretreated with β-blockers, Ca^{2+} channel antagonists or digoxin to slow AV conduction, which may otherwise become enhanced leading to a ventricular rate equivalent to the atrial rate. Hypotension may result from α-blockade or direct myocardial depression, which is exacerbated by hyperkalaemia.
- Non-cardiac – central nervous system toxicity known as 'cinchonism' is characterized by tinnitus, blurred vision, impaired hearing, headache and confusion.
- Drug interactions – digoxin is displaced from its binding sites so that its serum concentration is increased. Phenytoin will reduce quinidine levels (hepatic enzyme

induction) while cimetidine will increase quinidine levels (hepatic enzyme inhibition). The effects of depolarizing and non-depolarizing muscle relaxants are increased.

Kinetics

Quinidine is well absorbed from the gut and has an oral bioavailability of about 75%. It is highly protein bound (about 90%) and is metabolized by the liver to active metabolites, which are excreted mainly in the urine. The elimination half-life is 5–9 hours.

Ventricular tachyarrhythmias

Lidocaine

Lidocaine is a class Ib anti-arrhythmic agent.

Presentation

The 1% or 2% solutions (10–20 mg.ml^{-1}) are the preparations used in this setting.

Uses

Lidocaine is used to treat sustained ventricular tachyarrhythmias especially when associated with ischaemia (where inactivated Na$^+$ channels predominate) or re-entry pathways. An initial intravenous bolus of 1 mg.kg^{-1} is followed by an intravenous infusion of 1–3 mg.min^{-1} for an adult. This infusion rate should be slowed where hepatic blood flow is reduced as hepatic metabolism will also be reduced.

Mechanism of action

Lidocaine reduces the rate of rise of phase 0 of the action potential by blocking inactivated Na$^+$ channels and raising the threshold potential. The duration of the action potential and the refractory period are decreased as the repolarization phase 3 is shortened.

Side effects

- Cardiac – cardiovascular toxicity becomes apparent as plasma levels exceed 10 μg.ml^{-1} and are manifest as AV block and unresponsive hypotension due to myocardial depression. Some of the cardiac effects may be due to central medullary depression.
- Non-cardiac – these become apparent only when the plasma levels exceed 4 μg.ml^{-1}. Initially central nervous system toxicity is manifest as circumoral tingling, dizziness and parasthesia. This progresses to confusion, coma and seizures as plasma levels rise above 5 μg.ml^{-1}.

Kinetics

When used for the treatment of arrhythmias lidocaine is only given intravenously. It is 33% unionized and 70% protein bound. It is metabolized by hepatic amidases to products that are eliminated in the urine. Its elimination half-life is about 90 minutes so that in the presence of normal hepatic function a steady-state would be reached after about 6 hours in the absence of a loading dose. Its clearance is reduced in cardiac failure due to reduced hepatic blood flow.

Mexiletine

Mexiletine is an analogue of lidocaine with similar effects on ventricular tachyarrhythmias.

Presentation

It is presented as a colourless solution containing 250 mg mexiletine hydrochloride in 10 ml. The oral formulation is also available as modified release.

Uses

Mexiletine has similar indications to lidocaine particularly when arrhythmias are associated with ischaemia or digoxin.

Mechanism of action

Mexiletine reduces the rate of rise of phase 0 of the action potential by blocking Na^+ channels and raising the threshold potential. The duration of the action potential and the refractory period are decreased as the repolarization phase 3 is shortened.

Side effects

Mexiletine has a low therapeutic ratio and side effects are common.
- Cardiac – it may precipitate sinus bradycardia, supraventricular and ventricular tachyarrhythmias.
- Non-cardiac – up to 40% of patients have unacceptable nausea and vomiting and altered bowel habit. Confusion, diplopia, seizures, tremor and ataxia are also seen. Thrombocytopenia, rash and jaundice have also been reported.

Kinetics

Its oral bioavailability of 90% reflects good absorption from the upper part of the small bowel and minimal first-pass metabolism (about 10%). It is 65% plasma protein bound and has a volume of distribution of 6–13 $l.kg^{-1}$. It undergoes hepatic metabolism to a number of inactive metabolites. Up to 20% is excreted unchanged in the urine.

Both: supraventricular and ventricular tachyarrhythmias

Amiodarone

Amiodarone is a benzofuran derivative.

Presentation

It is presented as tablets containing 100–200 mg and as a solution containing 150 mg per ampoule. It should be diluted in 5% dextrose before administration.

Uses

Amiodarone is used in the treatment of SVT, VT and WPW syndrome. It is a complex drug with many actions and side effects.

A loading dose of 5 mg.kg^{-1} over 1 hour followed by 15 mg.kg^{-1} over 24 hours provides a starting point for its intravenous use, which should be adjusted according to response. When used orally treatment commences with 200 mg tds for 1 week, followed by 200 mg bd for a further week and thereafter 200 mg od.

Mechanism of action

While it has been traditionally designated a class III anti-arrhythmic, amiodarone also demonstrates class I, II and IV activity. By blocking K$^+$ channels it slows the rate of repolarization thereby increasing the duration of the action potential. The refractory period is also increased.

Side effects

The side effects of amiodarone will affect most patients if given for long enough although most are reversible if treatment is stopped.

- Pulmonary – patients may develop a pneumonitis, fibrosis or pleuritis. The reported incidence is 10% at 3 years with a 10% mortality rate. However, if treatment is stopped early enough the process may be reversed. There is some evidence to suggest that a high F$_i$O$_2$ may be a risk factor in the development of acute pulmonary toxicity when amiodarone is used in critically ill patients.
- Thyroid – both hyperthyroidism (in 0.9%) and hypothyroidism (in 6%) have been observed and both are usually reversible. It prevents the peripheral conversion of T4 to T3.
- Hepatic – cirrhosis, hepatitis and jaundice have all been observed. Liver function tests should be performed before and during long-term treatment.
- Cardiac – when large doses are given rapidly it may cause bradycardia and hypotension. It has a low arrhythmic potential. The QT interval may be prolonged.
- Ophthalmic – corneal microdeposits occur commonly but have little clinical significance, causing visual haloes and some mild blurring of vision. They are reversible.

Ophthalmic examination is recommended annually for those on long-term treatment.

- Gut – during the loading dose a metallic taste may be noticed. Minor intestinal upset is seen occasionally.
- Neurological – peripheral neuropathy and rarely myopathy have been reported.
- Dermatological – the skin becomes photosensitive and may remain so for a number of months after finishing treatment. A slate-grey colour particularly of the face may develop.
- Interactions – the effects of other highly protein bound drugs (phenytoin, warfarin) are increased and their doses should be adjusted. The plasma level of digoxin may rise when amiodarone is added due to displacement from plasma protein-binding sites and cause signs of toxicity. Caution should be exercised when used with drugs that slow AV conduction (β-blockers, verapamil) and it should not be given with other drugs that prolong the QT interval (phenothiazines, TCAs, thiazides) for fear of precipitating torsades de pointes.
- Miscellaneous – the intravenous preparation is irritant and should be administered via a central vein.

Kinetics

Amiodarone is poorly absorbed from the gut and has an oral bioavailability between 50% and 70%. In the plasma it is highly protein bound (>95%) and has a volume of distribution of 2–70 l.kg^{-1}. Muscle and fat accumulate amiodarone to a considerable extent. Its elimination half-life is long, varying from 20 to 100 days. Hepatic metabolism produces desmethylamiodarone, which appears to have some anti-arrhythmic activity. It is excreted by the lachrymal glands, the skin and biliary tract.

Flecainide

Presentation

Flecainide is available orally or intravenously and is an amide local anaesthetic with class Ic properties. The oral dose is 100 mg bd (maximum 400 mg daily). When used intravenously the dose is 2 mg.kg^{-1} over 10–30 minutes (maximum 150 mg). This may then be followed by an infusion, initially at 1.5 mg.kg^{-1}.h^{-1}, which is then reduced to 100–250 μg.kg^{-1}.h^{-1} for up to 24 hours (maximum 24-hour dose is 600 mg).

Uses

Flecainide has powerful anti-arrhythmic effects against atrial and ventricular tachyarrhythmias including WPW syndrome.

Mechanism of action

Flecainide prevents the fast Na^+ flux into cardiac tissue and prolongs phase 0 of the action potential. It has no effect on the duration of the action potential or the refractory period. Its effects are particularly pronounced on the conducting pathways.

Side effects

- Cardiac – flecainide may precipitate pre-existing conduction disorders and special care is required when used in patients with SA or AV disease or with bundle branch block. A paradoxical increase in ventricular rate may be seen in atrial fibrillation or flutter. When used to suppress ventricular ectopic beats following myocardial infarction it was associated with an increased mortality. Cardiac failure may complicate its use due to its negative inotropic effects. It raises the pacing threshold.
- Non-cardiac – dizziness, parasthesia and headaches may complicate its use.

Kinetics

Flecainide is well absorbed from the gut and has an oral bioavailability of 90%. It is about 50% plasma protein bound and has a volume of distribution of 6–10 l.kg^{-1}. Hepatic metabolism produces active metabolites, which along with unchanged drug are excreted in the urine.

Procainamide

Procainamide has similar effects to quinidine but is less vagolytic.

Uses

Procainamide has been used to treat both SVT and ventricular tachyarrhythmias. It is as effective as lidocaine in terminating VT. It may be given orally or intravenously. The oral dose is up to 50 mg.kg^{-1}.day^{-1} in divided doses and the intravenous dose is 100 mg slowly up to a maximum of 1 g. This may be followed by an infusion of 2–6 mg.min^{-1}, which should subsequently be converted to oral therapy.

Mechanism of action

Procainamide is a class Ia anti-arrhythmic and as such reduces the rate of rise of phase 0 of the action potential by blocking Na^+ channels. In addition, it raises the threshold potential and prolongs the refractory period without altering the duration of the action potential. It also antagonizes vagal tone but to a lesser extent than quinidine.

Side effects

These have limited its use.

- Cardiac – following intravenous administration it may produce hypotension, vasodilatation and a reduced cardiac output. It may also precipitate heart block. When used to treat SVT the ventricular response rate may increase. It may also prolong the QT interval and precipitate torsades de pointes.
- Non-cardiac – chronically a drug-induced lupus erythematosus syndrome with a positive anti-nuclear factor develops in 20–30% of patients (many of whom will be slow acetylators). Other minor effects include gastrointestinal upset, fever and rash. It reduces the antimicrobial effect of sulphonamides by the production of para-aminobenzoic acid.

Kinetics

Procainamide is well absorbed from the gut and has an oral bioavailability of 75%. Its short half-life of 3 hours necessitates frequent administration or slow release formulations. It is metabolized in the liver by amidases and by acetylation to the active N-acetyl procainamide. The latter pathway demonstrates genetic polymorphism so that patients may be grouped as slow or fast acetylators. The slow acetylators are more likely to develop side effects.

Disopyramide

Disopyramide is a class Ia anti-arrhythmic.

Presentation

It is available as tablets (including slow release) and as a solution containing 10 mg.ml^{-1}. The daily oral dose is up to 800 mg in divided doses; the intravenous dose is 2 mg.kg^{-1} over 30 minutes up to 150 mg, which is followed by an infusion of 1 mg.kg^{-1}.h^{-1} up to 800 mg.day^{-1}.

Uses

Disopyramide is used as a second-line agent in the treatment of both SVT and ventricular tachyarrhythmias. When used to treat atrial fibrillation or atrial flutter the ventricular rate should first be controlled with β-blockers or verapamil.

Mechanism of action

Disopyramide is a class Ia anti-arrhythmic and as such reduces the rate of rise of phase 0 of the action potential by blocking Na$^+$ channels. In addition, it raises the threshold potential and prolongs the refractory period, thereby increasing the duration of the action potential. It also has anticholinergic effects.

Side effects

- Cardiac – as plasma concentrations rise the QT interval is prolonged (occasionally precipitating torsades de pointes), myocardial contractility becomes depressed

while ventricular excitability is increased and may predispose to re-entry arrhythmias. Cardiac failure and cardiogenic shock occur rarely.
- Non-cardiac – anticholinergic effects (blurred vision, dry mouth and occasionally urinary retention) often prove unacceptable.

Kinetics

Disopyramide is well absorbed from the gut and has an oral bioavailability of 75%. It is only partially metabolized in the kidney, the majority of the drug being excreted in the urine unchanged. Its elimination half-life is about 5 hours but this increases significantly in patients with renal or cardiac failure.

Propafenone

Propafenone is similar in many respects to flecainide.

Presentation

It is available only as film-coated tablets in the UK although it has been used intravenously at a dose of 1–2 mg.kg^{-1}. The oral dose is initially 600–900 mg followed by 150–300 mg bd or tds.

Uses

Propafenone is used as second-line therapy for resistant SVT, including atrial fibrillation and flutter, and also for ventricular tachyarrhythmias.

Mechanism of action

Propafenone prevents the fast Na$^+$ flux into cardiac tissue and prolongs phase 0 of the action potential. The duration of the action potential and refractory period is prolonged especially in the conducting tissue. The threshold potential is increased and cardiac excitability reduced by an increase in the ventricular fibrillation threshold. At higher doses it may exhibit some β-blocking properties.

Side effects

Propafenone is generally well tolerated.
- Cardiac – owing to its weak β-blocking actions it should be used with caution in those with heart failure.
- Non-cardiac – it may produce minor nervous system effects and at higher doses gastrointestinal side effects may become more prominent. It may worsen myasthenia gravis. Propafenone increases the plasma levels of concurrently administered digoxin and warfarin. It may precipitate asthma due to its β-blocking properties.

Kinetics

Absorption from the gut is nearly complete and initially oral bioavailability is 50%. However, this increases disproportionately to nearly 100% as the enzymes involved in first-pass metabolism become saturated. It is more than 95% protein bound. Hepatic metabolism ensures that only tiny amounts are excreted unchanged. However, the enzyme responsible for its metabolism demonstrates genetic polymorphism so that affected patients may have an increased response.

Sotalol

Sotalol is a β-blocker but also has class I and III anti-arrhythmic activity.

Presentation

It is available as tablets and as a solution containing 40 mg in 4 ml. It is a racemic mixture, the D-isomer conferring the class III activity while the L-isomer has both class III and β-blocking actions.

Uses

Sotalol is used to treat ventricular tachyarrhythmias and in the prophylaxis of paroxysmal SVT. The oral dose is 80–160 mg bd and the intravenous dose is 50–100 mg over 20 minutes.

Mechanism of action

Sotalol prolongs the duration of the action potential so that the effective refractory period is prolonged in the conducting tissue. It is also a non-selective β-blocker and is more effective at maintaining sinus rhythm following DC cardioversion for atrial fibrillation than other β-blockers. The ventricular rate is also well controlled if the rhythm degenerates back into atrial fibrillation.

Side effects

- Cardiac – the most serious side effect is precipitation of torsades de pointes, which occurs in less than 2% of those being treated for sustained VT or VF. It is more common with higher doses, a prolonged QT interval and electrolyte imbalance. It may precipitate heart failure.
- Non-cardiac – bronchospasm, masking of symptoms of hypoglycaemia, visual disturbances and sexual dysfunction are all rare.

Kinetics

Sotalol is completely absorbed from the gut and its oral bioavailability is greater than 90%. It is not plasma protein-bound and is not metabolized. Approximately 90% is excreted unchanged in the urine while the remainder is excreted in bile. Renal impairment significantly reduces clearance.

Digoxin toxicity

Phenytoin

Although phenytoin is mainly used for its antiepileptic activity, it has a limited role in the treatment of arrhythmias associated with digoxin toxicity.

It depresses normal pacemaker activity while augmenting conduction through the conducting system especially when this has become depressed by digoxin. It also demonstrates class I anti-arrhythmic properties by blocking Na^+ channels.

Vasodilators

- **Sodium nitroprusside**
- **Nitrates**
- **Potassium channel activators**
- **Calcium channel antagonsis**
- **Miscellaneous**

Sodium nitroprusside (SNP)

Sodium nitroprusside is an inorganic complex and functions as a prodrug.

Presentation

It is presented in vials as a lyophilized reddish-brown powder containing 50 mg SNP. When reconstituted in 5% dextrose it produces a light orange- or straw-coloured solution with pH 4.5. If exposed to sunlight it will turn dark brown or blue because of liberation of cyanide (CN^-) ions at which point the solution should be discarded. Infusions may be protected from sunlight by aluminium foil or opaque syringes and giving sets.

Uses

Sodium nitroprusside is usually administered as a 0.005–0.02% (50–200 μg.ml^{-1}) intravenous infusion, the dose of 0.5–6 μg.kg^{-1}.min^{-1} being titrated to effect. The onset of action is within 3 minutes and because of its rapid breakdown its effects are short-lived. Various dose regimes are recommended and are all designed to avoid CN^- toxicity and thiocyanate (SCN) levels exceeding 100 μg.ml^{-1}. Up to 4 μg.kg^{-1}.min^{-1} may be used chronically while no more than 1.5 μg.kg^{-1}.min^{-1} is recommended during anaesthesia. It is not available orally.

Mechanism of action

Sodium nitroprusside vasodilates arteries and veins by the production of NO. This activates the enzyme guanylate cyclase leading to increased levels of intracellular cyclic GMP. Although Ca^{2+} influx into vascular smooth muscle in inhibited, its uptake into smooth endoplasmic reticulum is enhanced so that cytoplasmic levels fall, resulting in vasodilation.

Effects

- Cardiovascular – arterial vasodilation reduces the systemic vascular resistance and leads to a drop in blood pressure. Venous vasodilation increases the venous capacitance and reduces preload. Cardiac output is maintained by a reflex tachycardia. However, for those patients with heart failure the reduction in pre- and afterload will increase cardiac output with no increase in heart rate. The ventricular wall tension and myocardial oxygen consumption are reduced. It has no direct effects on contractility. Some patients develop tachyphylaxis, the exact mechanism of which is unclear.
- Respiratory – SNP may inhibit pulmonary hypoxic vasoconstriction and lead to increased shunt. Supplemental oxygen may help.
- Central nervous system – intracranial pressure is increased due to cerebral vasodilation and increased cerebral blood flow. However, cerebral autoregulation is maintained well below the normal limits during SNP infusion. In addition, cerebral function monitoring shows depressed cerebral function at a higher blood pressure when hypotension is induced by trimetaphan compared with SNP.
- Endocrine – plasma catecholamine and renin levels rise during SNP infusion.
- Gut – paralytic ileus has been reported following hypotensive anaesthesia induced by SNP. It is not clear if this is a direct effect or due to reduced mesenteric blood flow or simply due to opioids.
- General – the following effects are reversed when the rate of infusion is slowed: nausea and vomiting, dizziness, abdominal pain, muscle twitching and retrosternal pain.

Kinetics

SNP is not absorbed following oral administration. It has a short half-life and its duration of action is less than 10 minutes. However, the half-life of SCN is 2 days.

Metabolism

The metabolism of SNP is complicated (Figure 15.1). Initially within the red blood cell it reacts with oxyhaemoglobin to form NO, five CN^- ions and methaemoglobin. The methaemoglobin may then combine with CN^- to form cyanomethaemoglobin, which is thought to be non-toxic.

The remaining CN^- is then able to escape from the red blood cell where it is converted in the liver and kidney by the mitochondrial enzyme rhodanase with the addition of a sulphydryl group to form thiocyanate (SCN). Red blood cells contain the enzyme thiocyanate oxidase, which can convert SCN back to CN^-, but most SCN is excreted in the urine. SCN has an elimination half-life of 2 days but this may increase to 7 days in the presence of renal impairment. Alternatively CN^- combines with hydroxycobalamin (vitamin B_{12}) to form cyanocobalamin, which forms a non-toxic store of CN^- and can be excreted in the urine.

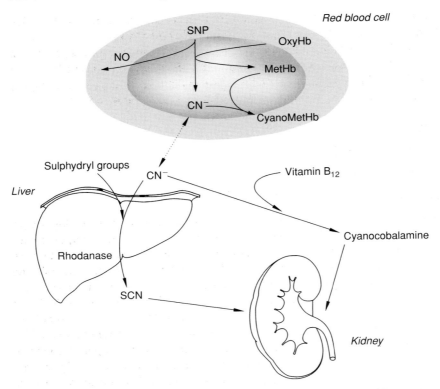

Figure 15.1. Metabolism of sodium nitroprusside (SNP). CN–, cyanide; SCN, thiocyanate.

Toxicity

The major risk of toxicity comes from CN^-, although SCN is also toxic. Free CN^- can bind cytochrome oxidase and impair aerobic metabolism. In doing so a metabolic acidosis develops and the mixed venous oxygen saturation increases as tissues become unable to utilize oxygen. Other signs include tachycardia, arrhythmias, hyperventilation and sweating. Plasma CN^- levels above 8 μg.ml^{-1} result in toxicity. It should be suspected in those who are resistant to SNP despite an adequate dose and in those who develop tachyphylaxis. It is more likely to occur in patients with hypothermia, severe renal or hepatic failure and those with vitamin B_{12} deficiency.

The management of CN^- toxicity involves halting the SNP infusion and optimizing oxygen delivery to tissues. Three treatments are useful:

- Dicobalt edetate, which chelates CN^- ions.
- Sodium thiosulphate, which provides additional sulphydryl groups to facilitate the conversion of CN^- to SCN. This is sometime used as prophylaxis.
- Nitrites – either sodium nitrite or amyl nitrite will convert oxyhaemoglobin to methaemoglobin, which has a higher affinity for CN^- than cytochrome oxidase.

While vitamin B_{12} is required to complex CN^- to cyanocobalamin, it is of little value in the acute setting. It is, however, sometimes used as prophylaxis.

SCN is 100 times less toxic than CN^- but its toxic effects may become significant if it is allowed to accumulate during prolonged administration especially in those with impaired renal function. Its accumulation is also more likely in those being given prophylactic sodium thiosulphate as it promotes the production of SCN.

Nitrates

Glyceryl trinitrate (GTN)

GTN is an organic nitrate.

Presentation

GTN is prepared in the following formulations: an aerosol spray delivering 400 μg per metered dose and tablets containing 300–600 μg, both used as required sublingually. Modified release tablets containing 1–5 mg for buccal administration are placed between the upper lip and gum and are used at a maximum dose of 5 mg tds while the 2.6–10 mg modified-release tablets are to be swallowed and used at a maximum dose of 12.8 mg tds. The transdermal patch preparation releases 5–15 mg/24 hours, and should be resited at a different location on the chest. The clear colourless solution for injection contains 1–5 mg.ml^{-1} and should be diluted to a 0.01% (100 μg.ml^{-1}) solution before administration by an infusion pump and is used at 10–200 μg.min^{-1}. GTN is absorbed by polyvinyl chloride; therefore, special polyethylene administration sets are preferred. GTN will explode if heated so transdermal preparations should be removed before DC cardioversion.

Uses

GTN is used in the treatment and prophylaxis of angina, in left ventricular failure associated with myocardial infarction and following cardiac surgery. It has also been used in the control of intra-operative blood pressure and for oesophageal spasm.

Mechanism of action

GTN vasodilates veins by the production of nitric oxide. This activates the enzyme guanylate cyclase leading to increased levels of intracellular cyclic GMP. Although Ca^{2+} influx into vascular smooth muscle is inhibited, its uptake into smooth endoplasmic reticulum is enhanced so that cytoplasmic levels fall resulting in vasodilation (Figure 15.2).

Effects

- Cardiovascular – in contrast to SNP and despite a similar mechanism of action GTN produces vasodilation predominantly in the capacitance vessels, that is, veins, although arteries are dilated to some extent. Consequently, it produces a reduction

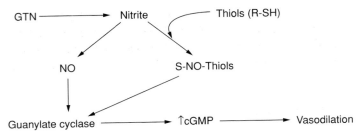

Figure 15.2. Metabolism of GTN.

in preload, venous return, ventricular end-diastolic pressure and wall tension. This in turn leads to a reduction in oxygen demand and increased coronary blood flow to subendocardial regions and is the underlying reason for its use in cardiac failure and ischaemic heart disease. The reduction in preload may lead to a reduction in cardiac output although patients with cardiac failure may see a rise in cardiac output. Postural hypotension may occur. At higher doses systemic vascular resistance falls and augments the fall in blood pressure, which while reducing myocardial work, will reduce coronary artery perfusion pressure and time (secondary to tachycardia). Coronary artery flow may be increased directly by coronary vasodilation. Tolerance develops within 48 hours and may be due to depletion of sulphydryl groups within vascular smooth muscle. A daily drug-free period of a few hours prevents tolerance. It has been suggested that infusion of acetylcysteine (providing sulphydryl groups) may prevent tolerance.

- Central nervous system – an increase in intracranial pressure and headache resulting from cerebral vasodilation may occur but is often only problematic at the start of treatment.
- Gut – it relaxes the gastrointestinal sphincters including the sphincter of Oddi.
- Haematological – rarely methaemoglobinaemia is precipitated.

Kinetics

GTN is rapidly absorbed from sublingual mucosa and the gastrointestinal tract although the latter is subject to extensive first-pass hepatic metabolism resulting in an oral bioavailability of less than 5%. Sublingual effects are seen within 3 minutes and last for 30–60 minutes. Hepatic nitrate reductase is responsible for the metabolism of GTN to glycerol dinitrate and nitrite (NO^{2-}) in a process that requires tissue thiols (R-SH). Nitrite is then converted to NO, which confers its mechanism of action (see above). Under certain conditions nitrite may convert oxyhaemoglobin to methaemoglobin by oxidation of the ferrous ion (Fe^{2+}) to the ferric ion (Fe^{3+}).

Isosorbide dinitrate (ISDN) and isosorbide mononitrate (ISMN)

ISDN is prepared with lactose and mannitol to reduce the risk of explosion. It is well absorbed from the gut and is subject to extensive first-pass metabolism in the liver to isosorbide 2-mononitrate and isosorbide 5-mononitrate (ISMN), both of which probably confer the majority of the activity of ISDN. ISMN has a much longer half-life (4.5 hours) and is used in its own right. It is not subject to hepatic first-pass metabolism and has an oral bioavailability of 100%. Both are used in the prophylaxis of angina.

Potassium-channel activators

Nicorandil

Nicorandil (nicotinamidoethyl nitrate) is a potassium-channel activator with a nitrate moiety and as such differs from other potassium-channel activators. It has been used in Japan since 1984 and was launched in the UK in 1994.

Presentation and uses

Nicorandil is available as tablets and the usual dose is 10–30 mg bd. It is used for the treatment and prophylaxis of angina and in the treatment of congestive heart failure and hypertension. It has been used experimentally via the intravenous route.

Mechanism of action

ATP-sensitive K^+ channels are closed during the normal cardiac cycle but are open (activated) during periods of ischaemia when intracellular levels of ATP fall. In the open state K^+ passes down its concentration gradient out of the cell resulting in hyperpolarization, which closes Ca^{2+} channels resulting in less Ca^{2+} for myocardial contraction.

Nicorandil activates the ATP-sensitive K^+ channels within the heart and arterioles. In addition, nicorandil relaxes venous capacitance smooth muscle by stimulating guanylate cyclase via its nitrate moiety, leading to increased intracellular cGMP.

Effects

- Cardiovascular – nicorandil causes venodilation and arterial vasodilation resulting in a reduced pre- and afterload. The blood pressure falls. Left ventricular end-diastolic pressure falls and there is an improved normal and collateral coronary artery blood flow, partly induced by coronary artery vasodilation without a 'steal' phenomenon. An increase in cardiac output is seen in patients with ischaemic heart disease and cardiac failure. It is effective at suppressing torsades de pointes associated with a prolonged QT interval. High concentrations in vitro result in a shortened action potential by accelerated repolarization. It also reduces the size of experimentally induced ischaemia, the mechanism of which is uncertain, so that an alternative, as yet undefined, cardioprotective mechanism has been postulated. Unlike nitrate therapy it is not associated with tolerance during prolonged administration. Contractility and atrioventricular conduction is not affected.
- Central nervous system – headaches, these usually clear with continued therapy.

- Metabolic – unlike other antihypertensives it has no effect on lipid profile or glucose control.
- Haematological – nicorandil inhibits in vitro ADP-induced platelet aggregation (in a similar manner to nitrates), which is associated with an increase of intraplatelet cGMP.
- Miscellaneous – giant oral apthous ulcers have been reported with its use.

Kinetics
Nicorandil is well absorbed from the gut with insignificant first-pass metabolism. The main metabolic route is denitration with 20% excreted as metabolites in the urine. The elimination half-life is 1 hour, although its actions last up to 12 hours, but neither is increased in the presence of renal impairment. It is not plasma protein-bound to any significant extent.

Calcium channel antagonists
Despite their disparate chemical structures, the Ca^{2+} channel antagonists are all effective in specifically blocking the entry of Ca^{2+} through L-type channels while leaving T-, N- and P-type Ca^{2+} channels unaffected. The L-type channel is widespread in the cardiovascular system and is responsible for the plateau phase (slow inward current) of the cardiac action potential. It triggers the internal release of Ca^{2+} and is regulated by cAMP-dependent protein kinase. The T-type channel is structurally similar to the L-type channel and is present mainly in cardiac cells that lack a T-tubule system, that is, SA node and certain types of vascular smooth muscle. They are not present in ventricular myocardium. N-type channels are only found in nerve cells.

Calcium channel antagonists have variable affinity for L-type channels in myocardium, nodal and vascular smooth muscle resulting in variable effects. They are all useful in the treatment of essential hypertension, although some are also particularly useful in the treatment of angina or arrhythmias.

Verapamil
Verapamil is a racemic mixture and a synthetic derivative of papaverine.

Presentation and uses
Verapamil is available as 20–240 mg tablets, some prepared as modified release and as an oral suspension containing 40 mg/5 ml. The colourless intravenous preparation contains 2.5 mg.ml^{-1}. It is used for certain supraventricular arrhythmias (not in atrial fibrillation complicating WPW syndrome) and angina. It has been used to treat hypertension although its negative inotropic properties limit its usefulness in this setting.

Table 15.1. Chemical classification of Ca^{2+} channel antagonists.

Class I	phenylalkylamines	verapamil
Class II	dihydropyridines	nifedipine, amlodipine, nimodipine
Class III	benzothiazepines	diltiazem

Mechanism of action

The L-isomer has specific Ca^{2+} channel blocking actions with a particular affinity for those at the SA and AV node, whereas the D-isomer acts on fast Na$^+$ channels resulting in some local anaesthetic activity.

Effects

- Cardiovascular – verapamil acts specifically to slow the conduction of the action potential at the SA and AV node resulting in a reduced heart rate. To a lesser extent it produces some negative inotropic effects and vasodilates peripheral vascular smooth muscle. It is a mild coronary artery vasodilator. Blood pressure falls. It may lead to various degrees of heart block or cardiac failure in those with impaired ventricular function and ventricular fibrillation in those with WPW syndrome.
- Central nervous system – it vasodilates the cerebral circulation.
- Miscellaneous – following chronic administration it may potentiate the effects of non-depolarizing and depolarizing muscle relaxants.

Kinetics

Verapamil is well absorbed from the gut but an extensive first-pass hepatic metabolism reduces the oral bioavailability to 20%. Demethylation produces norverapamil, which retains significant anti-arrhythmic properties. It is 90% plasma protein-bound and is mainly excreted in the urine following metabolism, although up to 20% is excreted in bile.

Nifedipine

Presentation and uses

Nifedipine is available as capsules containing 5–10 mg, the contents of which may be administered sublingually, and tablets containing 10–60 mg, some of which are available as sustained release. The onset of action is 15–20 minutes following oral and 5–10 minutes following sublingual administration. Swallowing the contents of an opened capsule may further reduce the onset time. It is used in the prophylaxis and treatment of angina, hypertension and in Raynaud's syndrome.

Effects

- Cardiovascular – nifedipine reduces tone in peripheral and coronary arteries, resulting in a reduced systemic vascular resistance, fall in blood pressure, increased

Table 15.2. Various pharmacological properties of some Ca^{2+} channel antagonists.

	Absorbed (%)	Oral bioavail- ability (%)	Protein binding (%)	Active metabolites	Clearance	Elimination half-life (h)
Verapamil	95	20	90	yes	renal	6–12
Nifedipine	95	60	95	no	renal	2–5
Diltiazem	95	50	75	yes	60% hepatic, 40% renal	3–6

coronary artery blood flow and reflex increases in heart rate and contractility. The cardiac output is increased. Occasionally these reflex changes worsen the oxygen supply/demand ratio.

Kinetics

Nifedipine is well absorbed following oral administration although hepatic first-pass metabolism reduces its oral bioavailability to 60%. It is 95% plasma protein-bound and has an elimination half-life of 5 hours following oral administration. It is predominantly excreted as inactive metabolites in the urine (Table 15.2).

Nimodipine

Nimodipine is a more lipid-soluble analogue of nifedipine and as such can penetrate the BBB. It is used in the prevention and treatment of cerebral vasospasm following subarachnoid haemorrhage and in migraine. It may be administered orally or intravenously.

Its action may be dependent on blocking a Ca^{2+}-dependent cascade of cellular processes that would otherwise lead to cell damage and destruction.

Diltiazem

Presentation and uses

Diltiazem is available as 60–200 mg tablets, some of which are available as slow release. It is also available in combination with hydrochlorothiazide. It is used for the prophylaxis and treatment of angina and in hypertension.

Effects

- Cardiovascular – diltiazem has actions both within the heart and in the peripheral circulation. It prolongs AV conduction time and reduces contractility but to a lesser extent than verapamil. It also reduces the systemic vascular resistance and the blood pressure falls although a reflex tachycardia is not usually seen. Coronary blood flow is increased due to coronary artery vasodilation.

Table 15.3. Main cardiovascular effects of some Ca^{2+} channel antagonists.

	Blood pressure	Heart rate	AV conduction time	Myocardial contractility	Peripheral and coronary artery vasodilation
Verapamil	↓	↓	↑	↓↓	↑
Nifedipine	↓	→↑	→↑	→↑	↑↑↑
Diltiazem	↓	↓	↑	↓	↑↑

Kinetics

Diltiazem is almost completely absorbed from the gut but hepatic first-pass metabolism reduces the oral bioavailability to 50%. Hepatic metabolism produces an active metabolite, desacetyldiltiazem, which is excreted in the urine. The urine also eliminates 40% of diltiazem in the unchanged form. Approximately 75% is plasma protein-bound.

Miscellaneous

Hydralazine

Presentation and uses

Hydralazine is available as 25–50 mg tablets and as a powder containing 20 mg for reconstitution in water before intravenous administration (5% dextrose should be avoided as it promotes its rapid breakdown). Hydralazine is used orally in the control of chronic hypertension and severe chronic heart failure in conjunction with other agents. It is used intravenously in acute hypertension associated with pre-eclampsia at 10–20 mg. This may take up to 20 minutes to work and repeat doses may be required.

Mechanism of action

The exact mechanism of action is uncertain but involves the activation of guanylate cyclase and an increase in intracellular cGMP. This leads to a decrease in available intracellular Ca^{2+} and vasodilation.

Effects

- Cardiovascular – its main effect is to reduce arteriolar tone and systemic vascular resistance, whereas the capacitance vessels are less affected. As a result postural hypotension is not usually a problem. Reflex tachycardia and an increase in cardiac output ensue but may be effectively antagonized by β-blockade.
- Central nervous system – cerebral artery blood flow increases as a result of cerebral artery vasodilation.

- Renal – despite an increase in renal blood flow, fluid retention, oedema, and a reduction in urine output is often seen. This may be overcome by concurrent administration of a diuretic.
- Gut – nausea and vomiting are common.
- Miscellaneous – peripheral neuropathy and blood dyscrasias. A lupus erythematosus type syndrome is occasionally seen after long-term use and may be more common in slow acetylators and women. It may require long-term corticosteroid therapy.

Kinetics

Hydralazine is well absorbed from the gut but is subject to a variable first-pass metabolism resulting in an oral bioavailability of 25–55% depending on the acetylator status of the individual. The plasma half-life is normally 2–3 hours but this may be shortened to 45 minutes in rapid acetylators. It is 90% protein-bound in the plasma. Up to 85% is excreted in the urine as acetylated and hydroxylated metabolites, some of which are conjugated with glucuronic acid. It crosses the placenta and may cause a foetal tachycardia.

Minoxidil

Presentation and uses

Minoxidil is prepared as 2.5–10 mg tablets, a 2% solution for intravenous use and a 5% lotion. It is used for severe hypertension and alopecia areata.

Its mechanism of action and principal effects are essentially the same as those of hydralazine. The mechanism by which it stimulates the hair follicle is poorly understood. It may also precipitate hypertrichosis of the face and arms and breast tenderness. It does not cause a lupus erythematosus-type reaction.

Kinetics

Minoxidil is well absorbed from the gut and has an oral bioavailability of 90%. It is not protein-bound in the plasma. Its plasma half-life is only 3 hours but its hypotensive effects may last for as long as 3 days. It undergoes hepatic glucuronide conjugation and is subsequently excreted in the urine.

Diazoxide

This vasodilator is chemically related to the thiazide diuretics.

Presentation and uses

Diazoxide is available as 50 mg tablets and as a solution for intravenous injection containing 15 mg.ml^{-1}. It is used intravenously to treat hypertensive emergencies associated with renal disease at 1–3 mg.kg^{-1} up to a maximum dose of 150 mg, which may be repeated after 15 minutes. It has also been used to treat intractable hypoglycaemia and malignant islet-cell tumours.

Mechanism of action

Its hypotensive effects are mediated through altered levels of cAMP in arterioles, producing vasodilation. It may also be due to a reduced Ca^{2+} influx. Its biochemical effects are due to inhibition of insulin secretion and increased release of catecholamines.

Effects

- Cardiovascular – diazoxide produces arteriolar vasodilation with little effect on capacitance vessels. As a result the blood pressure falls and there is an increase in heart rate and cardiac output. Postural hypotension is not a problem.
- Metabolic – it increases the levels of glucose, catecholamines, renin and aldosterone. It also causes fluid retention (despite its chemical relation to the thiazides), which may require treatment with a loop diuretic.
- Miscellaneous – the following effects may occur: nausea, especially at the start of treatment, extra-pyramidal effects including occulogyric crisis, thrombocytopenia and hyperuricaemia.

Kinetics

Diazoxide is well absorbed from the gut with an oral bioavailability of 80%, and is extensively protein-bound in the plasma (about 90%). The hyperglycaemic effects last about 8 hours while the hypotensive effects last about 5 hours. The plasma half-life, however, may last up to 36 hours. It is partly metabolized in the liver, being excreted in the urine as unchanged drug and as inactive metabolites.

Antihypertensives

- **Drugs affecting the renin–angiotensin–aldosterone system**
- **Adrenergic neurone blockade**
- **Centrally acting**
- **Ganglion blockade**
- **Diuretics**
- **Adrenoceptor antagonists**
- **Ca²⁺ channel antagonists**

Renin–angiotensin–aldosterone system

Physiology

The juxtaglomerular apparatus within the kidney consists of three distinct cell types:

- Juxtaglomerular cells form part of the afferent arteriole as it enters the glomerulus and are supplied by sympathetic nerves. They contain prorenin, which is converted to the acid protease renin before systemic release.
- The macula densa is a region of cells at the start of the distal convoluted tubule, which lie adjacent to the juxtaglomerular cells of the same nephron.
- Agranular lacis cells, which lie between the afferent and efferent arterioles adjacent to the glomerulus.

Under the following conditions the juxtaglomerular apparatus will cause the release of renin into the circulation:

- Reduced renal perfusion
- Reduced Na⁺ at the macula densa
- Stimulation of the renal sympathetic fibres via β_1-adrenoceptors

Renin (half-life 80 minutes) splits the decapeptide angiotensin I from the circulating plasma protein angiotensinogen, which is synthesized in the liver and is present in the α_2-globulin fraction of plasma proteins. Angiotensin-converting enzyme (ACE) converts angiotensin I to the active octapeptide angiotensin II, and also inactivates bradykinin. Angiotensin II is broken down in the kidney and liver to inactive metabolites and angiotensin III, which retains some activity (Figure 16.1).

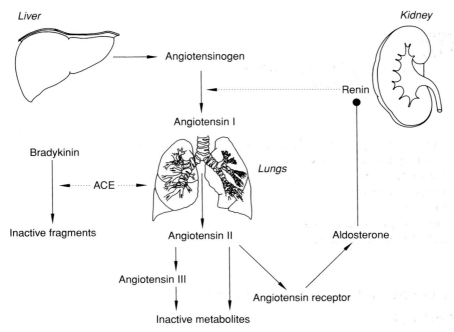

Figure 16.1. Renin–angiotensin–aldosterone system. ·····►, Enzyme action; ──•, negative feedback.

Angiotensin II

Mechanism of action

Two subtypes of angiotensin II receptor exist, AT_1 and AT_2. Angiotensin has a greater affinity for AT_1 receptors, which are G-protein-coupled.

Effects
- Potent vasoconstriction (about five times as potent as noradrenaline). Directly on arterioles and indirectly via central mechanisms.
- Blockade of noradrenaline re-uptake (uptake 1) at sympathetic nerves and sympathetic nervous system activation.
- Central effects – it increases thirst and the release of ADH and ACTH.
- It stimulates the release of aldosterone from the adrenal cortex and inhibits the release of renin from the juxtaglomerular cells.
- Reduced glomerular filtration rate.

259

ACE inhibitors and angiotensin II receptor antagonists are used widely in the treatment of hypertension. β-Blockers (cf. Chapter 13) reduce sympathetically mediated release of renin, which contributes to their antihypertensive effects.

Angiotensin-converting enzyme (ACE) inhibitors

ACE inhibitors are used in all grades of heart failure and in patients with myocardial infarction with left ventricular dysfunction where it improves the prognosis. They are used in hypertension especially insulin-dependent diabetics with nephropathy. However hypertension is relatively resistant to ACE inhibition in the black poulation where concurrent diuretic thereapy may be required. While most drugs should be continued throughout the peri-opereative period, ACE inhibitors and angiotensin II receptor antagonists should be omitted due to the increased frequency of peri-operative hypotension.

From a kinetic point of view ACE inhibitors may be divided into three groups:

Group 1. Captopril – an active drug that is metabolized to active metabolites.

Group 2. Enalopril, ramipril – prodrugs, which only become active following hepatic metabolism to the diacid moiety.

Group 3. Lisinopril – an active drug that is not metabolized and is excreted unchanged in the urine.

In other respects the effects of ACE inhibitors are similar and are discussed under captopril.

Captopril

Presentation

Captopril is available as 12.5–50 mg tablets that may also be combined with hydrochlorothiazide. The initial dose is 12.5 mg although 6.25 mg may be prudent for those with heart failure.

Mechanism of action

Captopril is a competitive ACE inhibitor and therefore prevents the formation of angiotensin II and its effects. Afterload is reduced to a greater degree than preload.

Effects

- Cardiovascular – captopril reduces the systemic vascular resistance significantly, resulting in a fall in blood pressure. The fall in afterload may increase the cardiac output particularly in those with heart failure. Heart rate is usually unaffected but may increase. Baroreceptor reflexes are also unaffected. Transient hypotension may occur at the start of treatment, which should therefore be initiated in the hospital for patients with anything more than mild heart failure.
- Renal – the normal function of angiotensin II to maintain efferent arteriolar pressure (by vasoconstriction) at the glomerulus in the presence of poor renal perfusion

is forfeit. Therefore renal perfusion pressure falls and renal failure may follow. As a result bilateral renal artery stenosis or unilateral renal artery stenosis to a single functioning kidney is considered a contraindication. Where normal renal perfusion is preserved, renal vasodilatation may occur leading to a naturesis.

- Metabolic – reduced aldosterone release impairs the negative feedback to renin production so that renin levels become elevated. It may also lead to hyperkalaemia and raised urea and creatinine, especially in those with even mildly impaired renal function.
- Interactions – captopril reduces aldosterone release, which may result in hyperkalaemia, so it should not be used with potassium-sparing diuretics. It has been associated with unexplained hypoglycaemia in Type I and II diabetes. These effects usually decrease with continued treatment. Non-steroidal anti-inflammatory drugs reduce captopril's antihypertensive effects and may precipitate renal failure.
- Cough – a persistent dry cough may be the result of increased levels of bradykinin, which are normally broken down by ACE. Non-steroidal anti-inflammatory drugs may alleviate this cough but at the expense of reduced antihypertensive effects.
- Miscellaneous – rare but serious effects may complicate its use and include angio-oedema (0.2%, more common in black patients), agranulocytosis and thrombocytopenia. Less serious side effects are more common and include loss of taste, rash, pruritus, fever and apthous ulceration. These are more common with higher doses and in patients with impaired renal function.

Kinetics

Captopril is well absorbed from the gut and has an oral bioavailability of 65%. It is 25% plasma protein bound. Approximately 50% is oxidized in the liver to the dimer and mixed sulphides all of which are eventually excreted in the urine. It has an elimination half-life of 4 hours, although this will be increased in the presence of renal impairment.

Enalopril

Kinetics

Enalopril is a prodrug, which is hydrolyzed in the liver and kidney to the active compound enaloprilat. It may be given orally (as enalopril) or intravenously (as enaloprilat). Its elimination half-life is 4–8 hours but increases to 11 hours in prolonged thereapy. It has a duration of action of approximately 20 hours.

Angiotensin II receptor antagonists (ARAs)

Losartan

Losartan is a substituted imidazole compound.

Presentation and uses
Losartan is available as 25–50 mg tablets and in combination with hydrochloroth-iazide. It is used in the treatment of hypertension where dry cough proves an unacceptable side effect of ACE inhibitor therapy.

Mechanism of action
Losartan is a specific angiotensin II receptor (type AT_1) antagonist at all sites within the body. It blocks the negative feedback of angiotensin II on renin secretion, which therefore increases, leading to increased angiotensin II. This has little impact due to comprehensive AT_1 receptor blockade.

Effects
These are broadly similar to those of the ACE inhibitors.
• Metabolic – as it does not block the actions of ACE, bradykinin may be broken down in the usual manner (by ACE). As a result, bradykinin levels are not raised and the dry cough seen with ACE inhibitors does not complicate its use.

Kinetics
Losartan is well absorbed from the gut but undergoes significant first-pass metabolism to an active carboxylic acid metabolite (which acts in a non-competitive manner), and several other inactive compounds. It has an oral bioavailability of 30% and is 99% plasma protein bound. Its elimination half-life is 2 hours while the elimination half-life of the active metabolite is 7 hours. Less than 10% is excreted unchanged in an active form in the urine. The inactive metabolites are excreted in bile and urine.

Contraindications
Like ACE inhibitors, Losartan is contraindicated in bilateral renal artery stenosis and pregnancy.

Comparing ARAs to ACE inhibitors
ARA use may become more widespread for the following reasons.
1. Blockade of the AT_1-receptor is the most specific way of preventing the adverse effects of angiotensin II seen in heart failure and hypertension, especially as angiotensin II may be synthesized by alternative non-ACE pathways.
2. The AT_2-receptor is not blocked, which may possess cardioprotective properties.
3. There is a much lower incidence of cough and angioedema and therefore improved compliance.

Adrenergic neurone blockade

This group of drugs interferes with the release of noradrenaline from adrenergic neurones.

Physiology

Noradrenaline is synthesized from tyrosine (see Chapter 12) within the adrenergic nerve terminal. It is held in storage vesicles and subsequently released into the neuronal cleft to act on adrenoceptors. Its actions are terminated by:

- Uptake 1 – noradrenaline is taken back into the nerve terminal by a high-affinity transport system. This provides the main route for terminating its effects. Within the neurone it is recycled and returned to storage vesicles. However, while in the cytoplasm some may be de-aminated by MAO.
- Uptake 2 – noradrenaline diffuses away from the nerve terminal into the circulation where it is taken up by extraneuronal tissues including the liver and metabolized by COMT.

Guanethidine

Presentation and uses

Guanethidine is available as tablets and as a colourless solution for injection containing 10 mg.ml^{-1}. It has been used as an antihypertensive agent but is currently used only for the control of sympathetically mediated chronic pain. The initial antihypertensive dose is 10 mg.day^{-1}, which is increased to a maintenance dose of $30–50 \text{ mg.day}^{-1}$. A dose of 20 mg is used when performing an intravenous regional block for chronic pain. Repeated blocks are usually required.

Mechanism of action

Guanethidine gains access to the adrenergic neurone by utilizing the uptake 1 transport mechanism. Following intravenous administration there is some initial hypotension by direct vasodilation of arterioles. Subsequently, it displaces noradrenaline from its binding sites, which may cause transient hypertension. Finally, guanethidine reduces the blood pressure by preventing the release of what little noradrenaline is left in the nerve terminal. Oral administration does not produce the same triphasic response, as its onset of action is much slower. It does not alter the secretion of catecholamines by the adrenal medulla.

Effects

- Cardiovascular – hypotension is its main action. Postural hypotension is common as it blocks any compensatory rise in sympathetic tone. Fluid retention leading to oedema may occur.
- Gut – diarrhoea is common.
- Miscellaneous – failure to ejaculate.

- Drug interactions – drugs that block uptake 1 (tricyclic antidepressants, cocaine) prevent guanethidine from entering the nerve terminal and disrupting noradrenaline storage. They therefore antagonize guanethidine.

Up-regulation of adrenoceptors follows the long-term use of guanethidine so that these patients are very sensitive to direct-acting sympathomimetic amines.

Kinetics

Following oral administration, guanethidine is variably and incompletely absorbed. Hepatic first-pass metabolism results in an oral bioavailability of 50%. It is not bound by plasma proteins and does not cross the BBB. It has an elimination half-life of several days. Elimination is by hepatic metabolism and excretion of unchanged drug and its metabolites in the urine.

Reserpine

Reserpine is no longer available in the UK. It is a naturally occurring alkaloid that was widely used to treat hypertension that failed to respond to β-blockers or diuretics.

Mechanism of action

Reserpine acts centrally and peripherally by preventing storage vesicles incorporating noradrenaline from neuronal cytoplasm leading to rapid de-amination by mitochondrial MAO and noradrenaline depleted neurones. Serotonin is also depleted.

Effects

- Cardiovascular – hypotension is mainly a result of a reduced cardiac output and systemic vascular resistance. Postural hypotension is rarely a problem, but nasal congestion is less well tolerated.
- Central nervous system – depression, lethargy, and nightmares are caused by reserpine's ability to cross the BBB. Extrapyramidal effects may also be seen. General anaesthetic requirements are decreased.
- Gut – diarrhoea and increased gastric acid secretions may lead to epigastric pain.
- Miscellaneous – sexual dysfunction, hyperprolactinaemia, gynaecomastia and galactorrhoea are seen rarely.
- Drug interactions – patients taking reserpine will exhibit increased sensitivity to direct-acting sympathomimetic amines (adrenoceptor up-regulation) but reduced sensitivity to indirect-acting sympathomimetic amines (depleted noradrenaline stores).

Kinetics

Following absorption from the gut, reserpine is metabolized slowly in the liver. Some metabolic products are excreted in the urine while most appear to be excreted unchanged in the bile. It has a half-life of many days. It crosses the placenta and BBB and also reaches breast milk.

Metirosine

Metirosine is a competitive inhibitor of tyrosine hydroxylase and can therefore prevent the synthesis of catecholamines. It should only be used to manage hypertension associated with phaeochromocytoma.

It may cause severe diarrhoea, sedation, extrapyramidal effects and hypersensitivity reactions.

Centrally acting

Methyldopa

Presentation and uses

Methyldopa is available as film-coated tablets containing 125–500 mg and as an oral suspension containing 50 mg.ml^{-1}. The rarely used intravenous preparation is colourless and contains 50 mg.ml^{-1} and uses sodium metabisulphite as the preservative. It is used at 250 mg tds increasing to a maximum of 3 g.day^{-1} to control hypertension, especially that associated with pregnancy.

Mechanism of action

Methyldopa readily crosses the BBB where it is decarboxylated to α-methyl-noradrenaline, which is a potent α_2-agonist. It retains limited α_1-agonist properties (α_2:α_1 ratio 10:1). Stimulation of presynaptic α_2-receptors in the nucleus tractus solitarii forms a negative feedback loop for further noradrenaline release so that α-methyl-noradrenaline reduces centrally mediated sympathetic tone, leading to a reduction in blood pressure.

Effects

- Cardiovascular – its main effect is a reduction in systemic vascular resistance leading to a fall in blood pressure. Postural hypotension is occasionally a problem. Cardiac output is unchanged despite a relative bradycardia. Rebound hypertension may occur if treatment is stopped suddenly but this is less common than with clonidine.
- Central nervous system – sedation is common, while dizziness, depression, nightmares and nausea are less common. The MAC of volatile anaesthetics is reduced.
- Haematological – a positive direct Coombs' test is seen in 10–20% of patients taking methyldopa. Thrombocytopenia and leucopenia occur rarely.
- Allergic – it may precipitate an auto-immune haemolytic anaemia. Eosinophilia associated with fever sometimes occurs within the first few weeks of therapy. A hypersensitivity reaction may cause myocarditis.

- Renal – urine may become darker in colour when exposed to air, due to the break-down of methyldopa or its metabolites.
- Hepatic – liver function may deteriorate during long-term treatment and fatal hepatic necrosis has been reported.
- Miscellaneous – it fluoresces at the same wavelengths as catecholamines so that assays of urinary catecholamines may be falsely high. Assays of VMA are not affected. It may cause constipation and gynaecomastia (due to suppressed prolactin release).

Kinetics

Methyldopa is erratically absorbed from the gut and has a very variable oral bioavailability and a slow onset of action. It is subject to hepatic first-pass metabolism, being converted to the O-sulphate. Less than 20% is bound to plasma proteins. Approximately 50% is excreted unchanged in the urine.

Clonidine

Clonidine is an α-agonist with an affinity for α_2-receptors 200 times that for α_1-receptors. Some studies identify it as a partial agonist.

Presentation and uses

Clonidine is available as 25–300 μg tablets and as a colourless solution for injection containing 150 μg.ml^{-1}. A transdermal patch is available but this takes 48 hours to achieve therapeutic levels. It is used in the treatment of hypertension, acute and chronic pain, the suppression of symptoms of opioid withdrawal and to augment sedation during ventilation of the critically ill patient.

Mechanism of action

The useful effects of clonidine rest on its ability to stimulate α_2-receptors in the lateral reticular nucleus resulting in reduced central sympathetic outflow, and in the spinal cord where they augment endogenous opiate release and modulate the descending noradrenergic pathways involved in spinal nociceptive processing. MAC appears to be reduced by stimulation of central postsynaptic α_2-receptors.

Transmembrane signalling of α_2-receptors is coupled to G_i, leading to reduced intracellular cAMP. K^+ channels are also activated.

Effects

- Cardiovascular – following intravenous administration the blood pressure may rise due to peripheral α_1 stimulation, but this is followed by a more prolonged fall in blood pressure. Cardiac output is well maintained despite a bradycardia. The PR interval is lengthened, atrioventricular nodal conduction depressed and the baroreceptor reflexes are sensitized by clonidine resulting in a lower heart rate for a given increase in blood pressure. Its effects on the coronary circulation are complicated as any direct vasoconstriction may be offset by a reduction in sympathetic tone and by the release of local nitric oxide. It stabilizes the cardiovascular responses to peri-operative stimuli. Rebound hypertension is seen more commonly when a dose of more than 1.2 g.day^{-1} is stopped abruptly. This is due to peripheral vasoconstriction and increased plasma catecholamines and may be exacerbated by β-blockade (leaving vasoconstriction unopposed). Increasing doses have a ceiling effect and are limited by increasing α_1 stimulation.

- Central nervous system – it produces sedation and a reduction of up to 50% in the MAC of volatile agents. It is anxiolytic at low doses but becomes anxiogenic at higher doses.
- Analgesia – clonidine has been used via the subarachnoid and epidural routes. It provides prolonged analgesia with no respiratory depression and appears to act synergistically with concurrently administered opioids. It does not produce motor or sensory blockade. Clonidine also appears to reduce post-operative opioid requirement when administered intravenously.
- Renal system – a number of mechanisms including inhibition of release of ADH have been implicated as the cause of diuresis during its use.
- Respiratory – in contrast to opioids it does not produce significant respiratory depression.
- Endocrine – the stress response to surgical stimulus is inhibited. Insulin release is inhibited although this rarely increases blood-sugar levels.
- Haematological – despite the presence of α_2-adrenoceptors on platelets, therapeutic doses of clonidine do not promote platelet aggregation and its sympatholytic effects block adrenaline-induced platelet aggregation.

Kinetics

Clonidine is rapidly and almost completely absorbed after oral administration, achieving an oral bioavailability of nearly 100%. It is 20% plasma protein bound and has a volume of distribution of about 2 l.kg^{-1}. The elimination half-life of clonidine is between 9 and 18 hours, with approximately 50% of the drug being metabolized in the liver to inactive metabolites, while the rest is excreted unchanged in the urine. The dose should be reduced in the presence of renal impairment.

Dexmedetomidine

Medetomidine is an α_2-agonist that has been used widely in veterinary practice for its sedation and analgesic properties.

Presentation and uses

Medetomidine is a racemic mixture but only the D-stereoisomer is active, so it has been developed as dexmedetomidine.

Mechanism of action

This is similar to that of clonidine although it is more potent and has a higher affinity for the α_2-receptor (α_2:α_1 ratio 1600:1). It is a full agonist.

Effects

These are broadly similar to those of clonidine.

Kinetics

Oral absorption is unpredictable but does avoid the initial hypertension that parenteral administration produces. It has an elimination half-life of 2 hours.

Atipamezole

Atipamezole is a selective α_2-antagonist that crosses the BBB to reverse the sedation and analgesia associated with clonidine and dexmedetomidine. At 2 hours its elimination half-life is similar to dexmedetomidine with obvious clinical benefit.

Ganglion blockade

This group of drugs competitively antagonizes nicotinic receptors at both parasympathetic and sympathetic ganglia and also at the adrenal cortex. Ganglion blockers do not inhibit nicotinic receptors at the neuromuscular junction although some muscle relaxants (tubocurare) may demonstrate some ganglion-blocking properties.

Trimetaphan

Trimetaphan is a quaternary ammonium compound.

Presentation and uses

Trimetaphan is available as a clear pale-yellow solution for intravenous injection containing 50 mg.ml^{-1}. It was used previously via the oral route to treat essential hypertension but drugs with better side-effect profiles have superseded it. Its sole current use is to induce hypotensive anaesthesia at 1–4 mg.min^{-1}.

Mechanism of action

Trimetaphan is a competitive antagonist at all nicotinic ganglionic receptors including those at the adrenal cortex and has a direct vasodilator effect on peripheral vessels. Histamine is also released but may not be significant in producing hypotension.

Effects

- Cardiovascular – the onset of hypotension is rapid when used by intravenous infusion. Pre- and afterload falls, and there may be a compensatory increase in heart rate to maintain cardiac output.

- Central nervous system – cerebral blood flow is not reduced as long as the preload is maintained with intravenous fluid and the mean blood pressure remains above approximately 50 mmHg. The cerebral metabolic rate is unchanged and it does not cross the BBB to any extent.
- Respiratory – histamine release may induce bronchospasm.
- Parasympathetic – owing to parasympathetic ganglion blockade the following effects are seen: constipation, urinary retention, dry mouth, mydriasis, increased intra-occular pressure and variable tachycardia. These may complicate recovery from anaesthesia.
- Miscellaneous – it inhibits plasma cholinesterase and prolongs the effects of depolarizing and non-depolarizing muscle relaxants, although this is variable.

Kinetics

Data are limited but it is mainly excreted unchanged in the urine. There may be some plasma hydrolysis. It crosses the placenta and has been associated with meconium ileus in neonates.

Hexamethonium (C6)

This quaternary ammonium compound has similar effects to trimetaphan. It is no longer used in the UK.

Diuretics

See Chapter 21.

Adrenoceptor antagonists

See Chapter 13.

Ca^{2+} channel antagonists

See Chapter 15 and 16.

Central nervous system

- **Hypnotics and anxiolytics**
- **Antidepressants**
- **Anticonvulsants**

Hypnotics and anxiolytics

Physiology

γ-Aminobutyric acid (GABA) is the main inhibitory neurotransmitter within the CNS and acts via two different receptor subtypes, $GABA_A$ and $GABA_B$:

- $GABA_A$ – this receptor is a **ligand-gated** Cl^- ion channel. It consists of five subunits (2α, β, δ and γ – each having a number of variants) arranged to form a central ion channel. GABA binds to and activates $GABA_A$ receptors and increases the opening frequency of its Cl^- channel, augmenting Cl^- conductance and thereby hyperpolarizing the neuronal membrane. Cl^- ion conductance is potentiated by the binding of BDZs to the α subunit of the activated receptor complex. $GABA_A$ receptors are essentially (but not exclusively) postsynaptic and are widely distributed throughout the CNS.

- $GABA_B$ – this receptor is **metabotropic** (i.e. acts via a G-protein and second messengers), and when stimulated it increases K^+ conductance, thereby hyperpolarizing the neuronal membrane. $GABA_B$ receptors are located both presynaptically on nerve terminals and postsynaptically in many regions of the brain, as well as in the dorsal horn of the spinal cord. Baclofen acts only via $GABA_B$ receptors to reduce spasticity.

BDZs modulate the effects of GABA at $GABA_A$ receptors. The specific α-subunit type determines the BDZ pharmacology – anxiolytic or sedative. Two BDZ receptor subtypes have been identified: BZ_1, found in the spinal cord and cerebellum – responsible for anxiolysis; and BZ_2, found in the spinal cord, hippocampus and cerebral cortex – responsible for sedative and anticonvulsant activity.

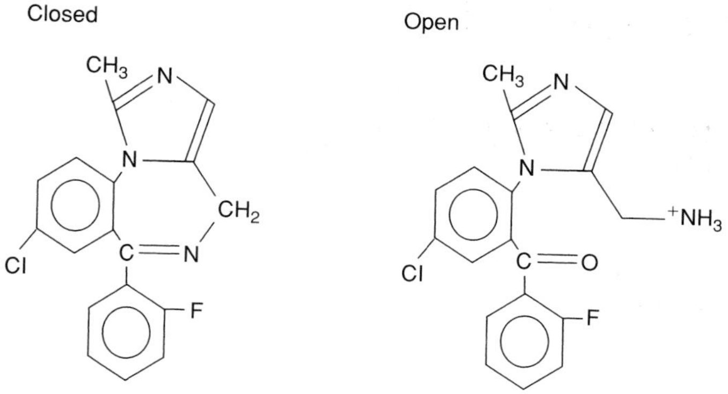

Closed

Open

Figure 17.1. Structures of midazolam.

Benzodiazepines (BDZs)

Uses

BDZs are used commonly in anaesthesia as premedication and to sedate patients during minor procedures. They are also used more widely as anxiolytics, hypnotics and anticonvulsants.

Structure

At its core BDZ have two ring structures. The first is a benzene ring (p93); the second has seven members (5 carbon and 2 nitrogen) and is called a di-azepine ring. However, for pharmacological activity, BDZs also have a carbonyl group at position 2 on the di-azepine ring, another benzene ring and a halogen on the first benzene ring.

Midazolam

Presentation

Midazolam is presented as a clear solution at pH 3.5. It is unique among the BDZs in that its structure is dependent on the surrounding pH. At pH 3.5 its di-azepine ring structure is open resulting in an ionized molecule, which is therefore water-soluble. However, when its surrounding pH is greater than 4 its di-azepine ring structure closes so that it is no longer ionized and therefore becomes lipid-soluble (Figure 17.1). Its pKa is 6.5, so that at physiological pH 89% is present in an unionized form and available to cross lipid membranes.

As it is water-soluble it does not cause pain on injection.

Table 17.1. Kinetics of some benzodiazepines.

	Diazepam	Midazolam	Lorazepam
Protein binding (%)	95	95	95
Elimination half-life (h)	20–45	1–4	10–20
Volume of distribution (l.kg^{-1})	1.0–1.5	1.0–1.5	0.75–1.30
Active metabolites	yes	yes	no
Clearance (ml.kg^{-1}.min^{-1})	0.2–0.5	6–10	1.0–1.5

Uses

Midazolam is used intravenously to sedate patients for minor procedures and has powerful amnesic properties. It is also used to sedate ventilated patients in intensive care.

Kinetics

Midazolam may be given orally (bioavailability approximately 40%), intranasally or intramuscularly as premedication. It has a short duration of action due to distribution. It is metabolized by hydroxylation to the active compound 1-α hydroxymidazolam, which is conjugated with glucuronic acid prior to renal excretion. Less than 5% is metabolized to oxazepam. It is highly protein bound (approximately 95%) and has an elimination half-life of 1–4 hours. At 6–10 ml.kg^{-1}.min^{-1} its clearance is larger than that of diazepam and lorazepam so that its effects wear off more rapidly following infusion.

Alfentanil is metabolized by the same hepatic P450 isoenzyme (3A3/4), and when administered together their effects may be prolonged.

Diazepam

Diazepam has a high lipid solubility, which facilitates its oral absorption and its rapid central effects. It is highly protein bound (approximately 95%) to albumin and is metabolized in the liver by oxidation to desmethyldiazepam, oxazepam and temazepam all of which are active. It does not induce hepatic enzymes. The glucuronide derivatives are excreted in the urine. It has the lowest clearance of the BDZs discussed here and its half-life is hugely increased by its use as an infusion (cf. context-sensitive half-time, p.77).

It may cause some cardiorespiratory depression. Liver failure and cimetidine will prolong its actions by reducing its metabolism. When administered with opioids or alcohol, respiratory depression may be more pronounced. In common with other BDZs it reduces the MAC of co-administered anaesthetic agents.

Lorazepam

Lorazepam shares similar pharmacokinetics and actions to other BDZs although its metabolites are inactive. It is used for premedication as an anxiolytic and amnesic.

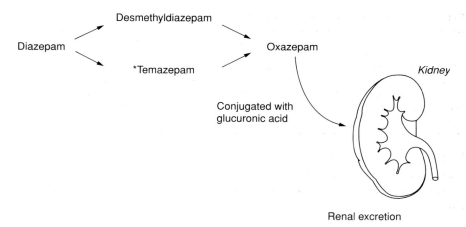

Figure 17.2. Metabolism of diazepam. *Less than 5% of temazepam is metabolized to oxazepam.

It may also be used in status epilepticus (50–100 μg.kg^{-1} i.v., s.l. or p.r. from 1 to 12 years, maximum dose 4 mg; >12 years, 4 mg).

It is well absorbed following oral or intramuscular administration, highly plasma protein bound (approximately 95%) and conjugated with glucuronic acid producing inactive metabolites, which are excreted in the urine (Figure 17.2).

Temazepam

Temazepam is used as a nighttime sedative and as an anxiolytic premedicant. It has no unique features within the BDZ family. It is well absorbed in the gut, is 75% protein bound and has a volume of distribution of 0.8 l.kg^{-1}. Eighty percent is excreted unchanged in the urine while glucuronidation occurs in the liver. Only a very small amount is demethylated to oxazepam. It has a half-life of about 8 hours and may result in some hangover effects.

Flumazenil

Flumazenil is an imidazobenzodiazepine.

Uses

Flumazenil is used to reverse the effects of BDZs, that is, excessive sedation following minor procedures or in the treatment of BDZ overdose. However, its use is cautioned in mixed drug overdose as it may precipitate fits. It is given by intravenous injection in 100 μg increments and acts within 2 minutes. Its relatively short half-life (about 1 hour) compared with many BDZs means that further doses or an infusion may be needed.

Mechanism of action

Flumazenil is a competitive BDZ antagonist. However, it has some agonist activity as well and its ability to precipitate seizures in certain patients may be a result of inverse agonist activity.

Effects

These include nausea and vomiting. It may also precipitate anxiety, agitation and seizures especially in epileptic patients.

Kinetics

Flumazenil is 50% plasma protein bound and undergoes significant hepatic metabolism to inactive compounds that are excreted in the urine.

Non-benzodiazepine hypnotics (the Z drugs)

Zopiclone, zaleplon and zolpidem are hypnotics that act via the BDZ receptor but cannot be classified as benzodiazepines structurally. They were developed in order to try to overcome some of the side effects of the BDZs, namely dependence and next day sedation.

Zopiclone has the longest elimination half-life of approximately 5 hours while zaleplon and zolpidem have elimination half-lives of 1 and 2 hours, respectively.

They have not had a major impact in the area of short-term hypnotics as they carry all the same side effects as the BDZs. Only where there has been a specific intolerance to a specific BDZ is switching to a Z drug recommended. Where general intolerance is a problem the patient is just as likely to expereince intolerance to the Z drugs.

Antidepressants

Four groups of drugs are used to treat depression:
- **Tricyclics**
- **Selective serotonin re-uptake inhibitors**
- **Monoamine oxidase inhibitors**
- **Atypical agents**

Tricyclics – TCAs (amitriptyline, nortriptyline, imipramine, dothiepin)

As its name suggests, this group of drugs was originally based on a tricyclic ring structure, although now many second-generation drugs contain different numbers of rings.

Uses

TCAs are used to treat depressive illness, nocturnal enuresis and as an adjunct in the treatment of chronic pain.

Table 17.2. Effects of various antidepressants.

	Anticholinergic effects	Sedation	Postural hypotension
TCA			
Amitriptyline	++++	++++	++
Imipramine	++	++	+++
Nortriptyline	++	++	+
Desipramine	+	+	+
SSRI			
Fluoxetine	+	nil	+

Mechanism of action

They competitively block neuronal uptake (uptake 1) of noradrenaline and serotonin (5-HT). In doing so they increase the concentration of transmitter in the synapse. However, the antidepressant effects do not occur within the same time frame, taking up to 2 weeks to work. They also block muscarinic, histaminergic and α-adrenoceptors, and have non-specific sedative effects (Table 17.2).

Effects

- Central nervous system – sedation and occasionally seizures in epileptic patients.
- Anticholinergic effects – dry mouth, constipation, urinary retention and blurred vision.
- Cardiovascular – postural hypotension especially in the elderly.

Kinetics

TCAs are well absorbed from the gut reflecting their high lipid solubility. They are highly plasma protein bound and have a high volume of distribution. Metabolism, which shows large interpatient variability, occurs in the liver and often produces active metabolites (e.g. imipramine to desipramine and nortriptyline).

TCA overdose

This is not uncommon in depressed patients. The features of tricyclic overdose include a mixture of:

- Cardiovascular effects – sinus tachycardia is common and there is a dose-related prolongation of the QT interval and widening of the QRS complex. Ventricular arrhythmias are more likely when the QRS complex is longer than 0.16 seconds. Right bundle branch block is also seen. The blood pressure may be high or low but in serious overdose hypotension may be refractory to treatment and culminate in pulseless electrical activity.

- Central effects – excitation, seizures (correlating with a QRS duration of more than 0.1 seconds) and then depression. Mydriasis is a feature, as is hyperthermia.
- Anticholinergic effects.

Treatment

This includes gastric lavage followed by activated charcoal. Supportive care may require supplementation with specific treatment. Seizures may be treated with benzodiazepines or phenytoin and ventricular arrhythmias with phenytoin or lidocaine. Inotropes should be avoided where possible as this may precipitate arrhythmias. Intravascular volume expansion is usually sufficient to correct hypotension. The anticholinergic effects may be reversed by an anticholinesterase, but this is not recommended as it may precipitate seizures, bradycardia and heart failure.

Selective serotonin re-uptake inhibitors – SSRIs (fluoxetine, paroxetine, sertraline, venlafaxine)

As their name suggests, SSRIs selectively inhibit the neuronal re-uptake of 5-HT. They are no more effective than standard antidepressants but do not have their associated side-effect profile. SSRIs are less sedative, have fewer anticholinergic effects and appear less cardiotoxic in overdose although they are associated with gastrointestinal side-effects (nausea and constipation).

Despite their side-effect profile, when combinations of serotonergic drugs are used the potentially fatal serotonergic syndrome may result, which is characterized by hyper-reflexia, agitation, clonus and hyperthermia. The commonest combination is an MAOI and SSRI – however, the phenylpiperidine opioids (particularly pethidine) have weak serotonin reuptake inhibitor properties and can also precipitate the syndrome.

Fluoxetine is an effective antidepressant causing minimal sedation. It is a 50:50 mix of two isomers that are equally active. It is well absorbed and metabolized in the liver by cytochrome P450 enzymes. In addition, there are non-saturable enzymes that prevent an unchecked rise in levels. However, the dose should be reduced in renal failure as accumulation may result. Side effects include nausea and vomiting, headache, insomnia, reduced libido and mania or hypomania in up to 1%.

Venlafaxine appears to block the re-uptake of both noradrenaline and 5-HT (and to a lesser extent dopamine) while having little effect on muscarinic, histaminergic or α-adrenoceptors.

Monoamine oxidase inhibitors – MAOIs

This group of drugs is administered orally for the treatment of resistant depression, obsessive compulsive disorders, chronic pain syndromes and migraine.

MAO is present as a variety of isoenzymes within presynaptic neurones and is responsible for the deamination of amine neurotransmitters. They have been classified as types A and B. Following their inhibition there is an increase in the level of amine neurotransmitters, which is thought to be the basis of their central activity. MAO-A preferentially deaminates 5-HT and catecholamines, while MAO-B preferentially deaminates tyramine and phenylethamine.

There are now two generations of MAOIs. The original generation inhibit MAO irreversibly and non-selectively (i.e. MAO-A and -B) while the new generation selectively and reversibly inhibit only MAO-A (RIMA). Neither group is used as first line therapy because of the potential for serious side effects and hepatic toxicity.

Non-selective irreversible MAOIs (phenelzine, isocarboxazid, tranylcypromine)

Phenelzine and isocarboxazid are hydrazines while tranylcypromine is a non-hydrazine compound. Tranylcypromine is potentially the most dangerous as it possesses stimulant activity.

Effects

In addition to controlling depression they also produce sedation, blurred vision, orthostatic hypotension and hypertensive crises following tyramine rich foods (cheese, pickled herring, chicken liver, Bovril and chocolate) and indirectly acting sympathomimetics. Hepatic enzymes are inhibited and the hydrazine compounds may cause hepatotoxicity. Interaction with pethidine may precipitate cerebral irritability, hyperpyrexia and cardiovascular instability. Interaction with fentanyl has also been reported.

Selective reversible MAOIs – RIMA (moclobemide)

Moclobemide causes less potentiation of tyramine than the older generation MAOIs and in general patients do not need the same level of dietary restriction. However, some patients are especially sensitive to tyramine and so all patients should be advised to avoid tyramine-rich foods and indirect-acting sympathomimetic amines.

It is completely absorbed from the gut but undergoes significant first-pass metabolism resulting in an oral bioavailability of 60–80%. It is metabolized in the liver by cytochrome P450 and up to 2% of the Caucasian and 15% of the Asian population have been shown to be slow metabolizers. The metabolites are excreted in the urine.

Linezolid is a new antibiotic indicated for methacillin-resistant *Staphlococcus aureus* and vancomycin-resistant enetrococci. It is also a MAOI and as such has the typical range of cautions and contraindications.

MAOIs and general anaesthesia

Those patients taking MAOIs and presenting for emergency surgery should not be given pethidine or any indirectly acting sympathomimetic amines (e.g. ephedrine). If cardiovascular support is indicated, direct-acting agents should be used but with extreme caution as they may also precipitate exaggerated hypertension. The elective case presents potential difficulties. If MAOI therapy is withdrawn for the required 14–21 days before surgery, the patient may suffer a relapse of their depression with potentially disastrous consequences. However, the newer agents may control depression more effectively and reduce the chance of a serious peri-operative drug interaction.

Indirectly acting sympathomimetic amines are heavily dependent on MAO for their metabolism and therefore may produce exaggerated hypertension and arrhythmias when administered with an MAOI. The directly acting sympathomimetic amines should also be used with caution although they are also metabolized by COMT and therefore are not subject to the same degree of exaggerated response.

MAOIs should be stopped for 2 weeks before starting alternative antidepressant therapy and 2 weeks should have elapsed from the end of tricyclic therapy to the start of MAOI therapy.

Atypical agents

Mianserin

Mianserin is a tetracyclic compound used in depressive illness, especially where sedation is required. It does not block the neuronal re-uptake of transmitters in contrast to the TCAs. It does, however, block presynaptic α_2-adrenoceptors, which reduces their negative feedback, resulting in increased synaptic concentrations of neurotransmitters.

It has very little ability to block muscarinic and peripheral α-adrenoceptors and as such causes less in the way of antimuscarinic effects or postural hypotension.

Its important side effects are agranulocytosis and aplastic anaemia, which are more common in the elderly.

Lithium carbonate

Lithium is used in the treatment of bipolar depression, mania and recurrent affective disorders. It has a narrow therapeutic index and plasma levels should be maintained at 0.5–1.5 mmol.l^{-1}. In excitable cells, lithium imitates Na$^+$ and decreases the release of neurotransmitters.

It may increase generalized muscle tone and lower the seizure threshold in epileptics. Many patients develop polyuria and polydipsia due to antidiuretic hormone antagonism. It may also produce raised serum levels of Na$^+$, Mg^{2+} and Ca^{2+}. Lithium prolongs neuromuscular blockade and may decrease anaesthetic requirements as it blocks brain stem release of noradrenaline and dopamine.

The thyroid gland may become enlarged and underactive and the patient may experience weight gain and tremor. Above the therapeutic level patients suffer with vomiting, abdominal pain, ataxia, convulsions, arrhythmias and death.

Anticonvulsants

Where possible a single agent should be used to treat epilepsy as it avoids the potential for drug interaction. In addition patients rarely improve with a second agent.

Phenytoin

Uses

Phenytoin has been used widely for many years in the treatment of grand mal and partial seizures, trigeminal neuralgia and ventricular arrhythmias following TCA overdose. It may be given orally or intravenously but the dose must be tailored to the individual patient as wide interpatient variation exists (about 9% of the population are slow hydroxylators) and blood assays are useful in this regard. It is incompatible with 5% dextrose, in which it becomes gelatinous. The normal therapeutic level is 10–20 μg.ml^{-1}.

Mechanism of action

The action of phenytoin is probably dependent on its ability to bind to and stabilize inactivated Na$^+$ channels. This prevents the further generation of action potentials that are central to seizure activity. It may also reduce Ca^{2+} entry into neurones, blocking transmitter release and enhancing the actions of GABA.

Effects

- Idiosyncratic – acne, coarsening of facial features, hirsutism, gum hyperplasia, folate-dependent megaloblastic anaemia, aplastic anaemia, various skin rashes and peripheral neuropathy.
- Dose-related – ataxia, nystagmus, parasthesia, vertigo and slurred speech. Rapid undiluted intravenous administration is associated with hypotension and heart block.
- Teratogenicity – it causes craniofacial abnormalities, growth retardation, limb and cardiac defects and mental retardation.
- Drug interactions – as phenytoin induces the hepatic mixed function oxidases it increases the metabolism of warfarin, BDZs and the oral contraceptive pill. Its metabolism may be inhibited by metronidazole, chloramphenicol and isoniazid leading to toxic levels. Furthermore phenytoin's metabolism may be induced by carbamazepine or alcohol resulting in reduced plasma levels.

Kinetics

The oral bioavailability is approximately 90% and it is highly plasma protein bound (90%). It undergoes saturable hepatic hydroxylation resulting in zero-order kinetics just above the therapeutic range. It can induce its own metabolism and that of other drugs. Its major metabolite is excreted in the urine.

Carbamazepine

Carbamazepine is also used in the treatment of trigeminal neuralgia. Its mode of action is similar to that of phenytoin. It may be given orally or rectally.

Effects

- Central nervous system – mild neurotoxic effects including headache, diplopia, ataxia, vomiting and drowsiness are common and often limit its use.
- Metabolic – it may produce an antidiuretic effect leading to water retention.
- Miscellaneous – drug-induced hepatitis, rashes in 5–10% and rarely agranulocytosis.
- Teratogenicity – it causes facial abnormalities, intrauterine growth retardation, microcephaly and mental retardation. The incidence increases with dose. Overall incidence is about 1/300–2000 live births.
- Drug interactions – as carbamazepine induces hepatic enzymes, it demonstrates many of the interactions seen with phenytoin. Levels of concurrently administered phenytoin may be elevated or reduced. Erythromycin can increase serum levels of carbamazepine.

Kinetics

Carbamazepine is well absorbed from the gut with a high oral bioavailability. It is approximately 75% plasma protein bound and undergoes extensive hepatic metabolism to carbamazepine 10,11-epoxide, which retains about 30% of carbamazepine's anticonvulsant properties. It powerfully induces hepatic enzymes and induces its own metabolism. Its excretion is almost entirely in the urine as unconjugated metabolites.

Sodium valproate

Uses

Sodium valproate is used in the treatment of various forms of epilepsy including absence (petit mal) seizures and in the treatment of trigeminal neuralgia.

Mechanism of action

Sodium valproate appears to act by stabilizing inactive Na^+ channels and also by stimulating central GABA-ergic inhibitory pathways. It is generally well tolerated.

Effects

- Abdominal – it may cause nausea and gastric irritation. Pancreatitis and potentially fatal hepatotoxicity are recognized following its use.
- Haematological – thrombocytopenia and reduced platelet aggregation.
- Miscellaneous – transient hair loss.
- Teratogenicity – it causes neural tube defects.

Kinetics

Sodium valproate is well absorbed orally, highly protein bound (approximately 90%) and undergoes hepatic metabolism to products (some of which are active), which are excreted in the urine.

Phenobarbitone is an effective anticonvulsant but its use is associated with significant sedation, which limits its use. It is a long-acting barbiturate that induces hepatic enzymes and interacts with other agents (warfarin, oral contraceptives, other anticonvulsants).

BDZs (see above) are widely used in the emergency treatment of status epilepticus and act by enhancing the chloride-gating function of GABA.

Other agents

Vigabatrin, gabapentin, lamotrigine and **pregabalin** are newer agents that are used in the control of persistent partial seizures.

Vigabatrin irreversibly inhibits GABA-transaminase, the enzyme responsible for the breakdown of GABA and therefore its duration of action is about 24 hours while its elimination half-life is only 6 hours. It is excreted unchanged in the urine. It interacts with phenytoin reducing its concentration by about 25% by an unknown mechanism. It may cause sedation, fatigue, headache, agitation and depression.

Lamotrigine acts on the presynaptic neuronal membrane and stabilizes the inactive Na^+ channel leading to a reduction in excitatory neurotransmitter release. It undergoes hepatic metabolism to an inactive conjugate. Its rate of metabolism is increased by other enzyme-inducing drugs (carbamazepine and phenytoin) but reduced by sodium valproate. It may precipitate headache, nausea, diplopia, ataxia and tremor. Approximately 0.1% of adults develop Stevens–Johnson or Lyell's syndrome. The incidence is higher in children.

Gabapentin's mode of action is uncertain but it may bind to Ca^{2+} channels within the brain. It is not plasma protein bound and has a terminal elimination half-life of 5–7 hours. It is excreted unchanged in the urine and does not interfere with other anticonvulsants as it does not affect hepatic enzyme systems. It is well tolerated. Gabapentin also has a role to play in the management of chronic pain.

Pregabalin is a potent ligand for the alpha-2-delta subunit of voltage-gated calcium channels in the central nervous system. Once bound there is a reduction in calcium influx leading to a reduction of excitatory neurotransmitter release. It is a structural analogue of gamma-aminobutyric acid (GABA – although it bears no pharmacological resemblance to GABA) and is prepared as the S-enantiomer. Its kinetics are predictable and its oral bioavailability is >90% and it readily crosses the BBB. Its terminal elimination half-life is 6 hours. In a manner similar to gabapentin it is not metabolized so that it does no interact with other anticonvulsants. It is excreted in the urine unchanged.

Antiemetics and related drugs

Nausea and vomiting has many causes including drugs, motion sickness, fear, pregnancy, vestibular disease and migraine. In previous decades anaesthesia was almost synonymous with vomiting, but with the advent of new anaesthetic agents and more aggressive treatment the incidence of vomiting has decreased. However, even the latest agents have failed to eradicate this troublesome symptom encountered in the peri-operative period.

Physiology

The vomiting centre (VC) coordinates vomiting. It has no discrete anatomical site but may be considered as a collection of effector neurones situated in the medulla. This collection projects to the vagus and phrenic nerves and also to the spinal motor neurones supplying the abdominal muscles, which when acting together bring about the vomiting reflex.

The VC has important input from the chemoreceptor trigger zone (CTZ), which lies in the area postrema on the floor of the fourth ventricle but is functionally outside the blood–brain barrier. The CTZ is rich in dopamine (D_2) receptors and also serotonin (5-HT) receptors. Acetylcholine (ACh) is important in neural transmission from the vestibular apparatus. Other input is summarized in Figure 18.1.

The treatment of nausea and vomiting is aimed at reducing the afferent supply to the VC. While the administration of antiemetics forms a vital part of treatment, attention should also be given to minimizing the administration of opioids by the use of non-steroidal anti-inflammatory drugs and avoiding unnecessary anticholinesterase administration. When propofol is used to maintain anaesthesia for minor surgery, where the use of opioids is limited, it may reduce the incidence of post-operative nausea and vomiting (PONV).

The following types of agents have been used:
- **Dopamine antagonists**
- **Anticholinergics**
- **Antihistamines**
- **5-HT$_3$ antagonists**
- **Miscellaneous**

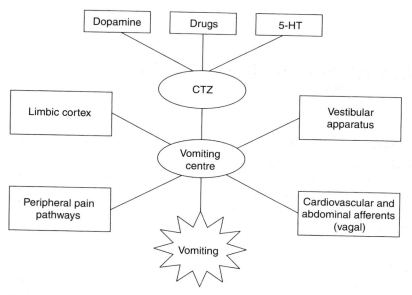

Figure 18.1. Summary of the various neural inputs that result in vomiting.

Dopamine antagonists

Phenothiazines

Phenothiazines are the main group of anti-psychotic drugs (neuroleptics) and have only a limited role in the treatment of vomiting. They are divided into three groups on the basis of structure, which confers typical pharmacological characteristics (Table 18.1).

Chlorpromazine

Chlorpromazine's proprietary name 'Largactil' hints at the widespread effects of this drug.

Uses

Chlorpromazine is used in schizophrenia for its sedative properties and to correct altered thought. Its effects on central neural pathways are complicated but are thought to involve isolating the reticular activating system from its afferent connections. This results in sedation, disregard of external stimuli and a reduction in motor activity (neurolepsy). It is sometimes used to control vomiting or pain in terminal care where other agents have been unsuccessful. It has also been shown to be effective in preventing PONV. It is occasionally used to treat hiccup.

Table 18.1. Groups of phenothiazines.

Propylamine	chlorpromazine
Piperidine	thioridazine
Piperazine	prochlorperazine, perphenazine

Mechanism of action

Chlorpromazine antagonizes the following receptor types: dopaminergic (D_2), muscarinic, noradrenergic (α_1 and α_2), histaminergic (H_1) and serotinergic (5-HT). It also has membrane-stabilizing properties and prevents noradrenaline uptake into sympathetic nerves (uptake 1).

Effects

- Central nervous system – extrapyramidal effects are due to central dopamine antagonism. The neuroleptic malignant syndrome occurs rarely. It has variable effects on hypothalamic function, reducing the secretion of growth hormone while increasing the release of prolactin (dopamine functions as prolactin release inhibitory factor). Temperature regulation is altered and may result in hypothermia.
- Cardiovascular – it antagonizes α-adrenoceptors resulting in peripheral vasodilation, hypotension and increased heat loss.
- Anticholinergic – it has moderate anticholinergic effects.
- Gut – appetite is increased and patients tend to gain weight (exacerbated by inactivity). While it has been shown to be an adequate antiemetic, its other effects have limited this role.
- Miscellaneous – contact sensitization. Direct contact should be avoided unless actually taking chlorpromazine. Cholestatic jaundice, agranulocytosis, leucopenia, leucocytosis and haemolytic anaemia are all recognized.

Kinetics

Absorption from the gut is good but due to a large hepatic first-pass metabolism (limiting its oral bioavailability to about 30%), it is often given parenterally. The large number of hepatic metabolites is excreted in the urine or bile, while a variable but small fraction is excreted unchanged in the urine.

Thioridazine

Thioridazine is not used to treat nausea and vomiting. It is used in schizophrenia and other psychoses where it is favoured in the elderly as it is only moderately sedative and is only rarely associated with extrapyramidal effects (Table 18.2).

Table 18.2. Effects of some dopamine antagonists.

	Chlorpromazine	Thioridazine	Prochlorperazine
Sedation	+++	++	+
Anticholinergic effects	++	+++	+
Extrapyramidal effects	++	+	+++

Prochlorperazine

Uses
Prochlorperazine is effective in the prevention and treatment of PONV and vertigo, as well as in schizophrenia and other psychoses.

Effects
- Central nervous system – extrapyramidal effects are seen more commonly in this class of phenothiazine. Acute dystonias and akathisia seem to be the most commonly encountered effects. Children and young adults are the most affected groups. When used peri-operatively it produces only mild sedation and may prolong the recovery time but the effects are not marked.
- Group specific – in common with other phenothiazines prochlorperazine may cause cholestatic jaundice, haematological abnormalities, skin sensitization, hyperprolactinaemia and rarely the neuroleptic malignant syndrome.

Kinetics
Absorption by the oral route is erratic and the oral bioavailability is very low due to an extensive hepatic first-pass metabolism. It may be given by suppository, intravenous or intramuscular injection.

Perphenazine has similar indications and kinetics to prochlorperazine, and has been shown to be effective in the prevention and treatment of PONV. It is associated with a higher incidence of extrapyramidal effects and increased post-operative sedation than prochlorperazine.

Butyrophenones

Droperidol
Droperidol is the only butyrophenone that is used in anaesthetic practice. However this agent is no longer available in the UK.

Uses

Droperidol has been shown to be effective in the prevention and treatment of PONV at doses from 0.25 to 5 mg, although the incidence of side effects increases with dose. It is also used in neurolept analgesia and in the control of mania.

Mechanism of action

Droperidol antagonizes central dopamine (D_2) receptors at the CTZ.

Effects

These are similar to those seen with phenothiazines.

- Central nervous system – sedation is more pronounced compared to the phenothiazines. The true incidence of extrapyramidal effects is unknown but increases with higher doses. They may develop more than 12 hours after administration and up to 25% of patients may experience anxiety up to 48 hours after administration. In sufficient dose it induces neurolepsis.
- Metabolic – it may cause hyperprolactinaemia.
- Cardiovascular – hypotension resulting from peripheral α-adrenoceptor blockade may occur.

Kinetics

Droperidol is usually given intravenously although it is absorbed readily after intramuscular injection. It is highly plasma protein bound (approximately 90%) and extensively metabolized in the liver to products that are excreted in the urine, only 1% as unchanged drug.

Domperidone

This D_2 antagonist is less likely to cause extrapyramidal effects as it does not cross the blood–brain barrier. Its use in children is limited to nausea and vomiting following chemotherapy or radiotherapy. It also increases prolactin levels and may cause galactorrhoea and gynaecomastia. The intravenous preparation was withdrawn following serious arrhythmias during the administration of large doses. It is only available as tablets or suppositories.

Benzamides

Metoclopramide

Uses

Metoclopramide is used as an antiemetic and a prokinetic. Approximately half of the clinical studies have demonstrated placebo to be as effective as metoclopramide as an antiemetic. However, metoclopramide appears to be most effective when 20 mg is given at the end of anaesthesia rather than at induction.

Mechanism of action

Metoclopramide exerts its antiemetic actions primarily through dopamine (D_2) receptor antagonism at the CTZ, although it does have prokinetic effects on the stomach (cf. Chapter 19). It also blocks 5-HT$_3$ receptors, which may account for some of its antiemetic properties.

Effects

- Central nervous system – metoclopramide crosses the blood–brain barrier and may precipitate extrapyramidal effects up to 72 hours after administration. Such effects are more common in young females (1 in 5000). Rarely it may precipitate the neuroleptic malignant syndrome. Sedation is seen more commonly during long-term administration. Agitation is occasionally seen following intramuscular premedication with 10–20 mg.
- Cardiovascular – hypotension, tachy- and bradycardias have been reported following rapid intravenous administration.

Kinetics

Metoclopramide is well absorbed from the gut although first-pass metabolism varies significantly producing a wide range in oral bioavailability (30–90%). It may be given intravenously. It is conjugated in the liver and excreted along with unchanged drug in the urine.

Anticholinergics

While so-called 'anticholinergic' agents are effective antagonists at muscarinic receptors, they have very little activity at nicotinic receptors and may therefore be thought of as essentially selective agents at normal doses.

The naturally occurring tertiary amines, atropine and hyoscine, are esters formed by the combination of tropic acid and an organic base (tropine or scopine) and are able to cross the blood–brain barrier. Their central effects include sedation, amnesia, anti-emesis and the central anticholinergic syndrome. Glycopyrrolate is a synthetic quaternary amine (therefore charged) with no central effects as it is unable to cross the blood–brain barrier.

Hyoscine

Hyoscine is a racemic mixture, but only l-hyoscine is active.

Uses

Hyoscine has traditionally been given with an intramuscular opioid as premedication, and in this setting has been shown to reduce PONV. It has also been used as a sedative and amnesic agent.

Table 18.3. Effects of some anticholinergics.

	Hyoscine	Atropine	Glycopyrrolate
Antiemetic potency	++	+	0
Sedation/amnesia	+++	+	0
Anti-sialagogue	+++	+	++
Mydriasis	+++	+	0
Placental transfer	++	++	0
Bronchodilation	+	++	++
Heart rate	+	+++	++

Effects

While hyoscine's main uses are derived from its central antimuscarinic effects, it also has peripheral antimuscarinic effects some of which can be useful and are summarized in Table 18.3.

Other central effects – it may precipitate a central anticholinergic syndrome, which is characterized by excitement, ataxia, hallucinations, behavioural abnormalities and drowsiness.

Kinetics

Its absorption is variable and its oral bioavailability lies between 10% and 50%. Transdermal administration is effective in reducing PONV and motion sickness despite very low plasma levels. It is extensively metabolized by liver esterases and only a small fraction is excreted unchanged in the urine. Its duration of action is shorter than that of atropine.

Atropine

Atropine is a racemic mixture, but only L-atropine is active.

Uses

Atropine is used to treat bradycardia and as an anti-sialagogue. It is also used to antagonize the muscarinic side effects of anticholinesterases. It is not used to treat PONV because of its cardiovascular effects.

Effects

- Central nervous system – it is less likely to cause a central cholinergic crisis than hyoscine and is less sedative.
- Cardiovascular – it may cause an initial bradycardia following a small intravenous dose. This may be due to its effects centrally on the vagal nucleus or reflect a partial agonist effect at cardiac muscarinic receptors.
- Respiratory system – bronchodilation is more marked than with hyoscine, leading to an increase in dead space. Bronchial secretions are reduced.

- Gut – it is a less effective anti-sialagogue than hyoscine. The tone of the lower oesophageal sphincter is decreased and there is a small decrease in gastric acid secretion.
- Miscellaneous – sweating is inhibited and this may provoke a pyrexia in paediatric patients. When administered topically it may increase intra-occular pressure, which may be critical for patients with glaucoma.

Kinetics

Intestinal absorption is rapid but unpredictable. It is 50% plasma protein bound and extensively metabolized by liver esterases. It is excreted in the urine, only a tiny fraction unchanged.

Glycopyrrolate

Gylcopyrrolate is indicated for anti-sialagogue premedication, the treatment of bradycardias and to protect against the unwanted effects of anticholinesterases. Its charged quaternary structure gives it a different set of characteristics compared to the tertiary amines. Intestinal absorption is negligible and the oral bioavailability is consequently less than 5%. It does not cross the blood–brain barrier and so it is devoid of central effects. It is minimally metabolized and 80% is excreted in the urine unchanged.

Antihistamines

Cyclizine

Cyclizine is a piperazine derivative. The parenteral preparation is prepared with lactic acid at pH 3.2. Consequently intramuscular and intravenous injection may be particularly painful.

Uses

Cyclizine is used as an antiemetic in motion sickness, radiotherapy, PONV and emesis induced by opioids. It is also used to control the symptoms of Ménière's disease.

Mechanism of action

Cyclizine is a histamine (H_1) antagonist, but also has anticholinergic properties that may contribute significantly to its antiemetic actions.

Effects

- Gut – it increases lower oesophageal sphincter tone.
- Anticholinergic – these are mild although it may cause an increase in heart rate following intravenous injection.
- Extrapyramidal effects and sedation do not complicate its use.

Kinetics

Cyclizine is well absorbed orally and has a high oral bioavailability (approximately 75%). Surprisingly little is known regarding the rest of the kinetics of this drug.

Promethazine

Promethazine has traditionally been used in combination with pethidine for intra-muscular premedication. However, it may also be used as an oral premed for children. It has significant anticholinergic properties and sedative effects. It is well absorbed from the gut but is subject to a significant first-pass hepatic metabolism so that its oral bioavailability is 25%. It has a duration of action of 3–6 hours and its metabolites are eliminated entirely in the urine.

5-HT₃ antagonists

Ondansetron

Ondansetron is a carbazole.

Presentation

Ondansetron is available as tablets (4–8 mg), a strawberry-flavoured lyophilisate (4–8 mg) to dissolve on the tongue, a suppository (16 mg) and as a clear solution containing 2 mg.ml^{-1} for slow intravenous injection.

Uses

Ondansetron is indicated for the treatment of nausea and vomiting associated with chemo- or radiotherapy and in the peri-operative period. It is ineffective for vomiting induced by motion sickness or dopamine agonists. It is licensed for children above 2 years of age.

Mechanism of action

The activation of 5-HT₃ receptors peripherally and centrally appears to induce vomiting. Chemo- and radiotherapy may cause the release of 5-HT from enterochromaffin cells. Peripheral 5-HT₃ receptors in the gut are then activated and stimulate vagal afferent neurones that connect to the VC, again via 5-HT₃ receptors. Thus ondansetron may antagonize 5-HT₃ both peripherally and centrally.

Effects

Ondansetron is well tolerated and its other effects are limited to headache, flushing, constipation and bradycardia following rapid intravenous administration.

Kinetics

Ondansetron is well absorbed from the gut with an oral bioavailability of about 60%. It is 75% protein bound and undergoes significant hepatic metabolism by hydroxylation and subsequent glucuronide conjugation to inactive metabolites. Its half-life is 3 hours. The dose should be reduced in hepatic impairment.

While ondansetron clearly has a place in the treatment of nausea and vomiting it has not universally been shown to be superior to low-dose droperidol or a phenothiazine. This together with its higher cost suggests it should be used only when conventional therapy is expected to or has failed.

Miscellaneous

Steroids

The role of dexamethasone as an antiemetic has traditionally been confined to chemotherapy induced nausea and vomiting. However more recently it has been used at a dose of 2.5–10 mg to prevent post-operative nausea and vomiting. Its mode of action in this area is uncertain.

Acupuncture

Several studies have demonstrated the effectiveness of acupuncture in the prevention of PONV. The acupuncture point lies between the tendons of flexor carpi radialis and palmaris longus about 4 cm from the distal wrist skin crease. It should be performed on the awake patient and is free from side effects.

Canabinoids

Nabilone acts at the VC and has been used as an antiemetic following chemotherapy.

Benzodiazepines

Lorazepam is used as an antiemetic during chemotherapy. It has amnesic and sedative properties. Its mode of action as an antiemetic is uncertain but it may modify central connections to the VC and prevent the anticipatory nausea that is seen with repeated doses of chemotherapy.

Drugs acting on the gut

- Antacids
- Drugs influencing gastric secretion
- Drugs influencing gastric motility
- Mucosal protectors
- Prostaglandin analogues

Antacids

Antacids neutralize gastric acidity. They are used to relieve the symptoms of dyspepsia and gastro-oesophageal reflux. They promote ulcer healing but less effectively than other therapies.

Aluminium and magnesium-containing antacids

Neither is absorbed from the gut significantly and due to their relatively low water solubility they are long-acting providing that they remain in the stomach. Aluminium-containing antacids have a slower action and produce constipation, while magnesium-containing antacids produce diarrhoea. Aluminium ions form complexes with some drugs (e.g. tetracycline) and reduce their absorption.

Sodium bicarbonate and sodium citrate

These antacids are water-soluble and their onset of action is faster than the aluminium- and magnesium-containing antacids. They are absorbed into the systemic circulation and may cause a metabolic alkalosis if taken in excess. Sodium bicarbonate releases carbon dioxide as it reacts with gastric acid, resulting in belching. Thirty milliliters of 0.3 M sodium citrate is often used with ranitidine to reduce gastric acidity before caesarean section. It should be given less than 10 minutes before the start of surgery due to its limited duration of action.

Drugs influencing gastric secretion

Physiology

Gastrin and ACh stimulate parietal cells (via gastrin and muscarinic receptors) to secrete H^+ into the gastric lumen. ACh is released from parasympathetic postganglionic fibres while gastrin is released from G-cells in the antral mucosa. However, the main stimulus for parietal cell acid secretion is via histamine receptor activation. Gastrin and ACh also stimulate the adjacent paracrine cells to produce and release histamine, which acts on the parietal cell, increasing cAMP and therefore acid secretion.

H$_2$ receptor antagonists

Cimetidine

Cimetidine is the only H$_2$ receptor antagonist with an imidazole structure.

Uses

It is used in peptic ulcer disease, reflux oesophagitis, Zollinger–Ellison syndrome and pre-operatively in those at risk of aspiration. It has not been shown to be of benefit in active haematemesis, although it does have a prophylactic role in those with critical illness.

Mechanism of action

Cimetidine is a competitive and specific antagonist of H$_2$ receptors at parietal cells.

Effects

- Gut – the gastric pH is raised and the volume of secretions reduced, while there is no change in gastric emptying time or lower oesophageal sphincter tone.
- Cardiovascular – bradycardia and hypotension follow rapid intravenous administration.
- Central nervous system – confusion, hallucinations and seizures are usually only seen when impaired renal function leads to high plasma levels.
- Respiratory system – low-grade aspiration of gastric content that has been stripped of its acidic, antibacterial environment will result in increased nosocomial pulmonary infections in critically ill ventilated patients.
- Endocrine – gynaecomastia, impotence and a fall in sperm count is seen in men due to its anti-androgenic effects.
- Metabolic – it inhibits hepatic cytochrome P450 and will slow the metabolism of the following drugs: lidocaine, propranolol, diazepam, phenytoin, tricyclic antidepressants, warfarin and aminophylline.

Kinetics

Cimetidine is well absorbed from the small bowel (oral bioavailability approximately 60%), poorly plasma protein bound (20%), partially metabolized (up to 60% if administered orally) in the liver by cytochrome P450 and approximately 50% excreted unchanged in the urine.

Ranitidine

Ranitidine is more potent than cimetidine.

Uses

Ranitidine has similar uses to cimetidine. However, because it does not inhibit hepatic cytochrome P450, it is often used in preference to cimetidine. It is used in combination with antibiotics to eradicate *H. pylori*. It is also used widely in labour with apparently no deleterious effects on the fetus or progress of labour.

Mechanism of action

Similar to that of cimetidine.

Effects

- Gut – similar to that of cimetidine.
- Cardiovascular – it may produce cardiac arrhythmias during rapid intravenous administration.
- Metabolic – it should be avoided in porphyria, although reports detailing this interaction are inconclusive. It has no anti-androgenic effects.
- Miscellaneous – rarely it may cause thrombocytopenia, leucopenia, reversible abnormalities of liver function and anaphylaxis.

Kinetics

Ranitidine is well absorbed from the gut, poorly protein bound (15%) and partially metabolized in the liver. It undergoes a greater degree of first-pass metabolism than cimetidine (oral bioavailability approximately 50%), while 50% of an administered dose is excreted unchanged in the urine.

Nizatidine and **famotidine** are newer H_2 antagonists with increased potency. Like ranitidine they do not inhibit hepatic cytochrome P450.

Proton pump inhibitors

Omeprazole

Uses

Omeprazole is used for similar indications to that of ranitidine but also in cases where H_2 blockade is insufficient. It may be given orally or intravenously.

Mechanism of action

A proton pump (K^+/H^+ ATPase) in the membrane of the parietal cell mediates the final common pathway of gastric acid secretion. Omeprazole reversibly blocks the proton pump and so achieves complete achlorhydria.

Effects

- Gut – the acidity and volume of gastric secretions is reduced, while no change is seen in lower oesophageal sphincter tone or gastric emptying.

- Metabolic – inhibition of hepatic cytochrome P450. This is limited, and although close monitoring is recommended with concurrent use of warfarin and phenytoin, their effects are rarely potentiated. The effects of diazepam may be increased via a similar mechanism.
- Miscellaneous – rashes and gastrointestinal upset are rare.

Kinetics

Omeprazole is degraded in gastric acid and so is prepared as a capsule with enteric-coated granules so that absorption occurs in the small intestine. It is a prodrug, becoming active within the parietal cell. It undergoes complete hepatic metabolism by cytochrome P450 to inactive metabolites, which are excreted in the urine (80%) and bile (20%).

Lansoprazole may be considered as an alternative to omeprazole.

Antimuscarinics

Pirenzipine is a selective antimuscarinic that was used in the treatment of gastric ulcers. It is relatively selective on the gut and decreases acid secretion but less effectively than H_2 blockers and the proton pump inhibitors. Its use has been discontinued.

Drugs influencing gastric motility

Metoclopramide

Metoclopramide is a dopamine antagonist with structural similarities to procainamide although it has no local anaesthetic properties.

Uses

Metoclopramide is used as a prokinetic and an antiemetic (see Chapter 18).

Mechanism of action

Its prokinetic actions are mediated by antagonism of peripheral dopaminergic (D_2) receptors and selective stimulation of gastric muscarinic receptors (which can be blocked by atropine).

Effects

- Central nervous system – extrapyramidal effects, the most common manifestations of which are akinesia and occulogyric crisis, are only seen when metoclopramide is given in high doses, in renal impairment, and to the elderly and the young. They can be treated with the anticholinergic agent benztropine. Metoclopramide may cause some sedation and enhance the actions of antidepressants. The neuroleptic malignant syndrome may also be triggered. Its central effects on the chemoreceptor trigger zone are discussed in Chapter 18.

- Gut – its peripheral actions result in an increased lower oesophageal sphincter tone and relaxation of the pylorus. It has no effect on gastric secretion.
- Cardiovascular – acute conduction abnormalities follow rapid intravenous administration, and acute hypertension occurs in phaeochromocytoma.
- Metabolic – it may precipitate hyperprolactinaemia and galactorrhoea, and should be avoided in porphyria. It inhibits plasma cholinesterase activity in vitro and may therefore prolong the effects of drugs metabolized by this enzyme.

Kinetics

Metoclopramide is well absorbed from the gut although first-pass metabolism varies significantly producing a wide range in oral bioavailability (30–90%). It may be given intravenously. It is conjugated in the liver and excreted along with unchanged drug in the urine.

Domperidone

This dopamine antagonist is less likely to cause extrapyramidal effects as it does not cross the blood–brain barrier. Its use in children is limited to nausea and vomiting following chemotherapy or radiotherapy. It also increases prolactin levels and may cause galactorrhoea and gynaecomastia. The intravenous preparation was withdrawn following serious arrhythmias during administration of large doses. It is only available as tablets or suppositories.

Mucosal protectors
Sucralfate

Sucralfate exerts a generalized cytoprotective effect by forming a barrier over the gut lumen. It protects ulcerated regions specifically. It does not alter gastric pH, motility or lower oesophageal sphincter tone, although it has been reported to have bacteriostatic effects.

Its actions are due to its local effects and virtually none is absorbed from the gut. Consequently it has no effect on the central nervous or cardiorespiratory systems.

Effects

- Gut – minor gastric disturbances. Enhanced aluminium absorption in patients with renal dysfunction or on dialysis. It may reduce the absorption of certain drugs (ciprofloxacin, warfarin, phenytoin and H_2 antagonists) by direct binding.

Prostaglandin analogues
Misoprostil

Misoprostil is a synthetic analogue of prostaglandin E_1.

Uses

It is used for the prevention and treatment of non-steroidal anti-inflammatory induced ulcers.

Mechanism of action

It inhibits gastric acid secretion and increases mucous secretion thereby protecting the gastric mucosa.

Effects

- Endocrine – it increases uterine tone and may precipitate miscarriage. Menorrhagia and vaginal bleeding have been reported.
- Gut – severe diarrhoea and other intestinal upset.
- Cardiovascular – at normal doses it is unlikely to produce hypotension but its use is cautioned where hypotension could precipitate severe complications (i.e. in cerebrovascular or cardiovascular disease).

Kinetics

Misoprostil is rapidly absorbed from the gut. Metabolism is by fatty acid-oxidizing systems throughout the body and no alteration in dose is required in renal or hepatic impairment.

Intravenous fluids

Body fluid compartments

Total body water makes up approximately 60% of total body weight. Two-thirds of body water is intracellular, the remaining third is divided between the intravascular (plasma, 20%) and interstitial (80%) compartment, that is, 3L intravascular, 12L interstitial, and 25L intracellular.

Intracellular

The composition of the intracellular volume is maintained by a metabolically active membrane. It has a low sodium concentration (10 mmol.l^{-1}) and a high potassium (150 mmol.l^{-1}) concentration.

Interstitial

The interstitial volume is that part of the extracellular volume that is not present in the plasma – it is the fluid that bathes the cells. During illness or injury its membrane becomes leaky allowing immunological mediators access and the formation of oedema. It has an electrolyte composition that is similar to the plasma with a high sodium concentration (140 mmol.l^{-1}) and a low potassium concentration (4 mmol.l^{-1}). It has less protein than the plasma and therefore a lower oncotic pressure.

Intravascular

The intravascular compartment has a composition similar to that of the interstitial space. When the red cell volume is added, the total blood volume is derived. Clearly the main function of the red cell is to transport oxygen from the lungs to the tissues. The plasma has a number of key functions, which include providing the fluid volume necessary to suspend the red cells, clotting and immunological functions.

Fluid replacement

In order to make appropriate choices about fluid replacement it is essential that the *processes of distribution* between the three compartments are understood. These principles can then be used to guide the use of the different types of fluid replacement available in order to achieve specific aims.

Processes of distribution

There are essentially three components to intravenous fluids: water, electrolytes (principally sodium) and large molecules (gelatins, starches, albumin). It is no surprise that each behaves differently because from a molecular point of view they are very dissimilar.

Water has no charge but can be encouraged to be polar and will distribute rapidly across all compartments in the body, resulting in a minimal increase in plasma volume. Sodium carries a charge and is distributed rapidly into the extracellular space, whereas potassium is transported into cells. Therefore, solutions with a high sodium content are distributed across the extracellular space resulting in a greater effect on plasma volume compared with 5% dextrose but still not a profound volume increase. By way of contrast, fluids with a significant component of large molecules remain largely contained in the plasma and as a result the contribution to the plasma volume is more significant.

However there are additional factors that govern fluid movement between the compartments, and these are linked in the Starling equation. They are:
- The shape and size of the molecules
- Hydrostatic pressure gradients (i.e. the actual pressure in certain anatomical spaces)
- Oncotic pressure gradients (i.e. the pressure generated by the components within these anatomical spaces)
- The time over which the fluid is given
- The endothelial barrier

The Starling equation

Fluid movement $= k[(P_c + \pi_p) - (P_i + \pi_p)]$

where k $=$ filtration constant for the capillary membrane
P_c $=$ capillary hydrostatic pressure
P_i $=$ interstitial hydrostatic pressure
π_p $=$ plasma oncotic pressure
π_i $=$ interstitial fluid oncotic pressure

So the administration of intravenous fluid depends on the specific aims in any given situation. For example when a patient is starved pre-operatively for a long period, it may become appropriate to administer maintenance fluid which consists of water and electrolytes. However if the patient is given bowel prep then the amount of water and electrolytes will need to be increased in order to maintain normality. Pyloric stenosis is a specific example in which careful fluid and electrolyte replacement are vital prior to surgery.

The picture may be complicated further as vascular permeability increases in burns, trauma, sepsis and surgery allowing immunological mediators to leave the intravascular space. Albumin follows resulting in a reduction of colloid oncotic pressure and the formation of oedema.

Crystalloids

Maintenance fluids only need to replace what is normally lost (i.e. ~70 mmol of sodium and ~2 litres of water). Smaller amounts of potassium and other electrolytes are also required.

Where crystalloids are used for volume expansion, 0.9% saline remains a common choice. However its chloride content is significantly higher than that found in plasma and this will promote a hyperchloraemic acidosis, which may also impair haemostasis and urine ouput.

Ringer's solutions were designed around the solutions used to bathe cultured cells. Hartmann added lactate, which allowed a reduced chloride concentration, and therefore prevented hyperchloraemic acidosis formation when used in vivo. However the addition of acetate instead of lactate may be advantageous in that it is metabolized not only in the liver and kidney but by all tissues so that its buffering capacity is retained during times of hypovolaemic shock. Both lactate and acetate are metabolized to bicarbonate.

Colloids

Gelatins

Gelatins are large molecular weight proteins that are commonly suspended in saline-like solutions. They are used for plasma replacement and initially increase colloid osmotic pressure. However the effects are not long lasting and therefore gelatins are not considered as serious volume expanders.

Formulation

The gelatins that were used initially had a very high molecular weight (100 000 Daltons), which provided a large colloid osmotic effect and subsequent plasma volume expansion, however at low temperatures the solution became gel-like. As a result lower molecular weight formulations were developed. These formulations only increase the plasma volume by the amount infused; they do not draw water in from the extracellular space.

Gelatins in use today are manufactured from bovine gelatin, which is heated, allowing the protein to denature, and cooled, allowing new inter-chain bonds to form. These bonds are either succinylated or urea cross-linked depending on the chemical conditons during cooling. The resultant product has a range of molecular weights, which is quoted in one of two ways: the weight average or the number average. The number average best reflects the mean osmotically active particle weight of a colloid and is the total weight of all the molecules divided by the total number of all the molecules. The weight average is a more complicated calculation, usually larger and usually quoted by the manufacturer.

Kinetics

More than 95% of infused gelatin is excreted unchanged in the urine. Unlike hydroxyethyl starches, gelatins are not stored in the reticulo-endotheial system. Their volume of dristribution varies greatly (minimum 120 ml.kg^{-1}) depending on the nature of the capillaries that alter in states of sepsis.

Side effects

The only signficant side effect is anaphylactic and anaphlactoid reactions, which occur in approximately 1 in 10 000 administrations.

The evidence on disturbances of coagulation is inconclusive.

Hydroxyethyl starches

Hydroxyethyl starch (HES) is a derivative of amylopectin that is a highly branched starch compound. When anhydroglucose residues are substituted with hydroxyethyl groups two important changes occur: first, increased solubility and second, reduced metabolism, which increases its half-life.

Formulation

There are many more preparations of HES than there are of gelatins. The types of preparation are based around concentration, molecular weights, the degree of substitution as described above and the C2:C6 ratio, which reflects the position of the substitution.

Kinetics

The high molecular weight HES solutions provide the longest plasma-volume-expanding effect but are also associated with unwanted effects. The low molecular weight HES solutions only have very limited duration of action, whereas the medium molecular weight HES solutions provide the best balance. However, high molecular weight HES solutions are now available in balanced electrolyte formulations, which are reported to reduce side effects.

Side effects

* **Coagulation** – the effects on coagulation are variable and depend on the molecular weight and degree of substitution of the HES. High molecular weight HES and/or those with a high degree of substitution may cause a type I von Willebrand-like syndrome and post-operative bleeding. Balanced electrolye preperations may eliminate these side effects.
* **Renal**–HES may be involved in the generation of renal tubular swelling as a result of reabsorption of macromolecules, which may lead to tubular obstruction,

Table 20.1. Composition of some intravenous fluids.

	Na⁺	Cl⁻	K⁺	Ca⁺⁺	Mg⁺⁺	Misc	Osmolality	pH
Saline 0.9%	154	154					308	5
Dextrose saline	31	31				Glucose 40 g	284	4.5
5% Dextrose						Glucose 50 g	278	4
Hartmann's	131	111	5	2		Lactate 29	281	6.5
Bicarbonate 8.4%	1000					HCO₃⁻ 1000		8
Gelofusine	154	125	0.4	0.4	0.4	Gelatin 40 g	274	7.4
Haemaccel 3.5%	145	145	5.1	6.25		Gelatin 35 g	301	7.3
Hespan 6%	154	154				Starch 60 g	310	5.5
Human albumin Solution 4.5%	100–160	100–160	<2			Albumin 45 g, citrate <15	270–300	6.9 +/− 0.5
Human albumin Solution 20%	50–120	<40	<10			Albumin 200 g	135–138	6.9 +/− 0.5

Osmolality units are mosmol/kg, all other units are mmol/l unless stated.

ischaemia and ultimately renal failure. This hyperoncotic acute renal failure is particularly likely in the severely dehydrated patient who receives large volumes of colloid.

- **Accumulation**–the reticuloendothelial system takes up HES and stores it. The degree of substitution and the total dose administered are the determining factors. It has been reported that following administration of large doses of HES, patients occur an itch, which may develop weeks later.
- **Anaphylaxis**–the incidence is in the order of 1 in 20 000.

Hydroxyethyl starch is clearly a very heterogenious group. Some of the older products have been associated with significant problems, but there is hope that the newer medium molecular weight products in balanced preperations may provide fewer problems.

Albumin

Albumin accounts for ~50% of the 5 available plasma proteins, the other 50% comprising α1-, α2-, β globulin and γ globulin. It is made up of 585 amino acids, has a molecular weight of 69 000 Da and is folded into a series of α helices, which form 3 domains each with a hydrophobic core and a polar outer exterior.

Hypoalbuminaemia in the critically ill has traditionally been corrected with infusions of albumin. However its use has become less widespread following work that showed no benefit over other colloids. Further research is required to clarify the situation.

Functions

Albumin exerts a greater colloid osmotic effect than its molecular weight alone might suggest due to its highly negative charge.

Albumin binds and transports drugs and endogenous molecules in the plasma. Acidic drugs (warfarin, aspirin, furosemide and amiodarone) tend to bind to albumin while basic drugs bind to α1-acid glycoprotein. Reductions in albumin concentration can increase the effects of drugs such as warfarin by increasing the free fraction. Albumin carries bilirubin, fatty acids, calcium and magnesium. Despite a low binding affinity, a significant amount of steroid is carried by albumin due to its abundance.

Kinetics

Albumin is synthesized in the liver and has a half-life of 20 days. Just under 50% is intravascular the remainder being present in the skin and muscle with lesser amounts in the gut, liver and subcutaneous tissue. In health albumin synthesis is balanced to match metabolism. Where metabolism or loss (renal or gastrointestinal) are significantly increased synthesis may not be able to keep up and hypoalbuminaemia ensues.

Bicarbonate

Bicarbonate serves various physiological functions including buffering and carbon dioxide carriage.

Its main use is to correct hyperkalaemia and in the treatment of certain types of metabolic acidosis.

Diuretics

The kidney is a complex organ maintaining fluid, electrolyte, and acid–base balance. It also serves an endocrine function by secreting renin and erythropoietin. Diuretics are drugs that act on the kidney to increase urine production and can be divided into the following groups:

- **Thiazides**
- **Loop diuretics**
- **Potassium sparing**
- **Aldosterone antagonists**
- **Osmotic**
- **Carbonic anhydrase inhibitors**

Thiazides (bendroflumethazide, chlorothiazide, metolazone)

Thiazides (which are chemically related to the sulphonamides) are widely used in the treatment of mild heart failure and hypertension, alone or in combination with other drugs. They have also been used in diabetes insipidus where they may increase the sensitivity of the collecting ducts to remaining ADH or cause Na^+ depletion and therefore reduced water absorption in the proximal tubule. In addition, they have been used in renal tubular acidosis. The main difference among the drugs is their rate of absorption from the gut due to differences in lipid solubility and rate of onset and duration of action due to differences in handling by the renal tubule.

Mechanism of action

Thiazides are moderately potent and act mainly on the early segment of the distal tubule by inhibiting Na^+ and Cl^- reabsorption. This leads to increased Na^+ and Cl^- excretion and therefore increased water excretion. The increased Na^+ load reaching the distal tubule stimulates an exchange with K^+ and H^+ so that thiazides tend to precipitate a hypokalaemic, hypochloraemic alkalosis. Thiazides also reduce carbonic anhydrase activity resulting in an increased bicarbonate excretion; however, this effect is small and of little clinical significance.

Metolazone has very powerful synergistic effects when combined with a loop diuretic and is useful in cases of renal failure.

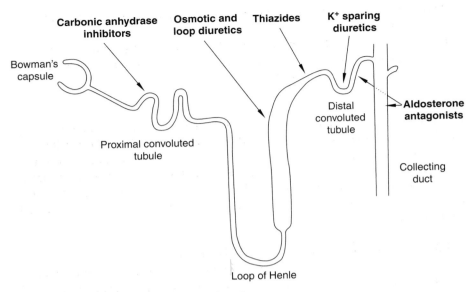

Figure 21.1. Main sites of action of the diuretics.

Effects

- Cardiovascular – thiazides appear to produce their antihypertensive effect by a reduction in plasma volume and systemic vascular resistance, which is maximally achieved at low dose.
- Renal – they reduce renal blood flow and may cause a reduction in glomerular filtration rate.
- Biochemical – their actions on the kidney lead to various biochemical imbalances. Hypokalaemia may provoke dangerous arrhythmias in those patients taking digoxin concurrently, although oral K^+ supplements usually maintain plasma levels within normal limits. Combination with a K^+ sparing diuretic may help to control plasma K^+. Hypercalcaemia may result from reduced renal Ca^{2+} excretion. Thiazides may also precipitate a hypochloraemic alkalosis, hyponatraemia and hypomagnesaemia. Thiazides and uric acid are secreted by the same mechanism within the renal tubules. This competition leads to reduced uric acid excretion and a rise in plasma levels, which may precipitate gout.
- Metabolic – reduced glycogenesis and insulin secretion coupled with enhanced glycogenolysis tends to raise plasma glucose levels. These effects are most noticeable in diabetic patients. Thiazides increase plasma cholesterol and triglyceride levels.
- Haematological – various blood dyscrasias are occasionally seen and include aplastic and haemolytic anaemia, leucopenia, agranulocytosis and thrombocytopenia.

- Miscellaneous – impotence, rash and photosensitivity occur rarely. Bendrofluazide may precipitate pancreatitis.
- Interactions – the hypokalaemia produced by thiazides may prolong the duration of action of non-depolarizing muscle relaxants. Non-steroidal anti-inflammatory drugs antagonize the effects of thiazides.

Kinetics

Bendroflumethazide is well absorbed from the gut in contrast with chlorothiazide, which is incompletely and variably absorbed. They both produce effects within 90 minutes of oral administration although bendroflumethazide has twice the duration of action at 18–24 hours. The lower lipid solubility of chlorothiazide results in elimination solely via the kidney – none being metabolized, unlike bendrofluazide, which is 70% metabolized in the liver to active metabolites, the rest being eliminated unchanged in the urine.

Loop diuretics (furosemide, bumetanide)

Loop diuretics (carboxylic acid derivatives) are used in severe heart failure to reduce peripheral and pulmonary oedema. They are also used in chronic and acute renal failure.

Mechanism of action

Loop diuretics inhibit Na^+ and Cl^- reabsorption in the thick ascending limb of the loop of Henle and to a lesser extent in the early part of the distal tubule. This impairs the action of the counter-current multiplier system and reduces the hypertonicity of the medulla, which reduces reabsorption of water in the collecting system. The thick ascending part of the loop of Henle has a large capacity for NaCl reabsorption, so when ion reabsorption is blocked the effects are marked.

Effects

- Cardiovascular – like thiazides they produce arteriolar vasodilatation which reduces systemic vascular resistance. The preload is also reduced ahead of any change that could be attributed to a diuresis.
- Renal – in contrast with the thiazides an increase in renal blood flow is seen with blood being diverted from the juxtaglomerular region to the outer cortex.
- Biochemical – the disturbances seen are similar to those induced by the thiazides and include hyponatraemia, hypokalaemia, hypomagnesaemia, and a hypochloraemic alkalosis. In contrast with the thiazides the loop diuretics may precipitate hypocalcaemia due to increased Ca^{2+} excretion. Hyperuricaemia is sometimes seen and occasionally precipitates gout.
- Metabolic – hyperglycaemia is less common than with thiazides. Loop diuretics increase plasma cholesterol and triglyceride levels although these usually return to normal during long-term treatment.

- Miscellaneous – deafness occasionally follows rapid administration of a large dose and is more common in patients with renal failure, and those on aminoglycoside therapy. Bumetanide is less ototoxic than furosemide but may also cause myalgia.
- Interactions – lithium levels may rise when given with loop diuretics.

Kinetics

Both furosemide and bumetanide are well absorbed from the gut although their oral bioavailability is different (65% and 95% respectively). Both drugs are highly plasma protein bound (>95%) and excreted largely unchanged in the urine.

Potassium sparing (amiloride)

Amiloride is a weak diuretic that is frequently used in combination with loop diuretics to prevent hypokalaemia.

Mechanism of action

At the distal convoluted tubule it blocks Na^+/K^+ exchange, creating a diuresis, and decreasing K^+ excretion.

Effects

- Metabolic – hyperkalaemia may sometimes follow its use. The hypokalaemic, hypochloraemic metabolic alkalosis seen with thiazide and loop diuretics is not a feature of K^+ sparing diuretics.

Kinetics

Amiloride is poorly absorbed from the gut, minimally protein bound and not metabolized.

Aldosterone antagonists (spironolactone)

Spironolactone is only available as an oral preparation. Potassium canrenoate is available parenterally and is metabolized to canrenone, which is also a metabolite of spironolactone.

Owing to its mode of action its effects take a few days to become established. It is used to treat ascites, nephrotic syndrome and primary hyperaldosteronism (Conn's syndrome).

Mechanism of action

Spironolactone is a competitive aldosterone antagonist. Normally aldosterone stimulates the reabsorption of Na^+ in the distal tubule, which provides the driving force for the excretion of K^+. When aldosterone is antagonized, K^+ excretion is significantly reduced while increased Na^+ excretion produces a diuresis. The diuresis produced is limited as only 2% of Na^+ reabsorption is under the control of aldosterone.

Effects

- Biochemical – hyperkalaemia is most common in patients with renal impairment. Angiotensin-converting enzyme (ACE) inhibitors also predispose to hyperkalaemia because they reduce aldosterone secretion. It may also produce hyponatraemia.
- Hormonal – gynaecomastia in men and menstrual irregularity in women are seen due to spironolactone's anti-androgenic effects. It is contraindicated in Addison's disease.

Kinetics

Spironolactone is incompletely absorbed from the gut and highly protein bound. It is rapidly metabolized and excreted in the urine.

Osmotic (mannitol)

The carbohydrate derivative mannitol is a polyhydric alcohol. Mannitol is used to reduce intracranial pressure (ICP) in the presence of cerebral oedema or during neurosurgery. It is also used to preserve peri-operative renal function in the jaundiced patient and those undergoing major vascular surgery. It is prepared in water as a 10 or 20% solution. For the treatment of raised ICP%, the initial dose is 1 $g.kg^{-1}$, which is then reduced to 0.1–0.2 $g.kg^{-1}$. However, if the serum osmolality rises above 320 $mosm.kg^{-1}$, further doses of mannitol should not be given due to an increased risk of renal failure.

Mechanism of action

Mannitol is freely filtered at the glomerulus but not re-absorbed in the tubules. It increases the osmolality of the filtrate so that by an osmotic effect the volume of urine is increased. It is unable to pass through an intact blood–brain barrier and by virtue of an increased plasma osmolality it draws extracellular brain water into the plasma. However, a head injury may give rise to a damaged blood–brain barrier. In this situation mannitol traverses the blood–brain barrier and will drag water with it, thereby increasing cerebral oedema.

Effects

- Cardiovascular – initially circulating volume is increased producing an increased preload and cardiac output. In susceptible patients this may precipitate heart failure.
- Renal – it produces an osmotic diuresis and increased renal blood flow that may result in a reduced intravascular volume.
- Central nervous system – it produces an acute reduction in ICP, which is not sustained during prolonged administration. It may also reduce the rate of formation of cerebrospinal fluid.
- Allergic – these responses occur rarely.

Kinetics

Mannitol is minimally absorbed from the gut. Following intravenous administration mannitol is distributed throughout the extracellular fluid space. It is freely filtered at the glomerulus and not reabsorbed, resulting in an elimination half-life of 100 minutes. It is not metabolized to any significant extent.

Carbonic anhydrase inhibitors (acetazolamide)

Acetazolamide is a weak diuretic that is more commonly used as prophylaxis against mountain sickness. When used as eye drops it inhibits aqueous humour production and is useful in the treatment of glaucoma.

Mechanism of action

Acetazolamide inhibits (non-competitively) carbonic anhydrase, which catalyzes the formation of H^+ and HCO_3^- from CO_2 and H_2O via H_2CO_3 in the proximal tubule. As a result less H^+ ions are available for excretion resulting in a metabolic acidosis, counteracting the respiratory alkalosis associated with mountain sickness.

Effects

- Biochemical — H^+ excretion is inhibited and HCO_3^- is not re-absorbed leading to an alkaline urine. Na^+ and water excretion are slightly increased providing an increased drive for K^+ secretion. Therefore, it produces an alkaline urine in the presence of a hyperchloraemic acidosis.

Kinetics

Acetazolamide has an oral bioavailability of more than 95%, is highly protein bound and is excreted unchanged in the urine.

Antimicrobials

Antimicrobial agents are used to kill or suppress the growth of microorganisms. The term antibiotic specifically refers to a chemical substance that is produced by microorganisms and has the capacity to kill or inhibit the growth of another microorganism.

Antimicrobials are used widely in intensive care where the selection and dissemination of resistance is a constant concern. Methicillin Resistant *Staphylococcus Aureus* (MRSA) and Vancomycin Resistant Enterococcus (VRE) have caused outbreaks in developed countries costing millions to control. Antimicrobial therapy should be directed by microbiological evidence wherever possible, empirical treatment should be rationalised to appropriate narrow spectrum cover and treatment should be discontinued at the earliest opportunity. The choice of agent must be influenced by unit protocols that will reflect the local pathogen prevalence and their known pattern of sensitivity.

This chapter can, therefore, only generalize about each agent's spectrum of activity and will refrain from suggesting appropriate treatment regimes. The following headings are used to discuss the various antimicrobials:
- **Antibacterial drugs**
- **Antifungal drugs**
- **Antiviral drugs**

Antibacterial drugs

β-Lactam antibacterial drugs

β-Lactam drugs can be subdivided into
- Penicillins
- Cephalosporins
- Carbapenems
- Monobactams

Penicillins

This group of antimicrobial drugs are based around the penicillin nucleus, which contains a fused β-lactam/thiazolidine ring.

β-lactam ring

Penicillins can be divided into:
- Narrow spectrum penicillins (benzylpenicillin)
- Narrow spectrum penicillins resistant to staphylococcal β-lactamase (flucloxacillin)
- Extended spectrum penicillins (ampicillin)
- Anti-pseudomonal penicillins (piperacillin)

Mechanism of action

Penicillins are bactericidal antibiotics that inhibit cell wall synthesis. The intact β-lactam ring binds to various proteins, the most important of which are transpeptidase and carboxypeptidase. Once these proteins are bound, peptidoglycan cross-linkage is prevented and the cell wall becomes weakened. The consequences of this vary according to the bacterial species being attacked.

Gram-positive cocci possess a thick peptidoglycan cell wall. When exposed to β-lactams, growth continues at a normal rate (with reduced cross-linkage) until the cell wall becomes weakened and lysis is inevitable. This is further assisted by the early release of a bacterial cellular component – lipoteichoic acid (a bacterial sugar alcohol phosphate). This component is intrinsically able to accelerate peptidoglycan breakdown and cell death. In spite of this, the use of β-lactams against susceptible gram-positive cocci rarely results in bacterial killing to the point of extinction. A significant number of β-lactam sensitive cells, known as *persistors*, will remain dormant until the antibiotic is removed. Extinction can be achieved, however, by the addition of a synergistic antibiotic such as an aminoglycoside, whose potency is further enhanced by the penicillin-induced peptidoglycan damage allowing gentamicin better intracellular penetration.

Gram-negative bacilli possess a thinner peptidoglycan wall surrounded by a lipopolysaccharide-lipoprotein envelope. Minimal damage to this layer weakens the cell wall and as a result of internal hydrostatic pressures, the bacteria become spherical (i.e. forms spheroplasts). Spheroplasts will lyse if placed in a hypo-osmolar environment, however, bacilli like *Haemophilus influenzae* (*H. influenzae*) have such a low intracellular osmolality that they rarely become osmotically challenged to the point where cell death occurs. When the antibiotic is removed, peptidoglycan integrity is restored; they reform bacilli and continue to divide normally.

Penicillin is also rendered ineffective by β-lactamase, which hydrolyzes the β-lactam ring. Various varieties of this enzyme exist with gram-positive β-lactamase being fundamentally different from the gram-negative types. Gram-negative β-lactamase is encoded on bacterial chromosomes and plasmids, which may be disseminated; the basis of acquired resistance.

Kinetics

Intestinal absorption is variable and certain penicillins are only available as parenteral preparations. Plasma half-lives are short (benzylpenicillin, 30 min; ampicillin, 2 hrs) and protein binding widely variable (ampicillin, 20%; flucloxacillin, 93%). Tissue penetration is generally good although inflammation is necessary for penicillins to pass into bone and through the blood-brain barrier. Penicillins are excreted by the kidneys in the unchanged form (60–90%), mainly by renal tubular secretion, but they are also excreted in bile (10%) and up to 20% is metabolized.

   Probenecid blocks renal tubular secretion so that when given in combination with penicillin the plasma concentration of the latter doubles. In addition probenecid inhibits active removal of penicillin from the CSF via the choroid plexus so that there is increased risk of CNS toxicity.

Use during continuous veno-venous haemodiafiltration (CVVHDF)

Penicillin dose adjustment is unnecessary for patients on CVVHDF with the exception of benzylpenicillin – the dose of which should be reduced by 30%. Penicillins combined with clavulanic acid (**Augmentin**^{TM}, **Timentin**^{TM}) or tazobactam (**Tazocin**^{TM}) require no dose adjustment for CVVHDF. However, if an anuric patient remains without filtration for a prolonged period then dose frequency reduction should be considered.

Side effects

- Hypersensitivity – allergy to penicillins occurs in up to 10% of the population, anaphylaxis occurs in 0.01%. Cross-reactivity exists between penicillins, cephalosporins and carbapenems in up to 10% of allergic people. Patients with a history of immediate reaction (urticaria, anaphylaxis or interstitial nephritis) should therefore avoid any of these β-lactams.
- Encephalopathy – benzylpenicillin is the most pro-convulsant β-lactam. Toxic CSF levels can be reached by intrathecal injection (maximum dose of benzylpenicillin is 12 mg), by using large doses in meningitic patients with renal impairment and by concomitant probenecid use.
- Gut – diarrhoea is common during oral therapy. Ampicillin is also associated with a low risk of pseudomembranous colitis (0.3–0.7%).
- Miscellaneous – ampicillin produces a maculopapular rash in 10% of all patients and 95% of patients with infectious mononucleosis. Bone marrow suppression has also been reported with penicillins.

Specific penicillins

Narrow spectrum penicillin

Benzylpenicillin (penicillin G) is inactivated by gastric acid and must be given parenterally. It is active against a wide variety of gram-positive pathogens, gram-negative cocci, and occasional gram-negative bacilli. Streptococci and Neisseria are extremely sensitive, whilst some *Proteus mirabilis* (*P. mirabilis*), Salmonella and *Enterococcus faecalis* (*E. faecalis*) are mildly so. *H. influenzae*, staphylococci, and Pseudomonas are resistant. Some anaerobic gram-positive cocci are sensitive but *Bacteroides fragilis* (*B. fragilis*) is resistant.

Narrow spectrum penicillins resistant to staphylococcal β-lactamase

Most staphylococci are resistant to benzylpenicillin as a result of β-lactamase production. However, the semi-synthetic penicillin **flucloxacillin** is moderately resistant and provides effective therapy in this setting. It is well absorbed from the gut but should be given intravenously for serious infections. It is less active against gram-positive cocci than benzylpenicillin but is effective against β-lactamase positive staphylococci. Metabolism produces both active and inactive metabolites. It may cause cholestatic jaundice several weeks after the end of a course of treatment.

Extended spectrum penicillins

Ampicillin is effective against the same range of organisms as benzylpenicillin (although slightly less active) as well as activity against some *H. influenzae*, Salmonella, *Escherichia coli* (*Esch. coli*), and *E. faecalis*. **Amoxycillin** has an identical spectrum to ampicillin but has better bioavailability and is bactericidal to susceptible gram-negative organisms at a lower concentration. Both are inactivated by β-lactamase. **Clavulanic acid** irreversibly inhibits a large range of β-lactamases and when combined with amoxycillin as Co-Amoxiclav reduces the minimum inhibitory concentration (MIC) against *H. influenzae*, *Branhamella catarrhalis* (*B. catarrhalis*), *Esch. coli*, *B. fragilis*, Klebsiella and *Staphylococcus aureus* (*Staph. aureus*) eight to sixty-four-fold. Clavulanic acid is weakly antimicrobial in its own right and may also be responsible for the rare occurrence of cholestatic jaundice several weeks after treatment has been stopped.

Anti-pseudomonal penicillins

The carboxypenicillin **ticarcillin** and the ureidopenicillins **azlocillin** and **piperacillin** have a broad spectrum (albeit with a lower activity than benzylpenicillin) and are particularly indicated for use against Pseudomonas, Citrobacter and Serratia. They are β-lactamase sensitive so ticarcillin is presented with clavulanic acid and piperacillin is presented with tazobactam (a β-lactamase inhibitor with no inherent antimicrobial activity.) Aminoglycosides have a synergistic effect against Pseudomonas when combined with this group of drugs. Ticarcillin in high doses has been shown to prolong bleeding time through platelet dysfunction. Its use in patients with a bleeding risk should be considered with care.

Cephalosporins

β-lactam ring

Cephalosporins possess a similar ring structure to penicillins but the thiazolidine ring is replaced by a six-membered hydrothiazine ring. The cephalosporins are extended-spectrum antimicrobials that are broadly categorized into successive generations. With each generation gram-positive cover is maintained but gram-negative cover is steadily improved. Some of the third-generation cephalosporins also demonstrate activity against Pseudomonas.

Mechanism of action

Cephalosporins are bactericidal and in common with all β-lactam antimicrobials exert their effect by disrupting peptidoglycan cell wall integrity (see above). The β-lactam ring in cephalosporins is more stable than that in penicillins and is less susceptible to β-lactamase, but once cleaved it becomes very unstable and rapidly decomposes to smaller fragments.

Pharmacokinetics

Cephalosporins distribute widely in the body, readily crossing inflamed membranes and the placenta. Third-generation agents penetrate CSF well especially if the meninges are inflamed (10% penetration), however, earlier generation agents penetrate less well and hardly at all if not inflamed. Protein-binding is variable (cefuroxime, 30%; ceftazidime, 20%) and plasma half-lives are generally short (1–1.5 hours). This contrasts markedly with ceftriaxone, which is 95% protein bound and has a prolonged half-life of 5.5–11 hours. Cephradine, cefuroxime and ceftazidime are not metabolized at all and are excreted unchanged in the urine. Cefotaxime is metabolized by the liver (the activity of the metabolites being 10% that of the parent compound) with only 50% appearing unchanged in the urine. Renal excretion utilizes both filtration and tubular secretion and probenecid does increase peak concentration and plasma half-life but to a lesser extent than penicillin.

Use during CVVHDF

Although the same dose should be given, dose interval adjustment is required for patients on CVVHDF. Cefuroxime should be given 8 hourly, cefotaxime 12 hourly, and ceftazidime 12–24 hourly. No interval adjustment is required for ceftriaxone.

Side effects

- Hypersensitivity – cross-reactivity with other β-lactams (see above).
- Haematological – a positive Coombs test has been reported with cefuroxime but without clinical consequences. Platelet abnormalities are much rarer than with ticarcillin, and ceftazidime has been associated with transient eosinophilia.
- Liver function – ceftazidime has been reported to cause abnormal liver function.

First-generation

Cefradine is active against β-lactamase producing staphylococcus, streptococcus and anaerobic gram-positive cocci. It has less activity against Neisseria while *H. influenzae* is resistant. It is used commonly when surgical prophylaxis for gram-positive organisms is required (classically orthopaedic surgery). Cefradine's lack of gram-negative cover makes it unsuitable for GI surgery.

Second-generation

This generation is more resistant to β-lactamase and has greater activity against *H. influenzae* and *Neisseria gonorrhoea* (*N. gonorrhoea*). **Cefuroxime** is active against Salmonella, Proteus sp., *Esch. coli*, Klebsiella, Citrobacter and Enterobacter. *E. faecalis*, Acinetobacter, Serratia and Pseudomonas remain resistant. Cefuroxime is commonly used for surgical prophylaxis during bowel surgery but lacks sufficient anaerobic cover to be used as a sole agent.

Third-generation

These drugs have improved gram-negative activity but their activity against some gram-positive bacteria (i.e. *Staph. aureus*) is less than the second-generation agents. **Cefotaxime** has the same gram-negative spectrum as cefuroxime except Acinetobacter, Serratia and some Pseudomonas are covered in addition. **Ceftazidime** is highly active against Pseudomonas, including strains resistant to aminoglycosides, but much less active against staphylococcus. **Ceftriaxone** has a long duration of action due to its long half-life and is administered once daily. These agents all have a very broad spectrum of activity and may encourage superinfection with resistant bacteria or fungi. Injudicious use of third-generation agents has been implicated in the encouragement of MRSA.

Carbapenems

Carbapenems have the broadest spectrum of any class of antimicrobial covering gram-positive and gram-negative aerobic and anaerobic organisms. They do not cover MRSA or *E. faecalis* and if used in isolation tend to generate Pseudomonas resistance; however, they still prove useful when treating neutropenic fever or life-threatening multi-resistant gram-negative sepsis.

Imipenem

This bactericidal carbapenem has a very broad spectrum of activity including many aerobic and anaerobic organisms especially Legionella, *Streptococcus faecium* (*Strep. Faecium*), Yersinia and all types of Pseudomonas (except *Pseudomonas maltophilia* (*P. maltophilia*). It is resistant to β-lactamase-producing organisms but is only moderately effective against *Clostridia perfringens* (*C. perfringens*). In spite of imipenem's broad spectrum some strains of Citrobacter, Enterobacter and Serratia are resistant (though not through the application of β-lactamase). Imipenem also induces β-lactamase expression in Pseudomonas which, does not alter susceptibility to imipenem but does impart substantial protection from other β-lactams.

Kinetics

Imipenem is partially metabolized by renal dehydropeptidase-I and is presented in combination with **cilastatin** (itself devoid of antimicrobial activity) to prevent this metabolism. As a result plasma and urine concentration are increased. It is mainly excreted unchanged in the urine and will accumulate in renal failure. When imipenem/cilastatin is used in patients on CVVHDF the dose must be halved and the dose-interval doubled to 12 hourly.

Side effects

Imipenem is generally well tolerated but may cause vomiting and diarrhoea (including pseudomembranous colitis), a positive Coombs' test, allergic reactions and convulsions. Imipenem has similar convulsive potential to benzylpenicillin but only presents problems in people with pre-existing CNS disorders or cases of relative overdose (renal insufficiency or concurrent probenecid use).

Meropenem

Meropenem is similar to imipenem but is not metabolized by renal dehydropeptidase-I and does not require combination with cilastatin. It is very resistant to β-lactamases although Pseudomonas has been reported to produce protective enzymes. Meropenem is less active than imipenem against gram-positive organisms but more active against gram-negative organisms that are moderately resistant to imipenem, however, the clinical significance of this is negligible.

Monobactams

Aztreonam

Aztreonam is a synthetic monobactam antimicrobial that is potently active against a wide range of gram-negative bacteria only. It has no useful activity against gram-positive or anaerobic organisms. Both Enterobacter and Pseudomonas are sensitive although it is often combined with gentamicin when treating severe Pseudomonal infections. It can be used in penicillin-allergic patients and has been used safely in patients with known IgE antibodies to benzylpenicillin.

Pharmacokinetics

Aztreonam is a parenteral preparation with a plasma half-life of 1–2 hours. It only has moderate CSF penetration and sputum penetration is poor (0.05%). Serous fluid penetration is better with good penetration into synovial fluid and bone. It undergoes minimal metabolism and is predominantly excreted unchanged in the urine. It can be used in patients on CVVHDF but the dose must be decreased by 50–70% (same dose interval.)

Side effects

Aztreonam is well tolerated but can cause an increase in bleeding time – INR and APTT should be monitored during use. Reversible marrow suppression has been reported as well as liver enzyme rises.

Macrolides

Macrolides have a range of activity similar to penicillin and may be used as alternative therapy in penicillin allergy. They cover most gram-positive organisms, Neisseria and Haemophilus, with activity against gram-positive and gram-negative anaerobes. However, they also have specific activity against Mycoplasma and Legionella for which they are indicated. **Erythromycin** represents the parent member of this group but more modern drugs are also now available. **Clarithromycin** causes less gastrointestinal upset and gives better cover against streptococci, Listeria and Legionella. **Azithromycin** provides better gram-negative cover (*Branhamella catarrhalis*, Neisseria and *H. influenzae* MIC being up to 8 times lower), improved bioavailability and longer half-life.

Mechanism of action

Macrolides are bactericidal or bacteriostatic depending on plasma concentration. They halt bacterial protein synthesis by binding to the 50S ribosomal subunit after formation of the initiation complex. Once bound the inhibition of translocation occurs at the first step.

Kinetics

Macrolides can be administered orally or parenterally. Erythromycin does irritate gastric mucosa and is also rapidly degraded in an acidic environment. CSF penetration is non-therapeutic even with inflamed meninges, but sputum and lung penetration is good. Protein binding is highly variable in this group with 70–90% of erythromycin and 12% of azithromycin being bound. Macrolides tend to be metabolized and excreted mainly via the liver; however, 40% of clarithromycin and 15% of erythromycin is excreted unchanged in the urine. Doses for both erythromycin and clarithromycin should be halved in patients on CVVHDF (protein binding of these drugs is saturable and they are not removed by dialysis) but dose adjustment for azithromycin is not required.

Erythromycin inhibits hepatic cytochrome P4503A, which is responsible for the metabolism of alfentanil and midazolam so that concurrent use leads to raised serum levels of these drugs.

Side effects

- Gut – nausea, vomiting and diarrhoea occur especially following intravenous injection due to a prokinetic effect. Various hepatic dysfunctions have been reported but are usually reversible.
- Cardiovascular – a prolonged QT interval is associated with erythromycin and clarithromycin and may precipitate ventricular tachycardia or torsades de pointes especially when taken with terfenadine.
- Interactions – the actions of theophylline, warfarin and digoxin may all be augmented when given with macrolides. Erythromycin should be avoided in porphyria.

Aminoglycosides

The aminoglycoside group contains a large number of naturally occurring and synthetic drugs including **gentamicin, netilmicin** and **tobramycin**. They cover a wide range of gram-negative enterobacteria and have gram-positive cover that includes staphylococci and to a limited extent streptococci. Aminoglycosides have no anaerobic activity but are synergistic with β-lactams and vancomycin. They are large polar molecules that need active transportation to gain entry into bacterial cells. This transportation is inhibited by divalent cations (calcium and magnesium), acidosis and low oxygen tensions. (Antimicrobial activity dramatically improves in urine if pH is raised.) Streptomycin is active against *Mycobacterium tuberculosis* and is only used in this setting. Neomycin is too toxic for systemic administration and may be used orally for pre-operative bowel sterilization (not absorbed).

Mechanism of action

Aminoglycosides are bactericidal antimicrobials that block protein synthesis by binding to the bacterial 30S ribosomal RNA subunit. Bacterial ribosomal RNA subunits are smaller than mammalian subunits and this difference is utilized by a number of antimicrobials that interfere with protein synthesis. Once bound to ribosomal RNA, aminoglycosides block tRNA attachment and mRNA is either not transcribed or totally misread (depending on aminoglycoside concentration). Enterococcal resistance in the UK is low and likely to be caused by enzyme-mediated deactivation. Altered cell permeability and altered ribosomal binding have also been found in resistant strains.

Kinetics

Owing to their low lipid solubility, aminoglycosides are not absorbed from the gut and must be given parenterally; aminoglycoside concentration being directly proportional to the rate of bacterial killing. They have low protein binding (20–30%), distribute predominantly in extracellular fluid and penetrate cells, CSF and sputum poorly. They are not metabolized and are excreted unchanged in the urine by filtration. Owing to their narrow therapeutic index, blood assays should be checked before and 1 hour after a dose to determine the most appropriate dose and the adequacy of its clearance.

Side effects

- Ototoxicity (vestibular and rarely auditory dysfunction) occurs when a significant amount of drug accumulates in the inner ear perilymph and is usually permanent. Perilymph penetration is related to peak aminoglycoside concentration and decreased removal due to high trough levels. This risk is increased in renal failure and with simultaneous use of furosemide.
- Nephrotoxicity is seen in up to 37% of intensive care patients treated with aminoglycosides and tends to be reversible on discontinuing treatment. Accumulation of the drug in the renal cortex leads to acute tubular necrosis that manifests within the first week of treatment. Synergistic toxicity is seen with some cephalosporins but the most likely independent risk factor is patient age. Netilmicin is the least toxic in this respect.
- Muscle weakness – aminoglycosides decreases the pre-junctional release of acetylcholine; reduces post-junctional sensitivity to acetylcholine and as a result increases non-depolarizing muscle relaxant potency. While intravenous calcium may reverse this effect, their use is still cautioned in myasthenia gravis.

Quinolones

Nalidixic acid is a synthetic 4-quinolone that is used for urinary tract infections. It provides no gram-positive or anaerobic cover and although it has a wide gram-negative spectrum, Pseudomonas is known to be resistant. Fluoroquinolones represent a much more significant category of antimicrobials. When compared to the 4-quinolones, this group has increased gram-positive cover and also includes Legionella, Mycoplasma, Rickettsia and Chlamydia. *Pseudomonas aeruginosa*

(*P. aeruginosa*) tends to be sensitive but resistance is acquired rapidly if used in isolation. **Ciprofloxacin** is the most commonly employed drug in this group and is active against a wide range of gram-negative and some gram-positive bacteria (streptococcus and enterococcus have moderate sensitivity). **Norfloxacin** is only available as an oral preparation for uncomplicated urinary tract infections and **Levofloxacin** has increased pneumococcal cover that lends itself for use in lower respiratory tract infections. **Ofloxacin** is more potent against both gram-negative and gram-positive organisms and has acquired less resistance. It is also indicated in lower respiratory tract infection as well as urinary sepsis.

Ciprofloxacin is also used as a first line treatment for anthrax infection and must be administered with rifampicin or clindamycin when infection is suspected. Penicillins and cephalosporins are not indicated if the potential for molecular biological manipulation of the presenting strain exists. Pneumonic plague also has bioterrorism potential and ciprofloxacin is similarly recommended as first-line treatment. Vaccines are available for both these conditions.

Mechanism of action

The quinolones are bactericidal antimicrobials that inhibit the α subunit of the DNA-gyrase enzyme. This enzyme is responsible for the negative supercoiling of bacterial DNA and when inactivated rapidly results in cell death.

Kinetics

Quinolones are well absorbed from the gut although this is reduced in the presence of magnesium, calcium/iron salts and sucralfate. They are widely distributed and have excellent CSF and tissue penetration. Protein binding lies between 15–40%. They undergo limited metabolism (active metabolites), and excretion is via urine and faeces mainly in the unchanged form (60–80% of ofloxacin is excreted in the urine). Dose reduction is only required in severe renal impairment and ciprofloxacin dose adjustment is unnecessary when patients are on CVVHDF.

Side effects
- Central nervous system – it should be used with caution in epileptic patients and it may cause restlessness, confusion and seizures.
- Gut – nausea, vomiting and abdominal pain can all occur.
- Haematological – haemolytic reactions can occur in patients with defects of glucose 6-phosphate dehydrogenase.
- Interactions – the half-life of concurrently administered theophylline is increased. It is recommended that where concurrent administration is necessary theophylline levels are measured.
- Allergic reactions and transiently altered liver function have been reported.

Glycopeptides

Glycopeptides are naturally occurring agents that are therapeutically important because of their gram-positive activity. They are active against most gram-positive bacteria including *Staph. aureus* (especially methicillin resistant), coagulase-negative staphylococci and gram-positive anaerobes such as Clostridia. They have very limited gram-negative action because the drugs are too large to penetrate the outer lipid layer of the bacteria. They are not used as first-line agents due to potential toxicity but are used for prophylaxis in patients at high risk of endocarditis who are allergic to penicillin. **Vancomycin** and **teicoplanin** are the only agents in this group available in the United Kingdom. They have very similar spectrum and differ mainly in pharmacokinetic and side-effect profiles.

Mechanism of action

These agents are bactericidal antimicrobials that work by inhibiting glycopeptide synthetase and thus preventing peptidoglycan formation in the bacterial cell wall.

Vancomycin

Vancomycin is a complex glycopeptide containing vancosamine and several amino acid moieties. Initial preparations were associated with a high incidence of nephro-toxicity and ototoxicity but the incidence of this has declined as the commer-cial preparations became more refined. Increased use of vancomycin has led to isolated cases of vancomycin-resistant *Staph. aureus* in the United Kingdom and vancomycin-resistant enterococcus has caused extensive outbreaks in other coun-tries.

Kinetics

Vancomycin is not absorbed from healthy intestine but is used orally for antibi-otic associated pseudomembranous colitis due to *Clostridium difficile* (*C. difficile*). Following intravenous administration there is marked individual variability in drug kinetics with an elimination half-life between 3 and 13 hours. Plasma protein-binding is quoted between 10% and 80% (the variation is probably due to methodological dif-ferences). It is well distributed to serous fluids but CSF penetration is very poor even in the presence of meningitis. Bone penetration is similarly poor with undetectable bone concentrations in 50% of patients treated for osteomyelitis. Ninety percent is eliminated in the urine as unchanged drug.

Intravenous administration should be monitored with blood assays to ensure ade-quate clearance bearing in mind that peak levels are governed predominantly by dose and trough levels by dose and interval. Maintaining trough levels between 10 and 15 mg.l^{-1} will ensure therapeutic efficacy whilst minimizing the chance of renal toxic-ity. If appropriate doses are administered within therapeutic trough levels, then peak levels will not exceed safe limits in adults and these levels are therefore not routinely measured.

Side effects

- Renal – nephrotoxicity is rare but is usually seen with concurrent administration of aminoglycosides or with pre-existing renal impairment. It usually resolves on withdrawal of vancomycin.
- Ototoxicity – very rare and usually associated with pre-existing hearing loss, renal impairment or concomitant treatment with another ototoxic drug. It is very uncommon if peak levels do not exceed 50 mg.l^{-1} and exceedingly rare if they do not exceed 30 mg.l^{-1}.
- Phlebitis – the intravenous preparation should be diluted when given peripherally.
- Histamine release – if administered too rapidly histamine release may cause hypotension, tachycardia and a widespread rash (known as the 'red man syndrome'). Administration should not exceed 10 mg.min^{-1}.
- Haematological – neutropenia and thrombocytopenia are rare and reversible.

Teicoplanin

Teicoplanin is a similar antibiotic to vancomycin but with a longer duration of action and 2–4 times the potency, allowing once daily administration. The preparation contains two components A$_1$ (a phosphoglycolipid) and A$_2$ (a complex of 5 glycopeptides). Resistance to teicoplanin is more common with up to 25% of *Staph. epidermidis* showing intermediate sensitivity.

Kinetics

Teicoplanin is not absorbed when given orally but can be given by intramuscular injection. It is 90% protein bound and has better distribution than vancomycin. Bone and CSF penetration are more reliable than with vancomycin but urine penetration is less. It is given twice daily for 48 hours to facilitate loading, then once daily thereafter (prolonged elimination half-life). In patients on CVVHDF the maintenance interval should be increased to once every 48 hours.

Side effects

Teicoplanin is better tolerated than vancomycin but side effects do include rash, eosinophilia, thrombocytopenia and fever. It has been used safely in patients known to exhibit red man syndrome after vancomycin.

Lincosamides

Clindamycin

Parenteral clindamycin phosphate is a semi-synthetic derivative that is highly active against gram-positive aerobes but demonstrates little activity against any gram-negative aerobic organisms. Anaerobic organisms are highly susceptible. It is notably active against a significant proportion of MRSA and covers Toxoplasma and *Plasmodium falciparum* (but not *Plasmodium vivax*).

Mechanism of action

Clindamycin is a bacteriostatic antimicrobial that inhibits bacterial protein synthesis by disrupting the function of the 50S ribosomal subunit. Resistance is inducible in gram-positive organisms that are normally sensitive and when present often imparts resistance to macrolides. Clindamycin has also been shown to inhibit the action of gentamicin on Enterobacter and *Staph. aureus.*

Kinetics

Clindamycin is widely distributed and highly protein bound (94%). It is hydrolyzed to four different forms (clindamycin base, clindamycose, demethyl and sulphoxide derivatives) with the sulphoxide derivative being the least active. CSF penetration is poor and clindamycin is not recommended for CNS infections. Bone and joint penetration, however, is very good and clindamycin is commonly employed to treat staphylococcal osteomyelitis. Drug metabolism is not fully elucidated but less than 10% of the drug is cleared in the urine. Although levels rise in renal failure, patients on CVVHDF should receive the same dose.

Side effects

Clindamycin is generally well tolerated although up to 30% of patients may suffer with diarrhoea. Pseudomembranous colitis (*C. difficile*) has been associated with clindamycin use but the incidence is less than 2%. Fever, rash and eosinophilia are more common (10%) and transient drop in neutrophil and platelet counts have also being described.

Rifamycins

Rifampicin

Rifampicin is a semi-synthetic antimicrobial with potent activity against gram-positive bacteria. It demonstrates marked activity against staphylococci and strep-tococci but *E. faecalis* is more resistant. Legionella sp., Neisseria and *H. Influenzae* are susceptible but other gram-negative organisms remain resistant. Most mycobac-teria (including *M. tuberculosis*) are sensitive to rifampicin; however *M. avium* tends to be resistant.

Mechanism of action

Rifampicin is bactericidal and binds to the β-subunit of DNA-dependant RNA poly-merase. This prevents bacterial DNA being transcribed into RNA and thus prevents protein synthesis. Resistance is readily inducible with rifampicin and this antimi-crobial should not be used as a single agent. Combination therapy needs careful consideration as some antimicrobials (ciprofloxacin) are antagonized by rifampicin.

Kinetics

Rifampicin is very lipid-soluble and correspondingly widely distributed. It penetrates CSF, abscesses and heart valves well and is 80% protein bound. It is metabolized by liver microsomes and excreted into the bile. Active transport of the drug into bile can become saturated and remaining drug will be excreted unchanged in the urine (where it imparts the characteristic red colour). Rifampicin also induces hepatic microsomes and other drug metabolism may be accelerated as a result (anticonvulsants, warfarin, steroids). Plasma levels are unaffected by renal failure and dose alteration for CVVHDF is unnecessary.

Side effects

Rifampicin is well tolerated causing transient gastrointestinal upset and a red discolouration of body fluids. Liver function is rarely impaired (more common with intermittent use) but should be monitored throughout therapy. It should be used with caution if liver function is known to be impaired. Rarely haemolytic anaemia and acute renal failure have also been reported.

Fusidanes

Fusidic acid

Fusidic acid is a naturally occurring bactericidal antibiotic that exhibits activity against gram-positive bacteria and some gram-negative organisms (bacilli are highly resistant). It has appreciable activity against *Staph. aureus*, MRSA and *Staph. epidermidis* but streptococci and pneumococci are relatively resistant.

Mechanism of action

Fusidic acid does not bind to bacterial ribosome but forms a complex with elongation factor and GTP. This complex is involved in protein translocation and will allow the incorporation of one amino acid residue before blocking further chain elongation. Consequently protein synthesis is inhibited and cell death follows. Clinical resistance remains uncommon especially if fusidic acid is administered with anti-staphylococcal penicillin. Mono-therapy is not recommended for this reason.

Kinetics

Fusidic acid is well distributed and highly protein bound (95%). Although it penetrates cerebral abscesses well, it is not active in the cerebral spinal fluid. Bone penetration is good and fusidic acid is often used to treat staphylococcal bone and joint sepsis. The drug is concentrated and excreted unchanged in the bile but little active drug appears in faeces. Similarly little drug activity is detected in urine and renal failure has little effect on plasma levels. Dose alteration while on CVVHDF is unnecessary.

Table 22.1. Guidelines for antibacterial prophylaxis.

Prevention aim	Type of surgery	Type of anaesthesia	Patient details	Options for prophylaxis (NB adult doses)
Endocarditis in patients with	Dental	Local/none	No recent penicillin	**Amoxycillin** (3 g p.o.) 1 h pre-op
• Valve lesion			Penicillin allergic or recent penicillin	**Clindamycin** (600 mg p.o.) 1 h pre-op
• Prosthetic valve				
• Septal defect			Previous endocarditis	**Amoxycillin** (1 g i.v.) and **gentamicin** (120 mg i.v.) then **amoxycillin** (500 mg p.o.) 6 h later
• PDA				
	General		*No special risk*	**Amoxycillin** (1 g i.v.) at induction, then **amoxycillin** (500 mg p.o.) 6 h later
				Amoxycillin (3 g p.o.) 4 h pre-op, then **amoxycillin** (3 g p.o.) asap post-op
			Special risk	**Amoxycillin** (1 g i.v.) and **gentamicin** (120 mg i.v.) at induction, then **amoxycillin** (500 mg p.o.) 6 h later
			Penicillin allergic or recent penicillin	**Vancomycin** (1 g i.v.) pre-op and **gentamicin** (120 mg i.v.) at induction
				Teicoplanin (400 mg i.v.) and **gentamicin** (120 mg i.v.) at induction

	Upper respiratory tract	Any	As for Dental
	Genito-urinary	Any	As for Dental/GA/ Special risk. NB if urine infected, ensure prophylaxis covers infecting organism
	Obstetrics, Gynaecology and GI procedures	Any	As for Genito-urinary (but prophylaxis only required for those at *special risk*)
Meningococcal meningitis	N/A	N/A	**Rifampicin** (600 mg p.o.) bd for 2 days **Ciprofloxacin** (500 mg p.o.) single dose **Ceftriaxone** (250 mg i.m.) single dose
Pneumococcal infection (in asplenia/sickle cell disease)	N/A	Any	**Penicillin V** (500 mg bd)
Infection in abdominal surgery	Upper GI surgery	Any	**Gentamicin** (120 mg i.v.) at induction **Cefuroxime** (1.5 g i.v.) 2 h pre-op
	Lower GI surgery	Any	**Gentamicin** and **metronidazole** **Cefuroxime** and **metronidazole**
	Hysterectomy	Any	**Metronidazole at induction**

Special risk = prosthetic valve or previous endocarditis. Recent pencillin = within the previous month

Side effects

Fusidic acid is well tolerated in general with occasional reports of rash or gastrointestinal symptoms. Rapid intravenous administration has been reported to cause transient hypocalcaemia (buffer effect) and parenteral use has been associated with abnormalities of liver function including jaundice. Thrombocytopenia is rare but has been associated with use.

Nitroimidazoles

Metronidazole

Metronidazole is a potent inhibitor of obligate anaerobes and protozoa (such as trichomonas and entamba). Clostridia, Bacteroides, *T. pallidum* and Campylobacter are all sensitive whilst anaerobic streptococci and lactobacilli are resistant. In spite of extensive use worldwide, resistance remains rare and in some countries has been shown to be undetectable.

Mechanism of action

The precise mechanism of action is still unclear but metronidazole possesses a nitro-group that becomes reduced (and charged) in anaerobic conditions. Such conditions are evident in the intracellular compartment of anaerobic organisms where the reduced nitro group becomes trapped by virtue of its charge. Bacterial DNA is then known to undergo strand breakage (mechanism unclear) and cell death follows.

Kinetics

Metronidazole does not bind to plasma proteins but is metabolized to active compounds. A third of the drug is metabolized to a hydroxy metabolite that is only eliminated slowly from plasma. The drug distributes widely in CSF, cerebral abscesses, prostate and pleural fluid. Seventy-five percent is excreted in urine (the majority in an unchanged form) and the drug is removed by dialysis. Dose adjustment while on CVVHDF is not required.

Side effects

Metronidazole is well tolerated with nausea or a metallic taste being most commonly described. Rare side effects include rashes, pancreatitis and peripheral neuropathy. It should not be combined with alcohol as a severe disulfuram-like reaction with flushing and hypotension will ensue.

Antifungal drugs

Polyenes

The majority of agents in this large group have no clinical application as they exhibit similar toxicity to mammalian and fungal cells. However, a small number of

Table 22.2. Summary of some antibacterial drugs.

Drug	Main uses	Notes
Benzylpenicillin	Streptococcal, Neisseria and Clostridia infection. Used in anthrax, leptospirosis, Lyme, tetanus and necrotising fasciitis.	Established resistance to some Pneumococcal, Gonococcal and Meningococcal infection. No longer drug of first choice in Meningococcal meningitis.
Flucloxacillin	Staphylococcal infection (joint, soft tissue, endocarditis, toxic shock syndrome).	May cause cholestatic jaundice.
Amoxycillin	Enterococcal infection and first-line treatment for Listeriosis. Useful agent for sensitive urological sepsis.	90% of *Staphylococci*, 50% *E. coli* and 15% *H. influenzae* resistant (less with co-amoxiclav). May cause cholestatic jaundice.
Piperacillin	Pseudomonal infection. Blind broad spectrum ICU cover (Tazocin).	Synergy with aminoglycosides, rarely used in isolation against Pseudomonas.
Cefradine (1st generation cephalosporin)	Surgical prophylaxis where predominant gram-positive cover required (orthopaedics).	*E. faecalis* and *H. influenzae* resistant.
Cefuroxime (2nd generation cephalosporin)	General surgery prophylaxis, peritonitis, pneumonia, joint infection, urinary sepsis.	Resistant to β-lactamase action. Improved cover against *H. influenzae*, Proteus, *N. gonorrhoea* and Klebsiella.
Cefotaxime (3rd generation cephalosporin)	Meningitis, nosocomial pneumonia, biliary infection, wound sepsis, urinary sepsis.	Less gram-positive cover than cefuroxime. Excellent CSF penetration. *E. faecalis* and listeria resistant. Improved cover for Pseudomonas, Serratia, Citrobacter and Acinetobacter.
Imipenem	Very broad antimicrobial spectrum. Role in blind treatment of severe sepsis in ICU. Used in neutropaenic sepsis.	Poor CNS penetration. Some MRSA insensitive. Synergy with aminoglycosides against *Pseudomonas*. Combined with Cilastatin.
Aztreonam	'Third'-line agent, reserved for use against multi-resistant organisms.	Gram-negative aerobic cover only. Hepatotoxic, rare cause of toxic epidermal necrolysis.

(*cont.*)

Table 22.2. (*cont.*)

Drug	Main uses	Notes
Tetracycline	Used to cover *Chlamydia*, brucellosis, Rickettsia, *Mycoplasma and Borrelia burgdorferi* (Lyme disease).	Intestinal chelation with Ca^{2+} and Mg^{2+} reduces absorption. May discolour teeth in children.
Erythromycin	Gram-positive infection in patients allergic to penicillin. First-line treatment of Legionella and Mycoplasma infection.	Irritant to peripheral veins. Potentially serious drug interactions (prolongs QT interval).
Gentamicin	Severe gram-negative sepsis (especially urinary). Endocarditis and surgical prophylaxis.	Blood assays required. Oto- and nephrotoxicity. *Streptococcus* and anaerobes are resistant.
Ciprofloxacin	Gram-negative sepsis, enteric fevers, biliary, urinary and joint sepsis. Increasing use in Legionella.	Excellent tissue penetration. First-line treatment for Anthrax and Pneumonic Plaque. Problematic resistance due to overuse.
Vancomycin	MRSA, other Staphylococcal and Streptococcal infection, endocarditis, pseudomembranous colitis.	Potentially toxic – blood assays required. Red man syndrome and neutropaenia associated. Poor penetration.
Clindamycin	Staphylococci, Streptococci, *E. faecalis* and anaerobic infection (joint, peritonitis, soft tissue).	Good penetration into bone. Useful when penicillin allergic. Role in necrotising fasciitis.
Rifampicin	Mycobacteria, Staphylococci Streptococci, and Neisseria infection.	Major role in treatment of TB. Monitor liver function. Restricted use.
Fusidic Acid	Staphylococcal infection (osteomyelitis, endocarditis and soft tissue).	Reserved for severe sepsis (adjunct). *E. faecalis*, Giardia and *P. falciparum* covered. Hepatotoxic.
Metronidazole	Exclusive anaerobic and parasitic cover (Entamoeba, Giardia, Trichomonas).	Avoid concomitant ethanol administration.

Table 22.3. Summary of antibacterial drug activity.

Pathogen \ Antibiotic	Benzyl penicillin	Flucloxacillin	Ampicillin	Augmentin	Piperacillin	Tazocin	Cefradine	Cefuroxime	Cefotaxime	Ceftazidime	Meropenem	Aztreonam	Erythromycin	Gentamicin	Ciprofloxacin	Vancomycin	Clindamycin	Rifampicin	Fusidic acid	Metronidazole
Strep. pyogenes	■	●	●	●	●	●	●	●	●	●	●		●		○	●	●	●		
Strep. pneumoniae	■	●	○	●	○	●	●	●	●	●	●		●		○	●	●	●		
Staph. aureus		■		●			●	○	●	●	●		○		○	●	●	●	●	
Staph. epidermidis				●				●	●	●	●			●	○	●	●	●	●	
MRSA											○				●	●	■	○	●	
B. anthracis	●		●	●							●				■		■			●
Listeria spp.			■								●			●	●	○				
Legionella spp.											●		■		●			●		
E. faecalis			■	●	●	●					●				●	●			●	
N. gonorrhoeae	○	○	○		●	●			●	●	●	●			■					
N. meningitidis	■	●	●	●	●	●	●	●	●	●	●	●			■			●	●	
H. influenzae			○	●	●	●	●	■	●	●	●	●		○	●			●	●	
Esch. coli			○	○	○	●	●	●	●	●	●	●		●	●					
Klebsiella spp.				●	●	●	○	●	●	●	●	●		●	●					
P. mirabilis			○	●	○	●	○	■	●	●	●	●		●	●					
Enterobacter spp.				●	●	●		■	●	●	●	●		●	●					
Salmonella spp.			○	●					●	●	●	●			■					
Shigella spp.			○	●					●	●	●	●			■					
Serratia spp.					●	■			●	●	●	●		●	●					
Citrobacter spp.					●	■		○	●	●	●	●		●	●					
P. aeruginosa					○	●			○	■	●	●		●	■		○			
B. fragilis				●	●	●					●						●		●	■
C. perfringens	■		●	●	●		●		○		●						●		●	●
C. tetani	■		●	●	●		●		○		●						●		●	●
C. difficile															●	●	●			■
T. pallidum	■												●							●

● Generally susceptible

○ Occasionally resistant

■ Potential first-line agent

Note: significant local variation will exist in microbial sensitivity, local guidelines should be consulted

important agents are available for systemic and topical therapy, the most important systemic intensive care agent being amphotericin B.

Amphotericin B

Amphotericin is a wide spectrum antifungal used in the treatment of serious systemic infections. Its spectrum of activity includes *Aspergillus*, *Candida* and *Cryptococcus*. It is often combined with flucytosine for cryptococcosis and occasionally for systemic candidosis. In common with most antifungal agents resistance is seldom acquired during treatment. Isolates of some *Candida* spp. (including *Candida krusei*) have been reported after prolonged treatment, especially from heart valve vegetations, and fungal endocarditis normally requires surgical intervention to cure.

Mechanism of action

Amphotericin reacts with **ergo**sterol in the fungal cell membrane, creating pores through which cell contents are lost. It reacts less with **chole**sterol and is not as toxic to human cells. As the dose is increased, the pore size created increases and cell damage occurs at a faster rate.

Kinetics

Amphotericin is only administered parenterally and is highly plasma protein bound. Tissue penetration is poor and negligible levels are found in CSF or urine. It appears to be metabolized by the liver and plasma levels do not rise in renal failure. However, due to its potential for nephrotoxicity, dose reduction is still considered in renally impaired patients. Liposomal preparations are available that allow higher doses to be given with less renal toxicity – they are considerably more expensive.

Side effects

- Renal – renal impairment is only reversible if treatment is stopped early. Renal toxicity can be limited if the dose is gradually increased over the first 48 hours.
- Miscellaneous – it may cause any of the following: gastrointestinal upsets, blood dyscrasias, febrile reactions, muscle pains, visual and hearing disturbances, convulsions, anaphylaxis and altered liver function tests. Some of these effects can be ameliorated by reducing the rate of administration or by the co-administration of steroids or antihistamines.

Azoles

This category can be further subdivided into triazoles (fluconazole and itraconazole) and imidazoles (ketoconazole and miconazole). They are active against a wide range of fungi and yeasts including *Candida* spp., *Coccidioides* spp., *Cryptococcus* spp. and *Histoplasma* spp. Itraconazole and miconazole also cover *Aspergillus* spp. infection. Resistance is rarely problematic but isolates are known to demonstrate resistance to more than one agent.

Mechanism of action

These agents all work by disrupting ergosterol synthesis. The blockade of 14-α demethylation during ergosterol manufacture leads to an alteration in membrane function. Higher concentrations of azoles also damage ergosterol directly leading to loss of membrane integrity, cell leakage and death.

Kinetics

These drugs are all absorbed well via the oral route with the exception of miconazole, which is available in a parenteral form (prepared in cremophor EL).

Fluconazole is minimally protein bound (12%) and penetrates CSF well. It is not metabolized in man and excreted unchanged in the urine. Itraconazole, ketoconazole and miconazole are all highly protein bound (99%) and do not penetrate CSF. They are not therapeutically active in urine but tissue levels are high. Ketoconazole and miconazole are metabolized by the liver and inactive metabolites excreted in bile. Itraconazole is degraded before inactive metabolites are excreted in bile. No dose adjustment for renal failure or CVVHDF is required with these antifungals.

Side effects

Drug interaction
- Cisapride metabolism is inhibited and high plasma concentrations increase the risk of prolonged QT syndrome and fatal arrhythmias.
- Warfarin effect is enhanced.

Ketoconazole
- Gastrointestinal symptoms (20%), rash and pruritus
- Hepatitis (rare)
- Steroid synthesis inhibition (subclinical adrenocortical deficiency)

Miconazole
- Thrombophlebitis
- Cardiac arrhythmias with rapid i.v. administration

Antiviral drugs

Viruses utilize the biochemical components of their host cell and it is, therefore, difficult to prevent viral replication without causing damage to the host cell.

Acyclovir

Acyclovir is used to treat infection due to *Herpes simplex* (type I and II) and *Varicella zoster.*

Mechanism of action

Acyclovir inhibits nucleic acid synthesis. Cells infected with *H. simplex* or *V. zoster* contain a virally encoded thymidine kinase that converts acyclovir to acyclovir monophosphate. This is then converted to an active triphosphate that inhibits viral DNA polymerase and acts as a chain terminator. The thymidine kinase present in uninfected cells has a low affinity for acyclovir and therefore only very small amounts of acyclovir triphosphate are produced. This variable affinity forms the basis of its selectivity. Whilst useful against *H. simplex* and *V. zoster* it does not eradicate them and is only effective if given at the start of an infection.

Kinetics

Intestinal absorption is erratic and the oral bioavailability is low at approximately 25%. Acyclovir is widely distributed with 15% being protein bound. It is partially metabolized to inactive compounds but largely undergoes active tubular excretion unchanged into the urine, but this can be blocked by probenecid. Dose reduction in renal failure is required and a dose of 3.5 $mg.kg^{-1}.day^{-1}$ has been suggested for patients on CVVHDF.

Side effects

- Renal – rapid intravenous administration may precipitate renal impairment.
- Thrombophlebitis – it is highly irritating to veins and may cause ulcers when extravasated.
- Central nervous system – tremors, confusion, seizures and coma during rapid intravenous administration are recognized.

Zidovudine

Zidovudine is used to treat the human immunodeficiency virus (HIV) in combination with other antiviral agents.

Mechanism of action

Zidovudine is a nucleoside reverse transcriptase inhibitor (or nucleoside analogue) that is converted by various kinase enzymes to zidovudine triphosphate, the active compound. This binds to HIV-reverse transcriptase and when it becomes incorporated into proviral DNA chain termination occurs. Its affinity for HIV-reverse transcriptase is 100 times greater than for host DNA polymerase.

Kinetics

Zidovudine is given orally or intravenously and distributes widely. It is transported by the choroid plexus into the CSF where levels are 50% plasma levels. It is conjugated in the liver and up to 80% is excreted in the urine as the glucuronide. Accumulation occurs in renal failure and dose reduction is required. Patients on CVVHDF should receive doses at the lower end of the dosage range.

Side effects

- Haematological – anaemia and neutropenia.
- Gut – gastrointestinal upset, anorexia, deranged liver function, steatorrhoea and lactic acidosis.
- Miscellaneous – headache, myalgia, parasthesia and pigmentation of nail beds and oral mucosa.

Drugs affecting coagulation

- **Anti-platelet drugs**
- **Heparins and protamine**
- **Oral anticoagulants**
- **Drugs affecting the fibrinolytic system**

Physiology

Haemostasis is complicated. Two models are currently used to explain what is thought to occur.

The classical model

This has three elements: platelets, the coagulation cascade and fibrinolysis. The first two are involved in preventing haemorrhage by thrombus formation, while fibrinolysis is an essential limiting mechanism.

Thrombus formation is initially dependent on platelet adhesion, which is triggered by exposure to subendothelial connective tissue. The von Willebrand factor, which is part of the main fraction of factor VIII, is essential in this process. Subsequent platelet aggregation and vasoconstriction is enhanced by the release of thromboxane A_2 (TXA_2) from platelets. Adjacent undamaged vascular endothelium produces prostacyclin (PGI_2), which inhibits aggregation and helps to localize the platelet plug to the damaged area. The localized primary platelet plug is then enmeshed by fibrin converting it to a stable haemostatic plug.

The coagulation cascade is formed by an intrinsic and extrinsic pathway, which converge to activate factor X and the final common pathway (Figure 23.1). The intrinsic pathway is triggered by the exposure of collagen, thereby activating factor XII, while the extrinsic pathway is triggered by leakage of tissue factors, activating factor VII.

Venous thrombus consists mainly of a fibrin web enmeshed with platelets and red cells. Arterial thrombus relies more on platelets and less on the fibrin mesh.

A crucial part of this process is its limitation to the initial site of injury. Circulating inhibitors, of which anti-thrombin III is the most potent, perform this function. In

Intrinsic and extrinsic pathways

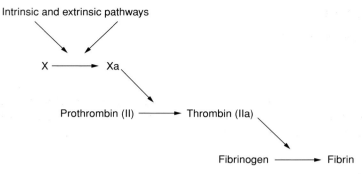

Figure 23.1. Final common pathway of the coagulation cascade.

addition, a fibrinolytic system is activated by tissue damage, converting plasminogen to plasmin, which converts fibrin into soluble degradation products.

The cell-based model

The cell-based model has been developed more recently in light of the perceived failings of the classical model, in particular its failure to explain haemostatic mechanisms in vivo. For example, factor XII deficiency does not result in an increased bleeding tendency in vivo despite abnormal in vitro tests; the bleeding tendency surrounding factor XI deficiency is not closely related to *in vitro* tests.

The cell-based model places greater importance on the interaction between specific cell surfaces and clotting factors. Haemostasis is proposed to actually occur on the cell surface, the type of cell with its specific range of surface receptors allowing different cells to play specific roles in the process.

The cell-based model proposes that coagulation is the sum of three processes each occurring on different cell surfaces rather than as a cascade. The three processes are **initiation, amplification** and **propogation**. Following vascular injury cells that bear tissue factor are exposed to the circulation and to circulating clotting factors thereby initating the process. The limited amount of thrombin generated is crucial in amplifying the procoagulant signal and causes platelets to become covered in activated co-factors. The whole process is propogated by the activation of clotting factors on the surface of the tissue factor bearing cells and platelets. As a result, large amounts of thrombin are formed leading to the formation of fibrin from fibrinogen, which consolidates the platelet plug and forms a stable clot. It is this propogation phase that is so deficient in haemophilia despite relatively normal initiation and amplification phases because of insufficient platelet surface thrombin production.

Anti-platelet drugs

Cyclo-oxygenase I inhibition

Aspirin

Uses

Aspirin reduces the risk of unstable angina progressing to acute myocardial infarction (MI) and reduces the mortality following acute MI. The risk of stroke is also reduced for patients with transient ischaemic attacks.

Mechanism of action

Aspirin acts by irreversible inhibition of cyclo-oxygenase (by acetylation) within the platelet resulting in reduced production of TXA_2. This may be achieved with only 75 mg daily. Its effects and kinetics are discussed in Chapter 9.

Platelet phosphodiesterase inhibition

Dipyridamole

Uses

Dipyridamole has been used with limited success in conjunction with warfarin to prevent thrombus formation on prosthetic valves. There is some evidence that when combined with aspirin, dipyridamol may further reduce the risk of stroke, compared to aspirin alone.

Mechanism of action

Dipyridamole inhibits platelet adhesion to damaged vessel walls (by inhibiting adenosine uptake), potentiates the affects of prostacyclin and at high doses inhibits platelet phosphodiesterase activity resulting in increased cAMP levels and lower intraplatelet calcium levels. Compared to aspirin it inhibits platelet adhesion to vessel walls more than platelet aggregation.

It is a potent coronary artery vasodilator and may be used in conjunction with thallium–201 during myocardial imaging.

Inhibition of ADP binding

Ticlodipine and clopidogrel

Like ticlopidine, clopidogrel is a thienopyridine derivative. Neutropenia may be seen with toclopidine (2.4%) and clopidogrel (0.02%). Thrombocytopenia may also accompany their use.

Uses

- Clopidogrel – When used for patients with peripheral vascular disease it reduces the risk of ischaemic stroke and myocardial infarction when compared to aspirin. It is also used following coronary artery stenting in combination with aspirin to prevent stent thrombosis. It is associated with less gastrointestinal bleeding than aspirin but severe rash is more common.
- Ticlodipine – Because of its side effects ticlodipine should only be used when aspirin has failed. It may be used to prevent stroke and during coronary stenting.

Mechanism of action

Clopidogrel and ticlodipine irreversibly prevent ADP from binding to its receptor on the platelet surface, thereby preventing the glycoprotein IIb/IIIa-receptor transforming into its active form.

Kinetics

Clopidogrel's effects are apparent 2 hours after an oral dose but its full effects are seen only after 3 to 7 days of treatment. Therapy should be stopped for a minimum of 7 days preoperatively to prevent excessive bleeding.

Glycoprotein IIb/IIIa-receptor anatagonists

Abciximab is a monoclonal antibody with a high affinity for the platelet glycoprotein IIb/IIIa receptor. It has a plasma half-life of 20 minuts but remains bound in the circulation for up to 15 days with some residual activity.

Eptifibatide is a cyclic heptapeptide with a lower receptor affinity and a plasma half-life of 200 minutes. Fifty percent undergoes renal clearance.

Tirofiban has intermediate receptor affinity and undergoes renal (65%) and faecal (25%) clearance.

Uses

They are used around the time of acute coronary events. They are used intravenously for a short duration during concurrent unfractionated heparin therapy with close control of APTT and or ACT. They carry the rare but serious complication of thrombocytopenia.

Mechanism of action

They act by inhibiting the platelet glycoprotein IIb/IIIa-receptor and as such block the final common pathway of platelet aggregation. However, they do not block platelet adhesion, secretion of platelet products, inflammatory effects or thrombin activation.

Miscellaneous

Dextran 40 and dextran 70

These are polysaccharides that contain chains of glucose. They are produced by the fermentation of sucrose by the bacterium *Leuconostoc mesenteroides*.

Uses

They are used as prophylaxis against peri-operative venous thrombosis and as plasma volume expanders.

Mechanism of action

Their anticoagulant activity appears to depend on reducing platelet adhesiveness and a specific inhibitory effect on the von Willebrand factor. They also reduce red cell aggregation and provide a protective coat over vascular endothelium and erythro-cytes. The dilution of clotting factors and volume expansion also improves micro-circulatory flow.

Other effects

These include fluid overload, allergic reactions and anaphylaxis. Dextran 70 can impair cross matching by rouleaux formation. Renal failure is a rare complication.

Epoprostenol (prostacyclin – PGI$_2$)

This is a naturally occurring prostaglandin.

Uses

Epoprostenol is used to facilitate haemofiltration by continuous infusion into the extracorporeal circuit.

Mechanism of action

Epoprostenol causes inhibition of platelet adhesion and aggregation by stimulating adenylate cyclase. The ensuing rise in cAMP reduces intracellular Ca^{2+}, effecting the change. It may also have a fibrinolytic effect. The recommended dose range is 2–12 $ng.kg^{-1}.min^{-1}$.

Side effects

These relate to its vasodilator properties (hypotension, tachycardia, facial flushing and headache).

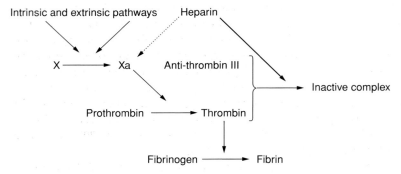

Figure 23.2. Actions of heparin. Heparin augments ($\longrightarrow$) the formation of the inactive 'anti-thrombin–thrombin' complex, while inhibiting ($\cdots\cdots\blacktriangleright$) factors Xa, IXa, XIa, and XIIa.

Heparins and protamine

Unfractionated heparin

Heparin is an anionic, mucopolysaccharide, organic acid containing many sulphate residues. It occurs naturally in the liver and mast cell granules and has a variable molecular weight (5000–25 000 Da).

Uses

Unfractionated heparin is used by continuous intravenous infusion to treat deep vein thrombosis (DVT), pulmonary embolus (PE), unstable angina and in critical peripheral arterial occlusion. Subcutaneous administration helps prevent venous thrombosis peri-operatively and in the critically ill. It is also used in the priming of extracorporeal circuits. There has been limited use in disseminated intravascular coagulation (DIC).

Mechanism of action

When anti-thrombin III combines with thrombin an inactive 'anti-thrombin–thrombin' complex is formed (Figure 23.2). The rate of formation of this complex is increased thousand-fold by heparin. At low concentrations factor Xa is inhibited, while factors IXa, XIa and XIIa are progressively inhibited as heparin concentrations rise. Platelet aggregation becomes inhibited at high concentrations and plasma triglyceride levels are lowered due to the release of a lipoprotein lipase from tissues, which reduces plasma turbidity.

Side effects

- Haemorrhage – this is the most common side effect and is due to a relative overdose.

- Thrombocytopenia – A non-immune based thrombocytopenia (type I) occurs within four days of anticoagulant doses of heparin. This rarely has clinical significance and the platelet count recovers without stopping heparin.

    This contrasts with the more severe (type II) immune-mediated thrombocytopenia, which occurs within 4 to 14 days of starting intravenous or subcutaneous heparin (fractionated and unfractionated). Heparin complexes with platelet factor 4, which is bound by IgG causing platelet aggregation and thrombosis. Half of these patients develop serious thrombosis after the platelet count starts to fall and mortality is high, mainly from pulmonary embolus. In addition 20% get arterial thrombosis leading to stroke and limb ischaemia.
- Cardiovascular – hypotension may follow rapid intravenous administration of a large dose.
- Miscellaneous – osteoporosis, due to complexing of mineral substance from bone, and alopecia have been reported. Heparin (including LMWH) can cause hyperkalaemia, which may be due to inhibition of aldosterone secretion. Patients with diabetes mellitus and chronic renal failure are particularly susceptible and the risk increases with the duration of therapy.

Kinetics

As the potency of commercial preparations varies, unfractionated heparin is presented as units.ml^{-1} rather than mg.ml^{-1}. It is ineffective orally and may only be given subcutaneously or intravenously. It has a low lipid solubility and does not cross the BBB or placenta. Owing to its negative charge it is highly bound in plasma to anti-thrombin III, albumin, proteases and fibrinogen. It is metabolized by hepatic heparinase and the products are excreted in the urine. During hypothermia (e.g. cardiopulmonary bypass) clearance is reduced. Its effects are reversed by protamine.

Low-molecular-weight heparins (LMWHs)

Enoxaparin, dalteparin, tinzaparin

These drugs are derived from the depolymerization of heparin by either chemical or enzymatic degradation. Their molecular weights vary from 2000 to 8000 Da.

Uses

LMWHs have proven benefit over unfractionated heparin in reducing the incidence of fatal PE after major orthopaedic surgery.

Advantages include:
- Single daily dose, due to a longer half-life
- Reduced affinity for von Willebrand factor
- Less effect on platelets
- Reduced risk of heparin induced thrombocytopenia
- Reduced need for monitoring

Mechanism of action

Compared with unfractionated heparin, LMWHs are more effective at inhibiting factor Xa and less effective at promoting the formation of the inactive 'antithrombin–thrombin' complex.

Protamine is not fully effective in reversing the effects of LMWH.

Monitoring heparin therapy

The activated partial thromboplastin time (APTT) measures the intrinsic system factors (VIII, IX, XI and XII) in addition to the factors common to both systems. Phospholipid, a surface activator (e.g. kaolin) and Ca^{2+} are added to citrated blood. The clotting time varies between laboratories but is about 28–35 seconds.

Monitoring LMWH is difficult as its main effects are inhibiting factor Xa, so the APTT is not altered.

Protamine

Protamine is a basic protein prepared from fish sperm. Its positive charge enables it to neutralize the anticoagulant effects of heparin by the formation of an inactive complex that is cleared by the reticulo-endothelial system. It is also used in the formulation of certain insulins.

It is given intravenously, 1 mg reversing 100 i.u. heparin.

Side effects

- Cardiovascular – hypotension (due to histamine release), pulmonary hypertension (complement activation and thromboxane release), dyspnoea, bradycardia and flushing follow rapid intravenous administration.
- Allergic reactions – patients having previously received insulin containing protamine and those allergic to fish may be at increased risk of allergic reactions.
- Anticoagulation – when given in excess it has some anticoagulant effects.

Oral anticoagulants

Warfarin

Uses

Warfarin is a coumarin derivative and is used for the prophylaxis of systemic thrombo-embolism in patients with atrial fibrillation, rheumatic valve disease or prosthetic valves. It is also used in the prophylaxis and treatment of DVT and PE.

Mechanism of action

Warfarin inhibits the synthesis of the vitamin K-dependent clotting factors: II (prothrombin), VII, IX and X. The precursors of these clotting factors are produced in

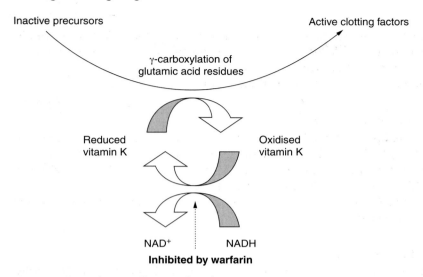

Inactive precursors   Active clotting factors

γ-carboxylation of
glutamic acid residues

Reduced
vitamin K

Oxidised
vitamin K

NAD⁺   NADH

Inhibited by warfarin

Figure 23.3. Mechanism of action of warfarin.

the liver and are activated by γ-carboxylation of their glutamic acid residues. This process is linked to the oxidation of reduced vitamin K. Warfarin acts by preventing the return of vitamin K to the reduced form (Figure 23.3).

Circulating factors will not be affected by the actions of warfarin, which therefore takes up to 72 hours to exert its full effect.

Side effects

- Haemorrhage
- Teratogenicity – this is more common and serious in the first trimester. During the third trimester it crosses the placenta and may result in foetal haemorrhage.
- Drug interactions – drugs that impair other aspects of coagulation (NSAIDs and heparin) will potentiate the effects of warfarin. Competition for plasma binding sites (NSAIDs) and inhibition of metabolism (cimetidine, alcohol, allopurinol, erythromycin, ciprofloxacin, metronidazole and TCAs) lead to potentiation of warfarin's effects. Barbiturates, rifampicin and carbemazepine induce hepatic enzymes and antagonize the effects of warfarin. Cholestyramine interferes with the absorption of fat-soluble vitamins and thereby potentiates the action of warfarin. The effects of warfarin are rapidly reversed by fresh frozen plasma. Vitamin K (1 mg) will also reverse its effects but more slowly, while 10 mg vitamin K will prevent anticoagulation for a number of days. Spinal and epidural anaesthesia is contraindicated in patients anticoagulated with warfarin.

Kinetics

Warfarin is completely absorbed from the gut and highly protein bound (>95%). It undergoes complete hepatic metabolism by oxidation and reduction to products that are subsequently conjugated and excreted in the urine.

Monitoring warfarin therapy

Prothrombin time (PT) is a measure of the extrinsic system (VII) and factors common to both systems. Tissue thromboplastin (a brain extract) and Ca^{2+} are added to citrated plasma. Clotting normally takes place in 10–14 seconds. The international normalized ratio (INR) is a ratio of the sample PT to a control international standard PT. Warfarin treatment should aim to increase the PT so that the INR is raised to between 2.0 and 4.5 depending on the clinical situation.

Ximelagatran

Ximelagatran is an oral direct thrombin inhibitor. It is a prodrug, which is converted to the active form – melagatran – in the liver. Melagatran is a potent competitive inhibitor of α-thrombin, which is highly selective for thrombin rather than other serine proteases.

It is taken twice a day and blood tests are not required to monitor its effects. However, in contrast to warfarin there is no antidote to reverse its effects should that become necessary. Overdose may be treated with prothrombin complex concentrates, fresh frozen plasma or recombinant factor VIIa. Ximelagatran may find its niche where warfarin is currently used and has proven efficacy in these areas (atrial fibrillation and venous thromboembolism). It requires no further precautions over LMWH when used alongside neuraxial blockade.

Kinetics

The oral bioavailability of meligatran after oral ximelagatran (compared with subcutaneous melagatran) is about 20%. It has a volume of distribution of 2 l/kg, and an elimination half-life of 3–5 hours, and as it is not metabolized further it is almost exclusively excreted via the kidneys. It has no interactions with drugs metabolized by the hepatic P450 system.

Drugs affecting the fibrinolytic system

Fibrinolytics

Streptokinase

Streptokinase is an enzyme produced by group C β-haemolytic streptococci.

Uses

Streptokinase is used to dissolve clot in arterial (acute MI, occluded peripheral arteries and PE) and venous (DVT) vessels.

Mechanism of action

Streptokinase activates the fibrinolytic system by forming a complex with plasminogen, which then facilitates the conversion of further plasminogen to active plasmin. The clot can then be lysed.

Side effects

- Haemorrhage – streptokinase is contraindicated in patients for whom a risk of serious bleeding outweighs any potential benefit of therapy (i.e. active internal bleeding, recent stroke, severe hypertension).
- Cardiovascular – it may precipitate reperfusion arrhythmias and hypotension during treatment of acute MI.
- Allergic reactions may occur as it is very antigenic. Where high antibody titres are expected (5 days to 12 months from previous exposure to streptokinase), an alternative should be sought.

Kinetics

Streptokinase is administered intravenously as a loading dose followed by an infusion. The loading dose is sufficient to neutralize any antibodies that are often present from previous exposure to streptococcal infection. The streptokinase–antibody complex is cleared rapidly and the streptokinase–plasminogen complex is degraded to a number of smaller fragments during its action.

Alteplase (rt-PA, tissue-type plasminogen activator) is a glycoprotein that becomes activated only when bound to fibrin, inducing the conversion of plasminogen to plasmin. Because of its mode of activation, systemic fibrinolysis occurs to a lesser extent than with streptokinase.

Urokinase was originally extracted from human adult male urine but is now prepared from renal cell cultures. Recombinant DNA technology is currently used to produce pro-urokinase. It is not antigenic and is used in the lysis of clots in arteriovenous shunts and in hyphaema (anterior chamber haemorrhage with refractory thrombi).

Antifibrinolytics

Aprotinin

Aprotinin is a polypeptide with 58 amino acids and has a molecular weight of 6512 Da. It is a naturally occurring proteolytic enzyme inhibitor acting on trypsin, plasmin and tissue kallikrein. It inhibits the fibrinolytic activity of the streptokinase–plasminogen complex. In addition it has been suggested that it preserves platelet function and decreases activation of the clotting cascade.

It has been used for the treatment of haemorrhage due to hyperplasminaemia at a dose of 500 000–1 000 000 units followed by 200 000 units per hour until the bleeding stops.

It has also been used in patients at high risk of bleeding during and after cardiopulmonary bypass. The dose here is 2 000 000 prior to sternotomy followed by 500 000 units per hour. In addition, 2 000 000 units is added to the cardiopulmonary bypass machine.

Side effects
- Hypersensitivity reactions including anaphylaxis.
- Coagulation – it prolongs the activated clotting time (ACT) of heparinized blood so that heparin/protamine protocols will need alteration during treatment with aprotinin.

Kinetics
Aprotinin is metabolized and eliminated by the kidney.

Tranexamic acid competitively inhibits the conversion of plasminogen to active plasmin. It is used to control bleeding due to excessive fibrinolysis, which may be local (prostatectomy or surgical procedures in haemophiliacs) or systemic (following intravenous fibrinolytic therapy or DIC). It is excreted essentially (95%) unchanged in the urine.

Drugs used in Diabetes

- Insulin
- Sulphonylureas
- Biguanides
- Other antidiabetics

Insulin

Physiology

Human insulin is a polypeptide of 51 amino acids and is formed by the removal of a connecting or 'C' peptide (34 amino acids) from pro-insulin. It has A and B chains, which are joined by two disulphide bridges. A third disulphide bridge connects two regions of the A chain.

Glucose forms the most potent stimulus for insulin release. It enters the β-cells of the islets of Langerhans in the pancreas, resulting in an increase in ATP, which closes K^+ channels. This causes depolarization and Ca^{2+} influx through voltage-sensitive Ca^{2+} channels, which triggers insulin release. By way of negative feedback the K^+ channels are re-opened. In health there is a continuous basal insulin release, which is supplemented by bursts when plasma glucose levels rise. Following its release it is carried in the portal circulation to the liver (its main target organ) where about one-half is extracted and broken down, as glucose is converted to glycogen.

Insulin binds to the α subunit of the insulin receptor, which consist of two α and two β subunits that span the cell membrane. Once bound, the whole complex is internalized. The mechanism by which this complex produces its effects is unclear but the tyrosine kinase activity of the β subunit appears important.

Insulin affects carbohydrate, fat and protein metabolism. It promotes hepatic (and extrahepatic) uptake of glucose and subsequently facilitates the actions of enzymes required to convert glucose into glycogen. Glycogenolysis is inhibited. Fat deposition is also increased by the promotion of hepatic fatty acid synthesis and subsequent storage as triglycerides. Lipolysis is inhibited. The storage of amino acids as proteins (anabolism) is promoted and catabolism inhibited.

Preparations

Insulin used to be extracted from porcine or beef pancreas but now is almost entirely produced by recombinant DNA technology using E. coli. Preparations are classified

Proinsulin

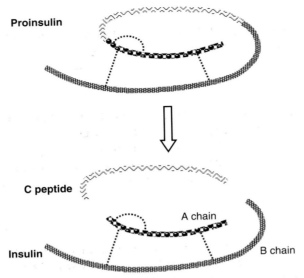

C peptide

A chain

Insulin

B chain

Figure 24.1. Convertion of pro-insulin to insulin and C peptide. (..... = disulphide bridge)

as short-, medium- or long-acting. In the UK the standard insulin concentration is 100 units.ml^{-1}.

- Short-acting – this is a simple solution of insulin that may be administered intra-venously for rapid effect. Following subcutaneous injection its duration of action may extend for up to 8 hours.
- Medium- and long-acting – when insulin is complexed with zinc or protamine, or produced as crystals rather than in its amorphous form, its solubility decreases and its absorption prolonged. This extends its duration of action to 16–35 hours.

Side effects

When calorie intake is insufficient hypoglycaemia will ensue. If untreated this will lead to coma and death. All insulins are immunogenic but despite this immunological resistance is rare. Beef insulin has three different amino acids compared to human insulin while pork insulin has only one; the latter is therefore less immunogenic. Localized lipodystrophy is also rare.

Sulphonylureas

Two generations of sulphonylureas exist and have slightly different characteristics:
- First generation – chlorpropamide, tolbutamide, acetohexamide.
- Second generation – glibenclamide, gliclazide, glipizide.

Uses

Sulphonylureas are used to control type II or non-insulin dependent diabetes (NIDDM), but should not replace dietary control.

Mechanism of action

In general these drugs work at the pancreas by displacing insulin from β-cells in the islets of Langerhans. For this reason they are ineffective in insulin-dependent diabetics who have no functioning β-cells. They may also induce β-cell hyperplasia, while reducing both glucagon secretion and hepatic insulinase activity. During long-term administration they also reduce peripheral resistance to insulin.

Kinetics

Sulphonylureas are all well absorbed from the gut and have oral bioavailabilities greater than 80%. Albumin binds these drugs extensively in the plasma. Chlorpropamide undergoes hepatic metabolism but to a much lesser extent than the others. A significant fraction is excreted unchanged in the urine and in the presence of renal failure its half-life is prolonged. The other drugs in this class are extensively metabolized in the liver to inactive metabolites (with the exception of glibenclamide whose active metabolites are probably of little clinical significance), which are subsequently excreted in the urine. Cimetidine inhibits their metabolism and, therefore, potentiates their actions. Drugs that tend to increase blood sugar (thiazides, corticosteroids, phenothiazines) antagonize the effects of the sulphonylureas and make diabetic control harder.

The second-generation sulphonylureas bind to albumin by non-ionic forces in contrast with tolbutamide and chlorpropamide that bind by ionic forces. Thus, anionic drugs such as phenylbutazone, warfarin and salicylate do not displace second-generation drugs to such an extent and may be safer during concurrent drug therapy.

Other effects

Side effects are generally mild but sometimes include gastrointestinal disturbances and rashes.

- Chlorpropamide – its long half-life and partial reliance on renal elimination results in a greater chance of hypoglycaemia, especially in the elderly. It may also cause facial flushing and vomiting following alcohol and rarely may enhance antidiuretic hormone secretion resulting in hyponatraemia. Photosensitivity may also occur.
- Tolbutamide – this drug has been associated with cholestatic jaundice, deranged liver function and blood dyscrasias.

Biguanides

Metformin

Metformin is the only currently available biguanide in the UK.

Mechanism of action

This is thought to include delayed uptake of glucose from the gut, increased peripheral insulin sensitivity (increasing peripheral glucose utilization) and inhibition of hepatic and renal gluconeogenesis.

Other effects

Gastrointestinal disturbances including diarrhoea sometimes occur but are generally mild. More significantly is its ability to precipitate severe lactic acidosis especially if taken by alcohol abusers or in the presence of renal impairment. It also lowers plasma cholesterol, triglycerides and low-density lipoproteins.

Kinetics

Metformin is slowly absorbed from the gut with a bioavailability of 60%. It is not bound by plasma proteins and is excreted unchanged in the urine. Renal impairment significantly prolongs its actions.

Other antidiabetics

Acarbose

Acarbose is a competitive inhibitor of intestinal α-glucosidase with a specific action on sucrase. Polysaccharides are therefore not metabolized into their absorbable monosaccharide form. This delay in intestinal glucose absorption reduces the postprandial hyperglycaemia normally seen in diabetics.

It is not absorbed significantly and has few other systemic effects. Owing to an increased carbohydrate load reaching the bacterial flora in the large bowel patients may experience borborygmi, flatulence and diarrhoea. Hepatic transaminases may be transiently raised.

Thiazolidinediones

Rosiglitazone and pioglitazone

Thiazolidinediones are oral antidiabetic agents with a high oral bioavailability. There effects may take weeks to be fully established due to their mechanism of action. Troglitazone was withdrawn due to hepatitis and consequently patients taking thiazolidinediones require liver function monitoring.

Mechanism of action

Thiazolidinediones activate peroxisome proliferator-activated receptor γ (PPARγ – situated within the cell nucleus) and thereby regulate a number of genes involved in glucose and lipid metabolism. As a result they act to improve insulin sensitivity.

Other effects

They may cause fluid retention and should not be given to those with significant heart failure.

Kinetics

Both drugs are extensively metabolized by hepatic cytochrome P450. Rosiglitazone metabolites are essentially inactive and mainly excreted in the urine. Some of the pioglitazone metabolites are active and are excreted in faeces and urine. Neither drug appears to have interactions with other drugs utilising the cytochrome P450 system.

Meglitinides

Repaglinide and metiglinide

Meglitinides are oral antidiabetic agents that may be of most use in treating patients with erratic eating habits as they are relatively short acting. They are taken just before meals.

Mechanism of action

Meglitinides block the potassium channels in beta cells in the pancreas, closing the ATP-dependent potassium channels and opening the cells' calcium channels. The resulting calcium influx causes the cells to secrete insulin.

Kinetics

Repaglinide has an oral bioavailability of 50%, is 98% plasma protein bound and is metabolized in the liver by CYP3A4 and therefore is potentially susceptible to drug interactions. Its elimination half-life is 1 hour.

Peri-operative care of the diabetic patient

A regional technique is often more appropriate as the patient will be able to eat and return to their normal drug regime more rapidly.

If a general anaesthetic is indicated the aim is to minimize the metabolic derangement by providing a balance of fluid, electrolytes, glucose and insulin. There is no single best way to achieve this and the approach chosen will reflect the type of diabetes, medication and proposed operation.

Diabetes	Type II
Medication	Long-acting tablets
Operation	Minor
Action	Transfer to short-acting tablets 1 week before surgery. Omit tablets on morning of operation. First on list. Treat as non-diabetic if blood sugar <7 mmol.l^{-1}. Restart tablets with first meal.
Diabetes	Type II
Medication	Long-acting tablets
Operation	Major
Action	Treat as Type I diabetes. Once eating convert to soluble insulin before meals and revert to tablets when total insulin requirement is <20 i.u.day^{-1}.
Diabetes	Type I
Medication	Insulin
Operation	Major or minor
Action	Alberti regime or insulin sliding scale

Alberti regime

Infusion of 500 ml 10% dextrose with 10 i.u. actrapid and 10 mmol KCl starting at 100 ml.h^{-1}. Blood sugar and potassium are measured every 2 hours and if adjustments are required a new infusion is prepared.

Insulin sliding scale

An infusion of 10% dextrose at 100 ml.h^{-1} is given alongside an infusion of soluble insulin. The starting hourly insulin rate is calculated by dividing the total daily units by 24. Blood sugar is measured hourly and the insulin rate is adjusted accordingly.

Corticosteroids and other hormone preparations

- **Glucocorticoids**
- **Drugs used in thyroid disease**
- **Oral contraceptives**
- **Hormone replacement therapy**

Glucocorticoids

The adrenal cortex releases two classes of steroidal hormones into the circulation:
- Glucocorticoids (from the zona fasciculata and zona reticularis)
- Mineralocorticoids (from the zona glomerulosa)

The main endogenous glucocorticoid in humans is hydrocortisone. Synthetic glucocorticoids include prednisolone, methylprednisolone, betamethasone, dexamethasone and triamcinolone. They have **metabolic, anti-inflammatory** and **immunosuppressive** effects.

Metabolic effects

Glucocorticoids facilitate gluconeogenesis (i.e. synthesis of glucose from a non-carbohydrate source, e.g. protein). Glycogen deposition and glucose release from the liver are stimulated but the peripheral uptake of glucose is inhibited. Protein catabolism is stimulated and synthesis inhibited.

When exogenous glucocorticoid is given in high doses or for prolonged periods, the altered metabolism causes unwanted effects. Increased protein catabolism leads to muscle weakness and wasting. The skin becomes thin leading to striae, and gastric mucosa becomes susceptible to ulceration. Dietary protein will not reverse these changes. Altered carbohydrate metabolism leads to hyperglycaemia and glycosuria. Diabetes may be provoked. Fat is redistributed from the extremities to the trunk, neck and face. Bone catabolism leads to osteoporosis.

Anti-inflammatory effects

Glucocorticoids reduce the production of tissue transudate and cell oedema in acute inflammation. Circulating polymorphs and macrophages are prevented from reaching inflamed tissue. The production of inflammatory mediators (prostaglandins, leukotrienes and platelet-activating factor) is suppressed by the stimulation of lipocortin, which inhibits phospholipase A_2. Normally phospholipase A_2 would facilitate the breakdown of membrane phospholipids to arachidonic acid, the precursor of inflammatory mediators, in particular prostaglandins.

These effects may reduce the patient's resistance to infection (latent tuberculosis may become reactivated), and the normal clinical features usually present may be absent until the infection is advanced.

Immunosuppressive effects

Glucocorticoids depress macrophage function and reduce the number of circulating T-lymphocytes. The transport of lymphocytes and their production of antibodies are also reduced. Interleukin 1 and 2 production is inhibited, which reduces lymphocyte proliferation.

Other effects

- Adrenal suppression – during long-term steroid therapy there is adrenal suppression due to negative feedback on corticotrophin-releasing hormone and ACTH (Figure 25.1). The adrenal gland becomes atrophic and remains so for many months after treatment has stopped. As a result the adrenal cortex cannot produce sufficient glucocorticoid when exogenous glucocorticoid is withdrawn abruptly or during periods of stress, that is, infection or surgery. If supplementary hydrocortisone is not administered in such patients peri-operatively, they are at risk of hypotension and possibly cardiovascular collapse (see below).
- Fluid retention – glucocorticoids have only weak mineralocorticoid activity. However, some do act on the distal renal tubule, leading to Na^+ retention and K^+ excretion. In very large doses, water retention may cause oedema, hypertension and cardiac failure. Mineralocorticoid (sodium retaining) activity is greatest with

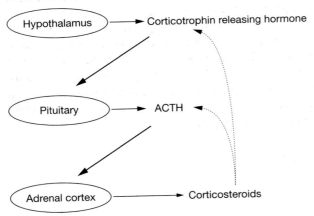

Figure 25.1. Feedback loops affecting corticosteroid production. $\longrightarrow$, Stimulates; $\cdots\cdots\blacktriangleright$, inhibits.

Table 25.1. Anti-inflammatory potential of various steroids.

Drug	Relative anti-inflammatory potency	Equivalent anti-inflammatory dose (mg)
Hydrocortisone	1	100
Prednisolone	4	25
Methylprednisolone	5	20
Triamcinolone	5	20
Dexamethasone	25	4

hydrocortisone and cortisone, lesser with prednisolone and least with methylprednisolone and dexamethasone.

- Vascular reactivity – glucocorticoids have a 'permissive action' on vascular smooth muscle, allowing them to respond efficiently to circulating catecholamines. Therefore, glucocorticoid deficiency leads to an ineffective response by vascular smooth muscle to circulating catecholamines. In sepsis there may be an inappropriately reduced production of cortisol so that higher levels of inotropic support are required. This may be improved by the administration of intravenous hydrocortisone.

Other 'permissive actions' of glucocorticoids include the calorigenic effects of glucagon and catecholamines, and the lipolytic and bronchodilator effects of catecholamines.

Peri-operative steroid supplementation

The magnitude of the surgical stimuls and the pre-operative dose of steroid need assessment in order to decide the most appropriate peri-operative supplementation regimen. Patients taking <10 mg prednisolone (or equivalent) pre-operatively have a normal hypothalamic-pituitary axis (HPA) and do not require peri-operative supplementation. Those taking >10 mg prednisolone require peri-operative supplementation in addition to their normal steroid. For minor surgery 25 mg hydrocortisone at induction is sufficient, for moderate surgery a further 100 mg hydrocortisone should be added over the first 24 hours post-operatively, which should be prolonged for up to 72 hours for major surgery. The HPA should be considered to be suppressed for up to 3 months and maybe longer after stopping steroids.

Drugs used in thyroid disease

Thyroid replacement

Thyroxine (T$_4$)

The thyroid gland synthesizes triiodothyronine (T$_3$) and thyroxine (T$_4$) by combining iodine with tyrosine residues present in thyroglobulin. The release of T$_3$ and T$_4$ is

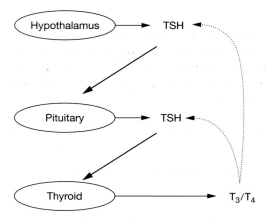

Figure 25.2. Feedback loops affecting thyroid hormone production. ⟶, Stimulates; ┄┄►, inhibits.

controlled by the hypothalamic thyrotropin-releasing hormone (TRH) and thyrotropin (TSH), which are inhibited in the presence of T_3 and T_4 (Figure 25.2).

Uses

Replacement hormone is required to treat hypothyroidism, which may be due to thyroid, hypothalamic or pituitary disease. Synthetic T_4 is the mainstay of oral replacement therapy but L-triiodothyronine (T_3) may be given intravenously (5–50 μg according to response) in hypothyroid coma as it has a faster onset. T_3 may also be given orally.

Mechanism of action

Free T_4 enters the cell via a carrier mechanism where most is converted to the more active T_3. Their main intracellular targets are receptors on the mitochondria and cell nucleus to which they bind inducing a conformational change.

Effects

- Cardiovascular – thyroid hormones exhibit positive inotropy and chronotropy. The cardiac output increases, while a reduced peripheral vascular resistance often leaves the mean arterial blood pressure unchanged. The increased myocardial oxygen demand may cause ischaemia in those with ischaemic heart disease.
- Respiratory – owing to an increased metabolic rate the minute volume increases.
- Central nervous system – they act as central stimulants and may evoke tremor. They also act to inhibit TSH and TRH by negative feedback.
- Metabolic – T_3 affects growth, development, lipid metabolism, intestinal carbohydrate absorption and increases the dissociation of oxygen from haemoglobin by increasing red blood cell 2,3-diphosphoglycerol (2,3-DPG).

Kinetics

When administered enterally both T_3 and T_4 are well absorbed from the gut. Once in the plasma they are more than 99% bound to albumin and thyroxine-binding globulin. Some T_4 is converted within the liver and kidneys to T_3 or to the inactive reverse T_3. Metabolism occurs in the liver and the conjugated products are excreted in bile. Up to 40% may be excreted unchanged in the urine.

Drugs used in the treatment of hyperthyroidism

Carbimazole

Carbimazole is a prodrug, being rapidly converted to methimazole in vivo.

Mechanism of action

Carbimazole prevents the synthesis of new T_3 and T_4 by inhibiting the oxidation of iodide to iodine and by inhibiting thyroid peroxidase, which is responsible for iodotryrosine synthesis and the coupling of iodotyrosines. Stored T_3 and T_4 is unaffected and so treatment with carbimazole requires weeks before the patient becomes euthyroid.

Side effects

These include rashes, arthralgia and pruritus. Agranulocytosis occurs rarely and may be heralded by a sore throat. It crosses the placenta and may cause foetal hypothyroidism; however, it is not contraindicated during breast feeding as only tiny amounts enter the breast milk.

Kinetics

Carbimazole is well absorbed from the gut and completely converted to methimazole during its passage through the liver. It increases the vascularity of and is metabolized within the thyroid gland. It is minimally plasma protein-bound.

Propylthiouracil

This oral preparation blocks the iodination of tyrosine and partially blocks the peripheral conversion of T_4 to T_3. There is no parenteral formulation and it is reserved for those patients intolerant of carbimazole. It has a slightly higher incidence of agranulocytosis.

Propranolol

Propranolol is a β-blocker with negative inotropic and chronotropic activity. It will help control the sympathetic effects of a thyrotoxic crisis. However, it also blocks the peripheral conversion of T_4 to T_3 and blocks hypersensitivity to the actions of catecholamines. It is relatively contraindicated for patients with heart failure or reversible airflow limitation. Guanethidine may be considered as an alternative in these cases.

Iodides

Iodide has been given as potassium iodide orally, sodium iodide intravenously and iodide containing radiographic contrast dyes. It is concentrated in the follicular cells where peroxidases oxidize it to iodine, which is then combined with tyrosine residues.

Iodide is required for normal thyroid function and when levels are too low or too high, thyroid function becomes abnormal. Large doses cause inhibition of iodide binding and hence reduced hormone production. This effect is greatest when iodide transport is increased, that is, in thyrotoxicosis. Iodide also reduces the effect of TSH on the thyroid gland and inhibits proteolysis of thyroglobulin. Thyroid vascularity is decreased, which is useful pre-operatively, but iodide is not used for prolonged periods as its actions tend to diminish with time.

Lithium may be considered in those with iodide sensitivity.

Oral contraceptives

The oral contraceptive pill (OCP) takes two forms: a combined oestrogen/ progesterone preparation and a progesterone-only preparation. The former is taken for 21 consecutive days followed by a 7 day break, while the latter is taken continuously.

Mechanism of action

The combined preparation inhibits ovulation by suppressing gonadotrophin-releasing hormone and inhibiting gonadotrophin secretion. The progesterone-only pill prevents ovulation in only 25% of women and appears to work by producing an unfavourable endometrium for implantation.

Side effects

- Major – these include cholestatic jaundice and an increased incidence of thrombo-embolic disease. The following are considered a contraindication for the combined OCP: a history of thrombo-embolism, obesity, smoking, hypertension or diabetes mellitus.
- Minor – these include breakthrough bleeding, weight gain, breast tenderness, headache and nausea. Hirsutism and depression may occur following the combined OCP. Side effects are lower in the progesterone-only pill.

Hormone replacement therapy

Hormone replacement therapy (HRT; oestrogen or oestrogen/progesterone combinations) is used to relieve menopausal symptoms, reduce osteoporosis and reduce the risk of cardiovascular disease.

Side effects

- Endometrial cancer – oestrogen therapy alone increases the risk of endometrial cancer and is therefore reserved for those who have had a hysterectomy. Women with a uterus require combined oestrogen/progesterone therapy.
- Breast cancer – oncerns have been raised regarding HRT and breast cancer and there may be a slightly higher risk of breast cancer with combined oestrogen/progesterone therapy compared to oestrogen alone.
- Deep vein thrombosis – HRT may increase the risk of deep vein thrombosis although the absolute risk is low. The mechanism is unclear, but HRT may provoke changes in relation to the haemostatic system, increasing age of patients and unmasking of thrombotic traits.

Peri-operative HRT

There is no evidence to support stopping HRT in the peri-operative period provided the usual thromboprophylaxis protocols are followed.

INDEX

Page numbers followed by "t" indicate tables and those followed by "f" indicate figures.